Illustrated Guide to Medical Terminology

Illustrated Guide to Medical Terminology

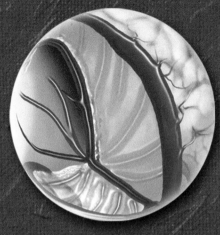

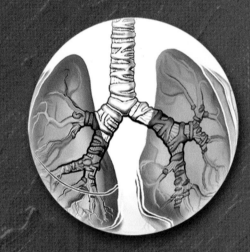

Juanita J. Davies

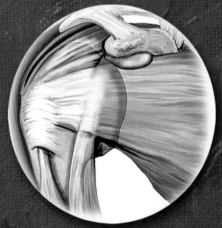

DELMAR
CENGAGE Learning

Australia • Brazil • Japan • Korea • Mexico • Singapore • Spain • United Kingdom • United States

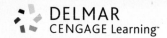

Illustrated Guide to Medical Terminology
Juanita J. Davies

Vice President, Health Care Business Unit:
 William Brottmiller

Acquisitions Editor: Matthew Seeley

Editorial Assistant: Nicole Bruno

Product Manager: Debra Flis

Marketing Director: Jennifer McAvey

Marketing Manager: Michele C. McTighe

Marketing Coordinator: Danielle Pacella

Technology Project Manager:
 Mary Colleen Liburdi

Production Director: Carolyn Miller

Production Manager: Barbara A. Bullock

Art & Design Coordinator: Alexandros Vasilakos

Content Project Manager: Thomas Heffernan

Project Editor: Ruth Fisher

For product information and technology assistance, contact us at
Cengage Learning Customer & Sales Support, 1-800-354-9706

For permission to use material from this text or product,
submit all requests online at **www.cengage.com/permissions**
Further permissions questions can be emailed to
permissionrequest@cengage.com

Library of Congress Control Number: 2006004729

ISBN-13: 978-1-4018-7919-8

ISBN-10: 1-4018-7919-5

Delmar
Executive Woods
5 Maxwell Drive
Clifton Park, NY 12065
USA

Cengage Learning is a leading provider of customized learning solutions with office locations around the globe, including Singapore, the United Kingdom, Australia, Mexico, Brazil, and Japan. Locate your local office at **www.cengage.com/global**

Cengage Learning products are represented in Canada by Nelson Education, Ltd.

To learn more about Delmar, visit **www.cengage.com/delmar**

Purchase any of our products at your local college store or at our preferred online store **www.ichapters.com**

Notice to the Reader

Publisher does not warrant or guarantee any of the products described herein or perform any independent analysis in connection with any of the product information contained herein. Publisher does not assume, and expressly disclaims, any obligation to obtain and include information other than that provided to it by the manufacturer. The reader is expressly warned to consider and adopt all safety precautions that might be indicated by the activities described herein and to avoid all potential hazards. By following the instructions contained herein, the reader willingly assumes all risks in connection with such instructions. The publisher makes no representations or warranties of any kind, including but not limited to, the warranties of fitness for particular purpose or merchantability, nor are any such representations implied with respect to the material set forth herein, and the publisher takes no responsibility with respect to such material. The publisher shall not be liable for any special, consequential, or exemplary damages resulting, in whole or part, from the readers' use of, or reliance upon, this material.

Printed in the United States of America
8 13

Dedication

To Jim

CONTENTS

CHAPTER 17 Male Reproductive System   **357**

CHAPTER 18 Female Reproductive System   **375**

CHAPTER 19 Endocrine System   **403**

DEVELOPMENT OF THE TEXT

Most learners find the structure of the body and its diseases very interesting to learn. However, over the years, I observed many of my students struggle with the written material to be learned. My colleagues said the same thing—they sensed frustration in many learners. More and more frequently, I found myself thinking that a comprehensive book with extensive illustrations and very simple writing would be very useful. That's what led me to write *Illustrated Guide to Medical Terminology*. I wanted to make it easy and enjoyable for every student to learn anatomy, physiology, medical terminology, and pathology.

The theme of this book is "Read, Look, and Listen so you can Speak and Write." This means that first you read the text, and then look at diagrams corresponding to what you have read. Often you are asked to write the names of parts on the diagrams. Then, you complete the review exercises and listen to terms from the chapter pronounced on the accompanying audio CD. You are asked to say the terms and then write them down. This process of reading the text, looking at the diagrams, writing in the structure names, completing the review exercises, listening to and repeating the correct pronunciation of terms, and finally writing the terms down on paper is the best way to learn. *Illustrated Guide to Medical Terminology* is ideal for visual and auditory learners, as well as learners whose first language is not English. I hope it serves you well.

TEXT ORGANIZATION

Illustrated Guide to Medical Terminology is organized based on the body-system approach. After more than 30 years of teaching, I feel confident that this is the most effective and learner-friendly way to teach terminology.

Chapter 1 outlines the proper way to analyze terms. Chapter 2 presents basic body organization and introduces the common anatomical roots. Chapter 3 introduces suffixes and Chapter 4 presents prefixes. Chapter 5 explains how the body is organized. The remaining 14 chapters are each devoted to a single body system.

CHAPTER ORGANIZATION

Each chapter begins with a very brief chapter outline in point form. This is followed by the learning objectives for the chapter, also in point form, and a brief introduction. In the body system chapters, an illustration of the body system to be studied immediately follows the introduction. The purpose is to provide a broad overview of the body system before details are presented. Each chapter has diagrams illustrating body structure, function, and disease. The text associated with the diagrams is as simple as possible. Regular review is accomplished by the use of sidebars that contain brief summaries. Memory devices designed to enhance learning are also included.

Vocabulary building is presented throughout each chapter. Near the end of each chapter is a list of common system-specific terms and their pronunciation. This list, used together with the accompanying audio CD, accomplishes the objective of having the learner listen to the correct pronunciation in order to speak and write the medical terms correctly. Quizzes with answers included throughout each chapter allow learners to test themselves on the content presented before moving on to new content in the chapter.

FEATURES DESIGNED TO ENHANCE LEARNING

This is the most comprehensive of the short-course medical terminology books on the market. The writing is simple and straightforward, even though the content is quite challenging. Despite the brevity of the textual material, each chapter tells a story so that the learner can chunk the information, which allows for ease of learning.

Be sure to read the **How to Use the Book** section on page xviii for detailed descriptions and images of the many features specifically developed to enhance your learning of medical terminology.

RESOURCES TO ACCOMPANY THIS BOOK

Audio CD

The audio CD in the back of the book contains pronunciations for terms that appear in the book. Each chapter includes a list of common terms and their pronunciation. This list should be used together with the audio CD. The learner listens to each term, practices the pronunciation, and then writes each term correctly.

Online Companion

The Online Companion web site at *www.delmarlearning.com/companions* is an instructor's resource that includes answers to review questions in the text, additional chapter quizzes with answer keys, course outline and syllabus.

Juanita Davies has taught anatomy and medical terminology for over 30 years. She has also written extensively on the subject of medical terminology. Her early work includes *A Programmed Learning Approach to Medical Terminology* and a computerized testbank containing 15,000 questions that students have been using since 1985. Her first book with Delmar, *Modern Medical Language,* is a combination of anatomy, medical terminology, pathology, signs and symptoms, diagnostic procedures, and treatment. Her second book, *Essentials of Medical Terminology,* combines anatomy with medical terminology. Her third book, *A Quick Reference to Medical Terminology,* is a basic handbook on medical terminology.

I am grateful for the many reviewers chosen by Delmar who examined my work and gave thoughtful feedback.

I am indebted to all of Delmar's publishing staff. Many of these individuals spent long hours guiding this book through a daunting publication process. A thank you goes to Marah Bellegarde, Acquisition Editor. Without Marah's suggestions, this book would not have begun. A very special thanks goes to Deb Flis, Product Manager, whose guidance shaped and molded this book. Her attention to detail was unparalleled. Alex Vasilakos, thank you for your hard work on art and design. I must mention, too, the help given by the many professionals who worked behind the scenes to help me write and refine this book.

Thank you to my husband, Jim, who spent many hours reading the manuscript. Your critiques were thorough, your suggestions imaginative.

Thank you to my daughter, Lisa, who spent many hours creating the layout for a sample chapter. Lisa, with your help I was always able to visualize what this manuscript could be on paper. Georgia, you were always there with words of encouragement, comfort, and support.

REVIEWERS

Delmar, Cengage Learning and the author would like to thank the following individuals for their valuable input.

Jennie Diaz-Ontiveros, CCMA
Medical Assistant Instructor
Tri-Cities Regional Occupational
Program
Whittier, California

Cassie Gentry, MEd, RHI, CHP
Chair, Department of Health Related
Professions
Program Director/Professor, Health
Information Technology
Community College of Southern
Nevada
Las Vegas, Nevada

Krista L. Hoekstra, RN, BSN
Practical Nursing Instructor
Hennepin Technical College
Brooklyn Park, Minnesota

Francine R. Page, LPN
Instructor, Medical Office
Technology Program
Health, Environmental, Natural &
Physical Science Division
Pikes Peak Community College
Colorado Springs, Colorado

June M. Petillo, MBA, RMC
Associate Professor and Director
of Medical Billing and Coding
Goodwin College
East Hartford, Connecticut

LEARNER-FRIENDLY APPROACH

The approach is simple—"Read, Look, and Listen in order to Speak and Write." This means that you first read the text and then look at diagrams corresponding to the text. You are often asked to write the names of parts on the diagrams. At the end of each chapter, complete the review exercises. Listen to terms from the chapter pronounced on the accompanying **audio CD.** Say the terms aloud and then write them down. This process of reading the text, looking at the diagrams, writing in the structure names, completing the review exercises, listening to and repeating the correct pronunciation of terms, and finally writing the terms down on paper maximizes your learning experience.

FULL-COLOR ILLUSTRATIONS

An illustration of the body system to be studied immediately follows the chapter introduction to provide a broad overview of the system before learning the details. Writing labels on the diagrams helps reinforce learning. Numerous diagrams illustrate body structure, function, and disease with the associated content presented as simply as possible.

LEARNING THE TERMS

Learning medical language is based on repetition. In each chapter, roots, suffixes, and prefixes are often repeated to reinforce learning. After each word element is introduced, it is followed by several examples of terms using that word element. This helps you remember the terms because you learn them in clusters using the same word element.

PRONUNCIATIONS

Pronunciations are presented phonetically beside every new term, and are repeated throughout the chapter.

Root		Meaning	
ather/o		fatty debris	
Term	**Term Analysis**		**Definition**
atheroma (ath-er-**OH**-mah)	-oma = mass; tumor		fatty mass or debris on the wall of the artery
atherosclerosis (ath-er-oh-skleh-**ROH**-sis)	-sclerosis = hardening		accumulation of fatty debris on the arterial wall

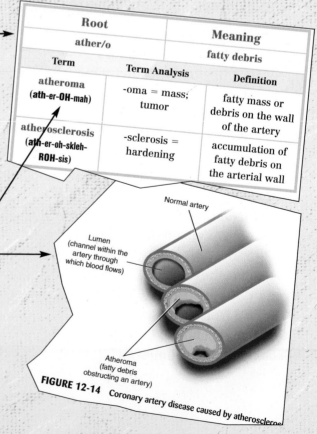

FIGURE 12-14 Coronary artery disease caused by atherosclerosis

Directional Terms

As stated above, we need directional terms to describe the position of body parts, particularly in relation to each other. Directional terms are also useful in communicating the location of diseases when they appear in the body.

All of the directional terms are listed in Table 5-1. To help you remember them, they are grouped in opposite pairs. For example, the terms "superior" and "inferior" are grouped because they are opposite sites: superior means "above," and inferior means "below." Figures 5-2 A–F illustrate the use of the terms.

HELPING YOU REMEMBER

To remember the meaning of supine, notice that supine has "up" as part of the word.

HELPING YOU REMEMBER

Suggestions are provided to help you remember a difficult term or concept presented in the chapter.

The body has two main cavities: the dorsal and the ventral. The dorsal cavity is also called the posterior cavity, because it at the back of the body. Posterior refers to the back. The ventral cavity is also called the anterior cavity, because it is at the front of the body. Anterior refers to the front. Each of these cavities has further subdivisions, which are shown in Figure 5-1.

Dorsal Cavity

The dorsal cavity is subdivided into two parts: the cranial cavity and vertebral cavity. The cranial cavity is inside the skull. The brain is contained in the cranial cavity. The vertebral cavity is in side the vertebral column, or spine. The spinal cord (a group of nerves) is contained in the vertebral cavity.

Ventral Cavity

The ventral cavity contains many internal organs including the heart, lungs, kidneys, digestive organs, and others. These internal organs are also called viscera (**VIS-er-ah**). A large muscle called the diaphragm (**DYE-ah-fram**) divides the ventral cavity into upper and lower cavities. The upper cavity is called the thoracic cavity. The lower cavity is the abdominopelvic (**ab-dom-ih-noh-PEL-vick**) cavity.

IN BRIEF

Regular review of what you have learned is accomplished through the use of sidebars that contain brief definitions of terms found on the same page.

IN BRIEF

The dorsal cavity is subdivided into the cranial and vertebral cavities.

The ventral cavity is subdivided into the thoracic and abdominopelvic cavities.

PRACTICE FOR LEARNING

Brief reviews ensure that you have mastered the content presented and are ready to move on to the next section of material.

PRACTICE FOR LEARNING: DIRECTIONAL TERMS

A. Write the opposite meaning of the following directional terms. The first one is done for you.

1. anterior _posterior_
2. lateral _____
3. proximal _____
4. deep _____
5. prone _____
6. dorsum _____

B. Underline the correct answer.

1. The neck is (inferior/superior) to the chin.
2. Your mouth is (medial/lateral) to your ear.

REVIEW EXERCISES

Numerous review exercises at the end of each chapter reinforce learning. **"Look-Alike and Sound-Alike Words"** lists medical terms and their definitions that are similar in spelling and sound. After studying these terms, practice using these words in context by completing the exercises that follow. **"Medical Terms in Context"** provides practice learning terms through mock medical reports.

6.5 REVIEW EXERCISES

Exercise 6-1 LOOK-ALIKE AND SOUND-ALIKE

Below is a list of look-alike and sound-alike words. Study the definitions of each set of words, then read the sentences carefully and circle the word in parentheses that correctly completes the meaning.

glands	organs that secrete chemicals
glans	the tip of the penis (glans penis)
patience	showing self-control
patients	a person under medical care
vesical	pertaining to the bladder (adj)
vesicle	blister (noun)

Exercise 8-6 MEDICAL TERMS IN CONTEXT

Define the bolded terms in context in the space below. Use your dictionary if necessary.

DISCHARGE SUMMARY

HISTORY OF PRESENT ILLNESS: The patient is a seven-year-old boy who showed signs of muscular weakness at age three to four years. The diagnosis of **muscular dystrophy** was made when the muscle **biopsy** confirmed **degeneration** of muscle fibers. He is still walking and was started on drug **therapy** four months ago.

PHYSICAL EXAMINATION: On examination, the patient is a pleasant young fellow. He has **proximal** muscle weakness. He has **hypertrophy** and some shortening of the **Achilles tendons**. General physical examination is within normal limits.

COURSE IN HOSPITAL: While in the hospital, an **intravenous** line started, and blood ~~were~~ taken for tests during a 24-~~riod. Th~~

"Pronunciation and Spelling Exercises" in each chapter helps you learn the common system-specific terms and their pronunciation.

5.9 PRONUNCIATION AND SPELLING

1. Listen to each word on the audio CD.
2. Pronounce each word carefully.
3. Spell each word in the space provided.

Word	Pronunciation	Spelling
epigastric	ep-ih-**GAS**-trick	
hypogastric	high-poh-**GAS**-trick	
iliac	**ILL**-ee-ack	
abdominal	ab-**DOM**-ih-nal	
cranial	**KRAY**-nee-al	

Illustrated Guide to Medical Terminology

CHAPTER 1

Basic Word Structure

LEARNING OBJECTIVES

After studying this chapter and completing the review exercises, you
should be able to:

1. Define a root, suffix, and prefix.
2. Recognize roots, suffixes, and prefixes in a medical term.
3. Learn the basic rules of medical word structure.
4. Write the meaning of the suffixes, roots, and prefixes found in this
    chapter.
5. Build medical terms.
6. Define medical terms.

INTRODUCTION

Medical words are made of parts. You need to learn what the parts are and what they mean in order to easily learn medical words. This chapter will teach you how to do that.

1.1 PARTS OF MEDICAL WORDS

Some medical words have only one part, but most have two or more. The main part is called a **root**.

Sample root: cardi

The last part of a word is the **suffix**.

Sample suffix: -al

The first part of the word is the **prefix**.

Sample prefix: peri-

Put these sample parts together and you get the word **pericardial** (**per-ih-KAR-dee-al**).

1.2 HOW TO LEARN MEDICAL WORDS

This is the way to learn medical words:

1. *Identify* the suffix, then the root, and then the prefix. Remember that most words have only two parts, so do not think you will find all three all the time. A few words only have one part.

2. *Define* the medical word by starting at the suffix. Find out what it means. Then go to the beginning of the word. It will be either a prefix or a root. Find out what it means. If there is another part, it will be a root. Once you have all the meanings, put them together.

PRACTICE FOR LEARNING: PARTS OF MEDICAL WORDS

Identify and write the part of **pericardial** indicated below. The answers are provided, but try to do the exercise first without looking at them.

Suffix _____ (means **pertaining to**)

Prefix _____ (means **around**)

Root _____ (means **heart**)

Now write the meaning of **pericardial** _____

Answers: suffix = -al, prefix = peri-, root = cardi. Pericardial means "pertaining to around the heart."

1.3 BASIC WORD STRUCTURE

Roots

A root is the main part of a medical word. It often refers to a body part.

Sample Roots:

aden   (root) means gland

hemat (root) means blood

oste   (root) means bone

arthr (root) means joint

Combining Vowel

In Section 1.2, you learned the term pericardial. In that example, the suffix -al joined the root **cardi** quite easily. Sometimes roots and suffixes do not go together so well. For example, if the root **hemat** was combined with the suffix -logy, the word would be hematlogy. This would be hard to pronounce, so a combining vowel is added. In this example, the combining vowel is "o." It is added to the end of the root to make the word hematology (**hee-mah-TOL-e-jee**), which is a lot easier to pronounce.

The combining vowel is usually "o." It can be used to connect a root to a suffix (as in the above example) or to join two roots. In the word osteoarthritis, the combining vowel joins the roots *oste* and *arthr.*

The combining vowel is used when the suffix starts with a consonant. If the suffix starts with a vowel, the combining vowel is **not** needed. For example, in the word arthritis (ar-**THRIGH**-tis), we do not add the combining vowel to *arthr* because the suffix -itis starts with a vowel.

PRACTICE FOR LEARNING: ROOTS AND COMBINING VOWELS

1. Define a root _____

2. Define a combining vowel _____

3. In the word **hematology,**

   a. _____ is the root.

   b. _____ is the combining vowel.

   c. _____ is the suffix.

4. A combining vowel is used when the suffix starts with a
   _____ .

5. A combining vowel is **not** used when the suffix starts with a
   _____ .

> *Answers:* **1.** The root is the main part of a medical word. It is often a body part. **2.** A combining vowel is a single letter, usually "o," added onto the end of the root. **3.** (a) hemat = root, (b) "o" = combining vowel, (c) -logy = suffix. **4.** consonant. **5.** vowel.

Combining Forms

You have already learned what a combining vowel is. The **combining form** is the name given to a root that is followed by a combining vowel. For example, the root *arthr,* written in its combining form, is:

arthr/o

The root is separated from the combining vowel by a slash (/). This is the standard way to write a combining form. It means that the combining vowel might be used in building medical words. Where the combining vowel is not needed for pronunciation, it is not used. In medical language, the root standing alone is almost always written in the combining form. So you should expect to see a root like **aden** written as **aden/o** almost all of the time.

PRACTICE FOR LEARNING: COMBINING FORMS

1. Define a combining form. Give an example.

   _____

   _____

2. What is the difference between the combining vowel and combining form?

   _____

   _____

   _____

   _____

> *Answers:* **1.** A combining form is the name given to a root that is followed by a combining vowel. Example: arthr/o. **2.** A combining vowel is a single letter, usually "o," added onto the end of a root. A combining form is the name given to a root that is followed by a combining vowel.

Suffixes

A suffix is the last part of a word. It can be attached to a root or a prefix. Whenever a suffix stands alone in this book, a hyphen comes before it.

Example 1:

adenoma (tumor of glands)
(ad-eh-NOH-mah)

aden/o   +   -oma
↑   ↑
root = gland   suffix = tumor; mass

Note: The combining vowel is dropped because the suffix starts with a vowel.

Example 2:

hematology (study of blood)
(hee-mah-TOL-eh-gee)

hemat/o   +   -logy
↑   ↑
root = blood   suffix = study of

Note: The combining vowel is **not** dropped because the suffix starts with a consonant.

Example 3:

osteoarthritis (inflammation of bone and joints)
(os-tee-oh-ar-THRIGH-tis)

oste/o   +   arthr/o   -itis
↑   ↑   ↑
root = bone   root = joint   suffix = inflammation

Note: The combining vowel joins two roots.

Prefixes

A prefix is the first part of a medical word. It can be attached to the beginning of the root or sometimes a suffix. Whenever a prefix stands alone in this book, it is followed by a hyphen. In example 4 below, the prefix is poly-.

Example 4:

polyadenoma (tumor of many glands)
(pahl-ee-ah-deh-NOH-mah)

poly-   aden/o   -oma
↑   ↑   ↑
prefix = many   root = gland   suffix = tumor

Example 5:

dysphasia (difficulty speaking)
(dis-**FAY**-zhee-ah)

dys-   +   -phasia
↑   ↑
prefix = difficulty   suffix = speech

PRACTICE FOR LEARNING: SUFFIXES AND PREFIXES

1. Underline the suffix in the following words:

   a. adenoma

   b. hematology

   c. osteoarthritis

   d. dysphasia

2. Underline the prefix in the following words:

   a. dysphasia

   b. polyadenoma

Answers: **1.** (a) -oma, (b) -logy, (c) -itis, (d) -phasia. **2.** (a) dys-, (b) poly-.

Basic Rules of Medical Word Structure

1. Use a combining vowel before a suffix that begins with a consonant.

Example 6:

hematology

hemat   +   o   +   -logy

(root + combining vowel + suffix)

2. Do not use a combining vowel before suffixes that start with a vowel.

Example 7:

adenoma

aden   +   oma

(root + suffix)

3. Use a combining vowel between two roots even if the second root begins with a vowel.

Example 8:

> osteoarthritis
>
> **oste** + **o** + **arthr** + **-itis**
>
> (root + combining vowel + root + suffix)

4. Define a medical word as follows: start with the suffix, then go to the beginning of the word, then to the middle of the word.

Example 9:

> osteoarthritis (inflammation of bones and joints)
>
> **oste/o** + **arthr** + **-itis**
>
> -itis = inflammation
>
> oste/o = bone
>
> arthr/o = joints

1.4 NEW ROOTS, SUFFIXES, AND PREFIXES

Use the following suggestions for learning word parts (roots, suffixes, and prefixes:

1. Pronounce the term repeatedly until it is easy for you.

2. Write it down. Ensure the spelling is correct.

3. Also write the definition. If possible, relate the word to a word, thought, or picture that will help you remember it.

HELPING YOU REMEMBER

Many students find that using memory tricks helps them remember. That works with medical terminology too. It can really help if you learn to mentally connect a word or word part with a feeling or a mental picture, especially if it is something that has personal meaning to you. For example, the first suffix below, -algia, means "pain." The best way to remember that suffix is to think of a particular pain you have experienced every time you see the suffix. So if someone who has broken a leg thinks of that every time she sees algia, she will never forget it. Use memory tricks whenever you can.

Roots	Meaning
aden/o	gland
arthr/o	joint
hemat/o	blood
oste/o	bone

Suffix	Meaning
-algia	pain
-itis	inflammation
-logy	study of
-oma	tumor; mass
-phasia	speech

Prefix	Meaning
dys-	difficult; pain; bad
poly-	many

1.5 REVIEW EXERCISES

Exercise 1-1   VOCABULARY

Build the medical term by filling in the blank with the correct word part or parts.

Example: *aden*itis   inflammation of a gland

1. _____itis   inflammation of a joint

2. _____logy   study of blood

3. aden_____   tumor of a gland

4. _____oma   tumor of bone

5. _____oma   tumor of many glands

6. _____itis   inflammation of bones and joints

Exercise 1-2 | DEFINITIONS

Define the following terms:

1. arthritis

   _____

2. adenoma

   _____

3. polyadenoma

   _____

4. osteoarthritis

   _____

5. hematology

   _____

Exercise 1-3 | WORD PARTS

Fill in the blanks with the correct word.

1. The three main parts of a medical word are the
   _____, _____, and
   _____.

2. The word part usually found at the end of a medical word is
   the _____.

3. When you define a medical word, you usually start at the
   _____, and then define the
   _____.

4. The root in hematology is _____.

5. The difference between the combining form and combining
   vowel is

   _____

   _____

   _____.

Exercise 1-4 — WORD PARTS

Circle True if the statement is true. Circle False if the statement is false.

1. The term "adenoma" has no suffix. True False

2. In the term "hematology," the combining form is used because the suffix starts with a consonant. True False

3. Usually, a combining vowel is not used between two roots. True False

4. The prefix poly- means "many." True False

Exercise 1-5 — DEFINITIONS (MEDICAL TO ENGLISH)

Give the meaning of the following word parts:

1. **hemat/o**

   _____

2. **arthr/o**

   _____

3. **aden/o**

   _____

4. **oste/o**

   _____

5. **-logy**

   _____

6. **-itis**

   _____

7. **oma**

   _____

8. **-phasia**

   _____

9. **dys-**

   _____

10. **poly-**

   _____

Exercise 1-6   DEFINITIONS (ENGLISH TO MEDICAL)

I. Write the root for the following:

  1. bone

    _____

  2. joint

    _____

  3. blood

    _____

  4. gland

    _____

II. Write the suffix for the following:

  1. inflammation

    _____

  2. speech

    _____

  3. study of

    _____

  4. tumor

    _____

III. Write the prefix for the following:

  1. difficult

    _____

  2. many

    _____

CHAPTER 2

Basic Body Structure

LEARNING OBJECTIVES

After studying this chapter and completing the review exercises, you should be able to:

1. Define anatomy and physiology.
2. Describe how the body is organized.
3. Define cells, tissues, organs, and systems.
4. Name 12 body systems and the common organs found in each system.
5. Define the roots that pertain to each body system.

INTRODUCTION

This chapter starts by introducing you to some basic concepts related to the study of the human body. It will prepare you to learn the roots you need to know for this and the following chapters on suffixes and prefixes.

The roots in this chapter are grouped according to body systems. You will find it much easier to remember each root if you associate it with a mental picture of the organs it refers to. The roots you encounter in this chapter will give you a foundation, a base for building medical terms. Note that the roots in the tables of this chapter are expressed in their combining forms, as described in Chapter 1.

2.1 ANATOMY AND PHYSIOLOGY

Two terms often used in this text are anatomy (ah-**NAT**-oh-mee) and physiology (**fiz-ee-OL-oh-jee**). Anatomy is the study of the structure or parts of the body. Physiology is the study of how a body part functions. For example, the biceps brachii (**BYE-seps BRAY-kee-eye**) muscle is located on top of the upper arm (Figure 2-1). It is made up of cells that are long and slender. These cells are called muscle fibers. The function of the biceps brachii is to flex the lower arm.

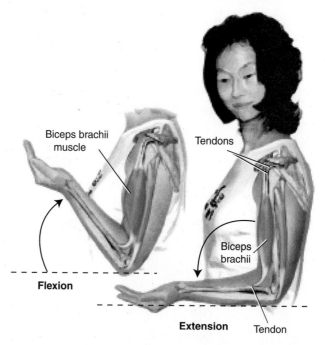

FIGURE 2-1 Anatomy: biceps brachii. Physiology: the function of the biceps brachii is movement such as flexion and extension of the lower arm. Tendons attach muscle to bone.

2.2 LEVELS OF ORGANIZATION

All life consists of living matter that can be seen only with a microscope. These structures are called **cells.** All cells are similar—although not identical—in structure. These microscopic structures carry on all of the functions of life such as the following:

- Taking in food and oxygen
- Producing heat and energy
- Eliminating wastes
- Responding to changes in the environment
- Reproducing

Trillions of cells make up the cellular level, which is the first level of organization of the body.

The next level is called **tissues.** Similar cells working together to perform a specific function combine to make up tissues. For example, muscle cells form muscle tissue. Nerve cells form nervous tissue. A **histologist** (**hiss-TOL-oh-jist**) is someone who specializes in the study of tissues. The major tissue types are:

- **Epithelial** (**ep-ih-THEE-lee-al**) **tissue:** Epithelial tissue covers external surfaces of the body, lines body structures, and forms glands. The skin is an example of an organ that is made up of epithelial tissue.

- **Connective tissue:** Connective tissue holds together body structures. Tendons and ligaments are examples of connective tissue.

- **Muscle tissue:** Muscle tissue is found in the heart, in body organs, and on top of bones.

- **Nervous tissue:** This tissue makes up nerves that conduct electrical impulses throughout the body.

The next level of organization is the **organs.** Tissues of all types combine to make up organs such as the muscles, nerves, liver, and heart.

Related organs make up **body systems,** such as the muscular and nervous systems.

All of the body systems combine to form the human being. These levels of organization are illustrated in Figure 2-2.

IN BRIEF

Cells
↓
Tissues
↓
Organs
↓
Body Systems
↓
Human Being

PRACTICE FOR LEARNING: ANATOMY AND PHYSIOLOGY

Choose the correct answer from the choices in parentheses.

1. The study of body structure is (anatomy/physiology).

2. The third structural level of body organization is (tissues/organs/cells/body systems).

3. Tissue that holds body structures together is (epithelial/connective).

4. Tissue covering the external surfaces of the body is (epithelial/connective).

5. A specialist in the study of tissue is a(n) (histologist/anatomist).

Answers: **1.** anatomy. **2.** organs. **3.** connective. **4.** epithelial. **5.** histologist.

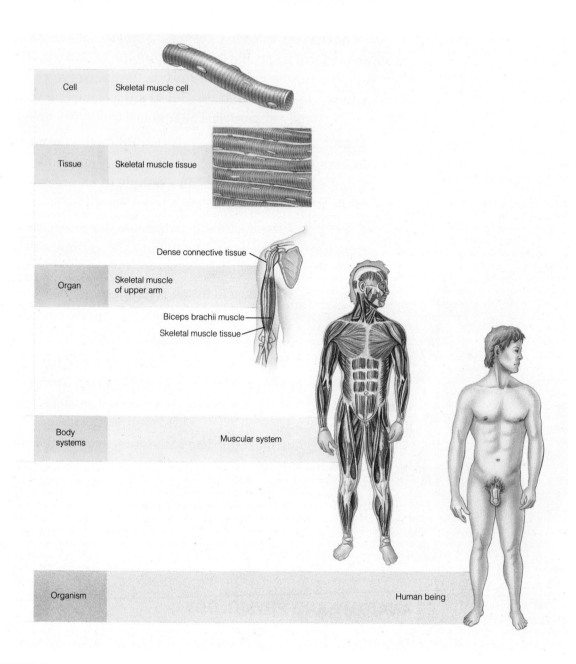

FIGURE 2-2 Levels of organization.

2.3 BODY SYSTEMS

Twelve body systems make up the human body: integumentary, skeletal, muscular, nervous, endocrine, cardiovascular, lymphatic and immune, respiratory, digestive, urinary, male reproductive, and female reproductive. These systems work together to perform all of the necessary functions of life. Figures 2-3 to 2-14 illustrate the most common features of all of these systems. A list of the common anatomical roots of each system is given for each figure.

2.4 COMMON ANATOMICAL ROOTS

Body as a Whole

Root	Meaning
bi/o	life
cephal/o	head
cervic/o	neck
cyt/o	cell
hist/o; histi/o	tissue
lip/o	fat
path/o	disease
viscer/o	internal organs

Integumentary System

Root	Meaning
cil/o; pil/o	hair
derm/o; dermat/o; cutane/o	skin
onych/o; ungu/o	nail

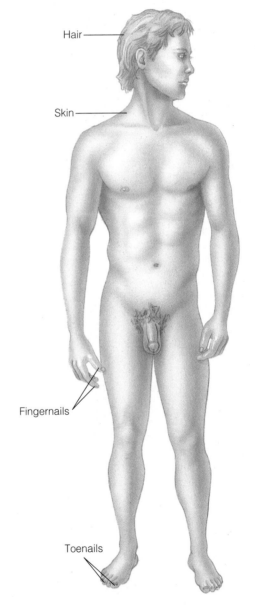

Hair

Skin

Fingernails

Toenails

**Integumentary system
(The Skin)**

FIGURE 2-3 The skin and related structures. Common structures: skin, hair, and nails.

Skeletal System

Root	Meaning
arthr/o	joint
chondr/o	cartilage
oste/o	bone

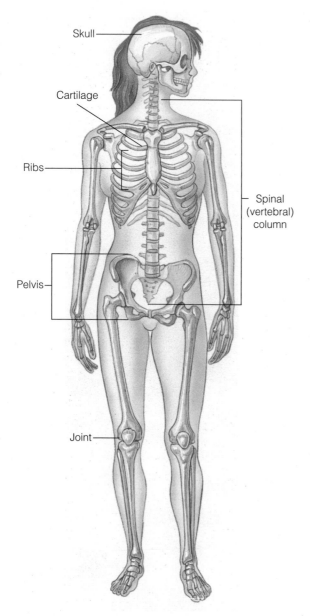

Skull

Cartilage

Ribs

Spinal
(vertebral)
column

Pelvis

Joint

Skeletal system

FIGURE 2-4 Skeletal system. Common structures: skull, vertebrae, pelvis, cartilage, ribs, joints.

Muscular System

Root	Meaning
my/o; muscul/o	muscle
tend/o; tendin/o	tendon

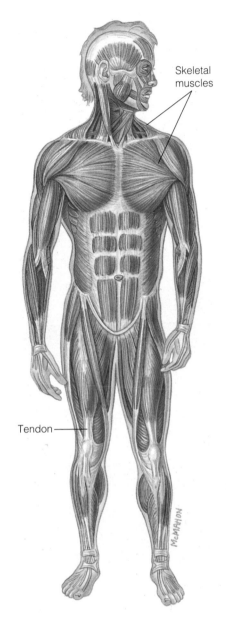

Skeletal muscles

Tendon

Muscular system

FIGURE 2-5 Muscular system. Common structures: muscles, tendons. Tendons attach muscle to bone.

Nervous System, Eyes, Ears

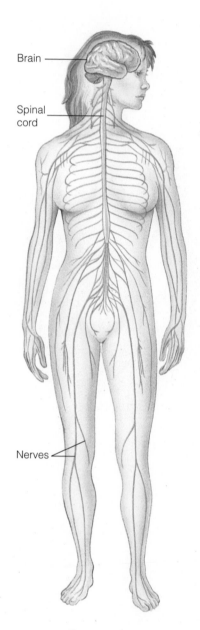

Nervous system

Root	Meaning
cerebr/o; encephal/o	brain
myel/o	spinal cord (also bone marrow)
neur/o	nerve
ophthalm/o; ocul/o	eye
ot/o	ear

FIGURE 2-6 Nervous system, eyes, ears. Common structures: brain, spinal cord, nerves, eyes, ears.

Endocrine System

Root	Meaning
aden/o	gland
adren/o	adrenal gland
pituitar/o	pituitary gland
thyroid/o	thyroid gland

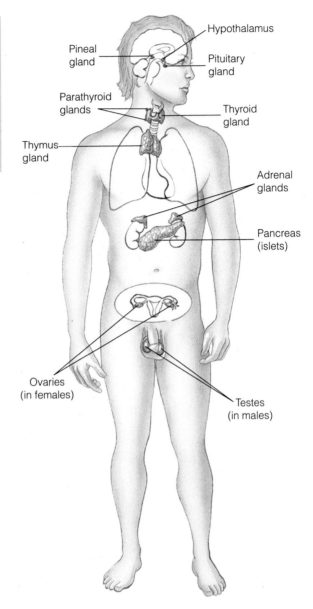

Endocrine system

FIGURE 2-7 Endocrine system. Common structures: pineal gland, hypothalamus, pituitary gland, thyroid gland, thymus gland, pancreas (islets), ovaries, testes, adrenal glands, parathyroid glands.

Cardiovascular System

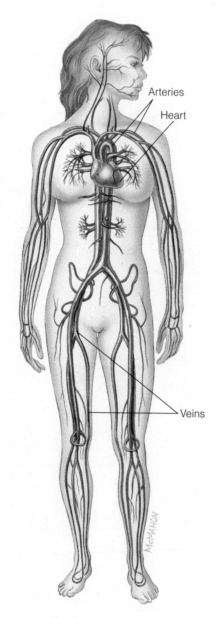

Arteries

Heart

Veins

Cardiovascular system

Root	Meaning
angi/o; vascul/o; vas/o	vessel
arteri/o	artery
cardi/o	heart
hem/o; hemat/o	blood
ven/o; phleb/o	vein

FIGURE 2-8 Cardiovascular system. Common structures: heart, arteries, veins.

Lymphatic and Immune Systems

Root	Meaning
lymphaden/o	lymph gland; lymph node
lymphangi/o	lymph vessel
splen/o	spleen
tonsill/o	tonsil

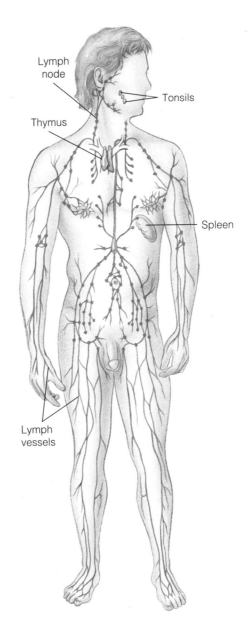

Lymphatic and immune systems

FIGURE 2-9   Lymphatic and immune systems. Common structures: tonsils, lymph nodes, spleen, lymph vessels, thymus.

Respiratory System

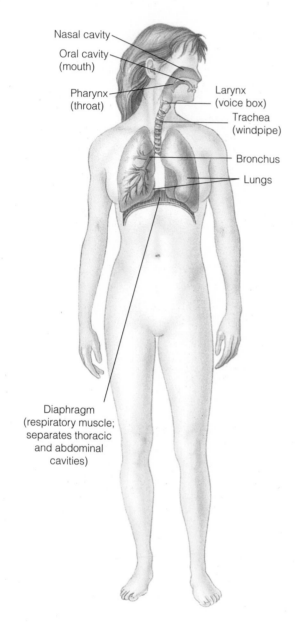

Nasal cavity

Oral cavity (mouth)

Pharynx (throat)

Larynx (voice box)

Trachea (windpipe)

Bronchus

Lungs

Diaphragm (respiratory muscle; separates thoracic and abdominal cavities)

Respiratory system

Root	Meaning
bronch/o	bronchus
laryng/o	larynx; voice box
naso; rhin/o	nose
pharyng/o	pharynx; throat
pneum/o; pneumon/o	lung
thorac/o	chest
trache/o	trachea; windpipe

FIGURE 2-10   Respiratory system. Common structures: oral cavity, nasal cavity, pharynx, larynx, trachea, bronchus, lungs, diaphragm.

Digestive System

Root	Meaning
abdomin/o	abdomen
col/o	colon; large intestine
enter/o	small intestine
esophag/o	esophagus
gastr/o	stomach
gloss/o; lingu/o	tongue
hepat/o	liver
or/o; stomat/o	mouth
pharyng/o	pharynx; throat (also part of the respiratory tract)

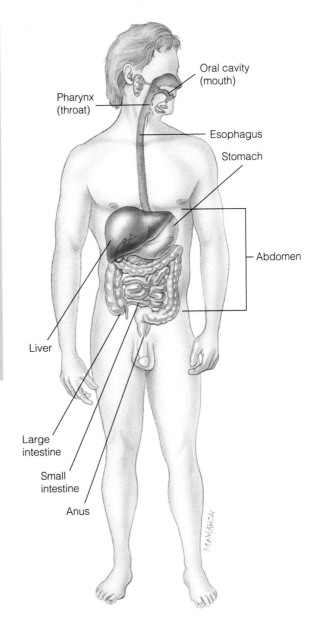

Digestive system

FIGURE 2-11 Digestive system. Common structures: oral cavity, pharynx, esophagus, stomach, small intestine, large intestine, anus, abdomen, liver.

Urinary System

Root	Meaning
cyst/o	bladder
ren/o; nephr/o	kidney
ureter/o	ureters
urethr/o	urethra

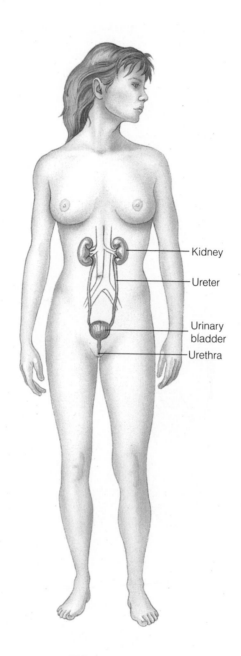

— Kidney

— Ureter

— Urinary bladder

— Urethra

Urinary system

FIGURE 2-12 Urinary system. Common structures: kidneys, ureters, urinary bladder, urethra.

Male Reproductive System

Root	Meaning
orchid/o; test/o	testicle; testis
prostat/o	prostate
vas/o	ductus deferens; vas deferens

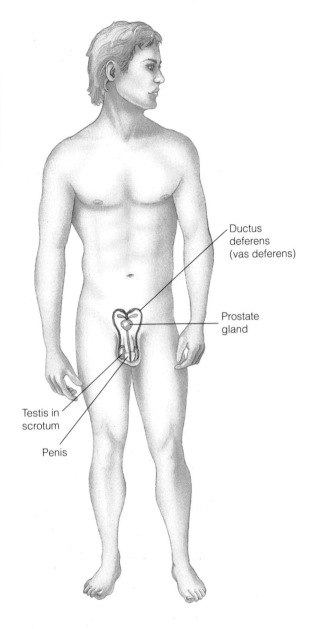

Ductus deferens (vas deferens)

Prostate gland

Testis in scrotum

Penis

Male Reproductive system

FIGURE 2-13 Male reproductive system. Common structures: prostate gland, testis, penis, ductus deferens.

Female Reproductive System

Root	Meaning
colp/o; vagin/o	vagina
gynec/o	female
mast/o; mamm/o	breast
oophor/o; ovari/o	ovary
salping/o	fallopian tube; uterine tube
hyster/o	uterus

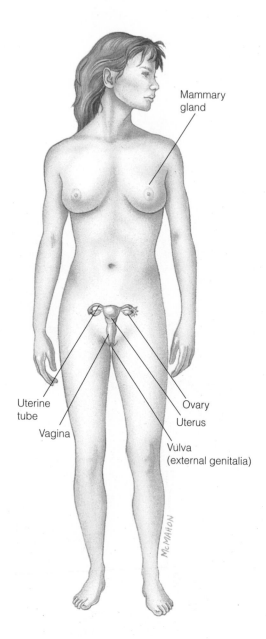

Mammary gland

Uterine tube

Vagina

Ovary

Uterus

Vulva (external genitalia)

Female Reproductive system

FIGURE 2-14 Female reproductive system. Common structures: mammary gland, uterine tube, ovary, uterus, vagina, vulva (external genitalia).

2.5 REVIEW EXERCISES

Exercise 2-1   DEFINITIONS

Give the meaning of the following roots.

1. abdomin/o _____

2. aden/o _____

3. adren/o _____

4. angi/o _____

5. arteri/o _____

6. arthr/o _____

7. bi/o _____

8. bronch/o _____

9. cardi/o _____

10. cephal/o _____

11. cerebr/o _____

12. cervic/o _____

13. chondr/o _____

14. cil/o _____

15. col/o _____

16. colp/o _____

17. cutane/o _____

18. cyst/o _____

19. cyt/o _____

20. dermat/o _____

21. encephal/o _____

22. enter/o _____

23. esophag/o _____

24. gastr/o _____

25. gloss/o _____

26. gynec/o _____

27. hem/o _____

28. hepat/o _____

29. hist/o _____

30. hyster/o _____

31. laryng/o _____

32. lingu/o _____

33. lip/o _____

34. lymphaden/o _____

35. lymphangi/o _____

36. mamm/o _____

37. mast/o _____

38. my/o _____

39. myel/o _____

40. nas/o _____

41. nephr/o _____

42. neur/o _____

43. ocul/o _____

44. onych/o _____

45. oophor/o _____

46. ophthalm/o _____

47. or/o _____

48. orchid/o _____

49. oste/o _____

50. ot/o _____

51. ovari/o _____

52. path/o _____

53. pharyng/o _____

54. phleb/o _____

55. pil/o _____

56. pneum/o _____

57. prostat/o _____

58. ren/o _____

59. rhin/o _____

60. salping/o _____

61. splen/o _____

62. stomat/o _____

63. tend/o _____

64. test/o _____

65. thorac/o _____

66. tonsill/o _____

67. trache/o _____

68. ungu/o _____

69. ureter/o _____

70. urethr/o _____

71. vagin/o _____

72. vas/o _____

73. vascul/o _____

74. ven/o _____

75. viscer/o _____

76. vulv/o _____

Exercise 2-2 | ROOTS

Give the root for each of the following.

1. fat _____

2. life _____

3. head _____

4. neck _____

5. cell _____

6. tissue _____

7. disease _____

8. internal organs _____

9. hair _____

10. skin _____

11. nail _____

12. joint _____

13. cartilage _____

14. bone _____

15. muscle _____

16. tendon _____

17. brain _____

18. spinal cord _____

19. nerve _____

20. eye _____

21. ear _____

22. gland _____

23. adrenal gland _____

24. pituitary gland _____

25. thyroid gland _____

26. vessel _____

27. artery _____

28. heart _____

29. blood _____

30. vein _____

31. lymph node _____

32. lymph vessel _____

33. spleen _____

34. tonsil _____

Exercise 2-3

SHORT ANSWERS

Answer the following in the space provided.

1. Define anatomy and physiology.

   _____

   _____

2. Name 12 body systems and at least two organs in each.

   _____

   _____

   _____

   _____

   _____

   _____

_____

_____

_____

_____

_____

_____

CHAPTER 3

Common Suffixes

LEARNING OBJECTIVES

After studying this chapter and completing the exercises, you should be able to do the following:

1. Spell and define common suffixes.
2. Identify suffixes used to convert medical nouns to adjectives.
3. Pronounce, spell, define, and write medical terms found in this chapter.

INTRODUCTION

In Chapter 1 you learned two important things about suffixes:

- The suffix is always at the end of a medical word.
- The suffix is the first thing to look at when you try to understand a medical word.

This chapter starts by listing new roots and prefixes. The next section introduces you to the most common suffixes. Each suffix and its meaning are listed first, followed by words using the suffix. These examples will help you remember the meaning of the suffixes. When you have learned them, you will be able to understand a great number of medical words.

3.1 NEW ROOTS AND PREFIXES

Use these additional roots and prefixes when studying the terms in this chapter.

Root	Meaning
electr/o	electric
radi/o	x-rays
tom/o	to cut

Prefix	Meaning
dia-	through; complete
pro-	before

3.2 LEARNING THE TERMS

Use the following suggestions for learning medical terms:

1. Pronounce the term repeatedly until it is easy for you.

2. Write it down. Ensure the spelling is correct.

3. Also write the definition. If possible relate the word to a word, thought, or picture that will help you remember it.

4. Analyze the term with the method taught in this text.

Suffix		Meaning
-algia		pain
Term	**Term Analysis**	**Definition**
cephalgia (sef-**AL**-jee-ah)	cephal/o = head	headache; pain in the head
otalgia (oh-**TAL**-jee-ah)	ot/o = ear	earache; pain in the ear

Suffix		Meaning
-cyte		cell
Term	**Term Analysis**	**Definition**
adipocyte (**AD**-ih-poh-**sight**)	adip/o = fat	fat cell

Suffix	Meaning
-ectomy	**surgical removal; excision**

Term	Term Analysis	Definition
hysterectomy (**hiss**-ter-**ECK**-toh-mee)	hyster/o = uterus	surgical removal or excision of the uterus
mastectomy (mas-**TECK**-toh-mee)	mast/o = breast	surgical removal or excision of the breast

NOTE: Excision means to cut out

Suffix	Meaning
-gnosis	**knowledge**

Term	Term Analysis	Definition
diagnosis (**dye**-ag-**NOH**-sis)	dia- = through; complete	determining what disease or condition is present through a study of the signs and symptoms, and laboratory, x-ray, and other diagnostic procedures *Example: After complete investigation, a diagnosis of osteoarthritis was made.*
prognosis (prahg-**NOH**-sis)	pro- = before	forecast of the outcome of the disease

NOTE: The prognosis is either good or bad. If the patient is likely to recover from the disease, the prognosis is good. If the patient is not likely to recover from the disease, the prognosis is bad.

(continued)

		*Example: The patient was admitted with a diagnosis of osteoarthritis. His **prognosis** was good.*

Suffix		Meaning
-gram		record; write
Term	**Term Analysis**	**Definition**
angiogram (**AN-jee-oh-gram**)	angi/o = vessel	record (image) of a blood vessel is produced using x-rays and contrast medium (Figure 3-1).

NOTE 1: An image is produced of the body structure, thereby creating a record of that structure.

NOTE 2: Contrast medium is a dye that is placed into the patient's body to improve the visibility of the x-ray.

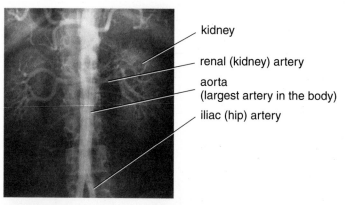

kidney

renal (kidney) artery

aorta (largest artery in the body)

iliac (hip) artery

FIGURE 3-1 Angiogram of abdominal arteries. In an angiogram, the arteries show up white because contrast medium has been placed into the body.

myelogram (**MY-eh-loh-gram**)	myel/o = spinal cord	record (image) of the spinal cord taken by x-rays

Term	Term Analysis	Meaning
mammogram (**MAM**-oh-gram)	mamm/o = breast	record (image) of the breast is produced using x-rays (Figure 3-2).

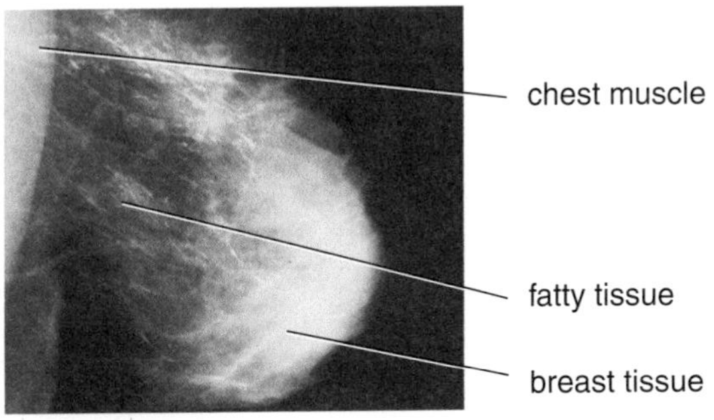

chest muscle

fatty tissue

breast tissue

FIGURE 3-2   Mammogram: record of the breast.

Term	Term Analysis	Meaning
venogram (**VEE**-noh-gram)	ven/o = vein	record (image) of a vein is produced using x-rays and contrast medium.

Suffix	Meaning	
-graph	instrument used to record	
Term	**Term Analysis**	**Definition**
cardiograph (**KAR**-dee-oh-**graf**)	cardi/o = heart	instrument used to record the heart's activity
electro-cardiograph (ee-**leck**-troh-**KAR**-dee-oh-**graf**)	electr/o = electric cardi/o = heart	instrument used to record the electrical activity of the heart (Figure 3-3A and B)

(continued)

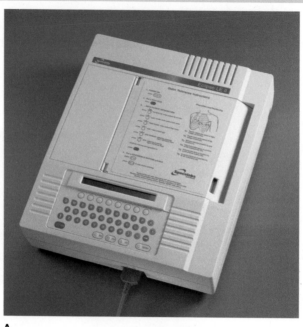

A

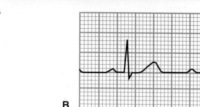

B

FIGURE 3-3 A. Electrocardiograph: instrument that
records the electrical activity of the heart. (Courtesy of
Spacelabs Medical Inc.) B. Electrocardiogram: record
of the electrical activity of the heart.

Suffix	Meaning	
-graphy	process of recording; process of producing images	
Term	**Term Analysis**	**Definition**
cardiography (**kar**-dee-**OG**-rah-fee)	cardi/o = heart	process of recording the heart's activity
computed tomography (kom-**PYOO**-ted) (toh-**MOG**-rah-fee)	tom/o = to cut	an x-ray beam rotates around the patient taking multiple images of an organ at different depths (Figure 3-4 A, B,

and C). The information is computer analyzed and converted to a picture of the body part.

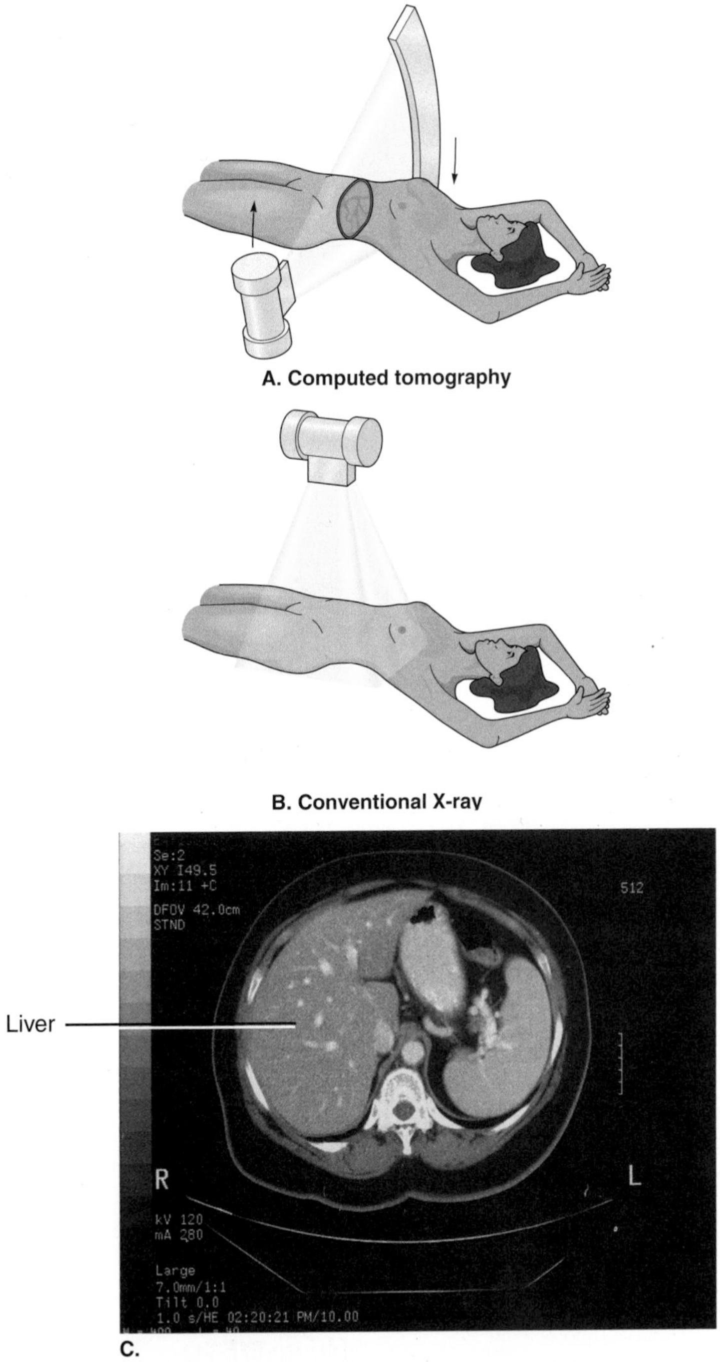

A. Computed tomography

B. Conventional X-ray

Liver

C.

FIGURE 3-4 Computed tomography and conventional x-ray procedure. A. Computed tomography. B. Conventional x-ray. C. Computed tomography (CT) scan shows blood vessels of the liver.

Term	Term Analysis	Definition
mammography (mam-**OG**-rah-fee)	mamm/o = breast	process of producing images of the breast (See Figure 3-5)

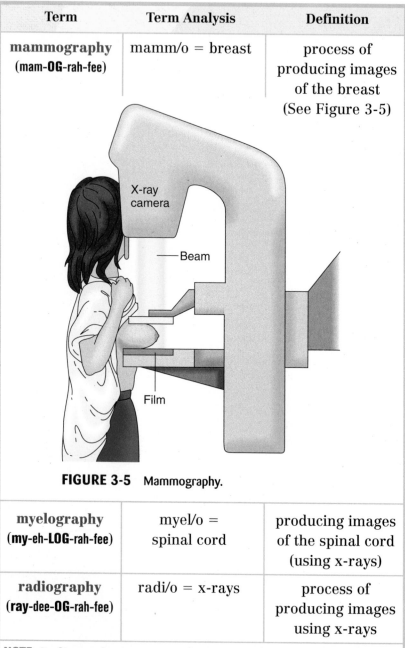

FIGURE 3-5 Mammography.

Term	Term Analysis	Definition
myelography (**my**-eh-**LOG**-rah-fee)	myel/o = spinal cord	producing images of the spinal cord (using x-rays)
radiography (ray-dee-**OG**-rah-fee)	radi/o = x-rays	process of producing images using x-rays

NOTE: Radiography is a general term. It refers to images that are taken of any internal body structure using x-rays.

Suffix	Meaning	
-itis	inflammation	
Term	**Term Analysis**	**Definition**
enteritis (**en**-ter-**EYE**-tis)	enter/o = small intestine	inflammation of the small intestine
stomatitis (**sto**-mah-**TYE**-tis)	stomat/o = mouth	inflammation of the mouth

Term	Term Analysis	Definition
tonsillitis (ton-sih-**LYE**-tis)	tonsill/o = tonsil	inflammation of the tonsils

Suffix	Meaning
-logy	study of

Term	Term Analysis	Definition
cardiology (**kar**-dee-**OL**-oh-jee)	cardi/o = heart	study of the heart
dermatology (**der**-mah-**TOL**-oh-jee)	dermat/o = skin	study of the skin

Suffix	Meaning
-logist	specialist; one who studies

Term	Term Analysis	Definition
gynecologist (**guy**-neh-**KOL**-oh-jist)	gynec/o = woman	specialist in the study of the diseases and treatment of female disorders
ophthalmologist (**ahf**-thal-**MOL**-eh-jist)	ophthalm/o = eye	specialist in the study of the diseases and treatment of eye disorders

Suffix	Meaning
-oma	tumor; mass

Term	Term Analysis	Definition
adenoma (**ad**-eh-**NOH**-mah)	aden/o = gland	tumor of a gland
osteoma (**os**-tee-**OH**-mah)	oste/o = bone	tumor of bone
hematoma (**hem**-ah-**TOH**-mah)	hemat/o = blood	mass or collection of blood outside a blood vessel; a bruise

Suffix	Meaning
-osis	abnormal condition

Term	Term Analysis	Definition
nephrosis (neh-**FROH**-sis)	nephr/o = kidney	abnormal condition of the kidney

Suffix	Meaning
-pathy	disease

Term	Term Analysis	Definition
nephropathy (nef-**ROP**-pah-thee)	nephr/o = kidney	disease of the kidney
neuropathy (new-**ROP**-pah-thee)	neur/o = nerve	disease of the nerve

Suffix	Meaning
-plasty	surgical reconstruction

Term	Term Analysis	Definition
rhinoplasty (**RYE**-noh-**plas**-tee)	rhin/o = nose	surgical reconstruction of the nose; nose job
arthroplasty (**AR**-throh-**plas**-tee)	arthr/o = joint	surgical reconstruction of a joint

Suffix	Meaning
-rrhage; -rrhagia	bursting forth

Term	Term Analysis	Definition
hemorrhage (**HEM**-or-idj)	hem/o = blood	bursting forth of blood; bleeding
gastrorrhagia (**gas**-troh-**RAY**-jee-ah)	gastr/o = stomach	bleeding from the stomach

Suffix	Meaning
-rrhaphy	to suture (to sew)

Term	Term Analysis	Definition
colporrhaphy (kol-**POR**-ah-fee)	colp/o = vagina	suturing the wall of the vagina (Figure 3-6)

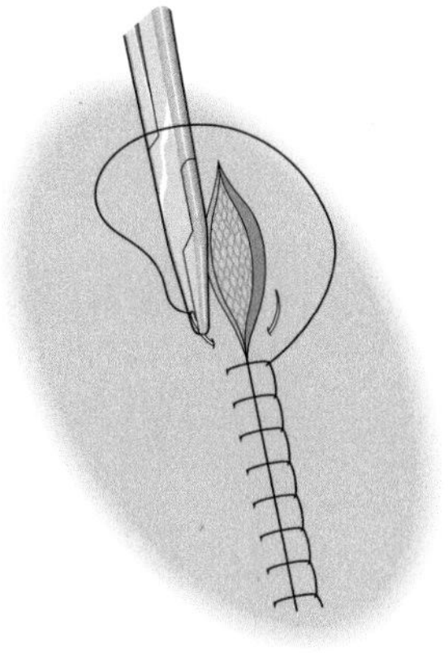

Continuous sutures

FIGURE 3-6   To suture (sew). The edges of the wound are brought together by suturing.

Suffix	Meaning
-rrhea	flow; discharge

Term	Term Analysis	Definition
otorrhea (**oh**-toh-**REE**-ah)	ot/o = ear	discharge from the ear

Suffix	Meaning
-rrhexis	rupture

Term	Term Analysis	Definition
splenorrhexis (**splee**-nor-**ECKS**-sis)	splen/o = spleen	ruptured spleen

Suffix	Meaning
-scope	instrument used to view inside a body cavity or organ

Term	Term Analysis	Definition
arthroscope (**AR**-throh-skope)	arthr/o = joint	instrument used to view the inside of a joint (Figure 3-7)

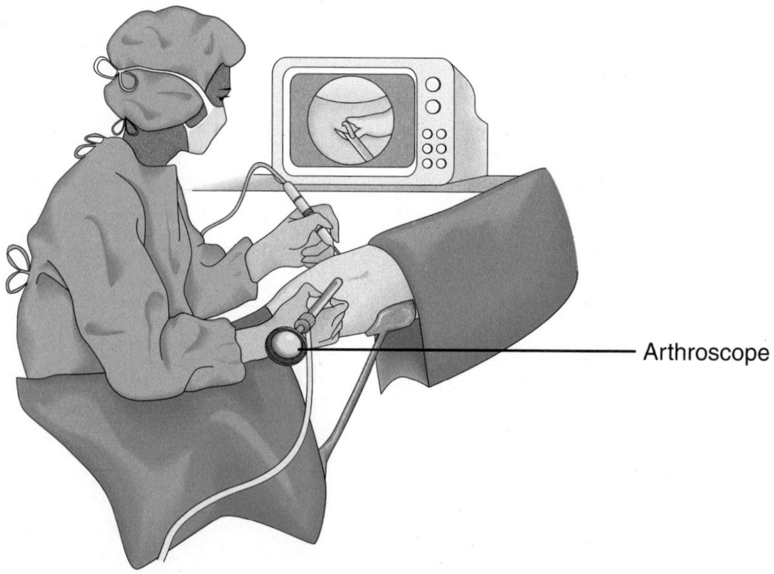

FIGURE 3-7 Arthroscope in use during an arthroscopy.

Term	Term Analysis	Definition
gastroscope (**GAS**-troh-skope)	gastr/o = stomach	instrument used to view the inside of the stomach

Suffix	Meaning
-scopy	the process of viewing inside a body cavity or organ

Term	Term Analysis	Definition
endoscopy (en-**DOS**-koh-pee)	endo- = within	process of visually examining the inside of a body cavity or organ using an endoscope (Figure 3-8)

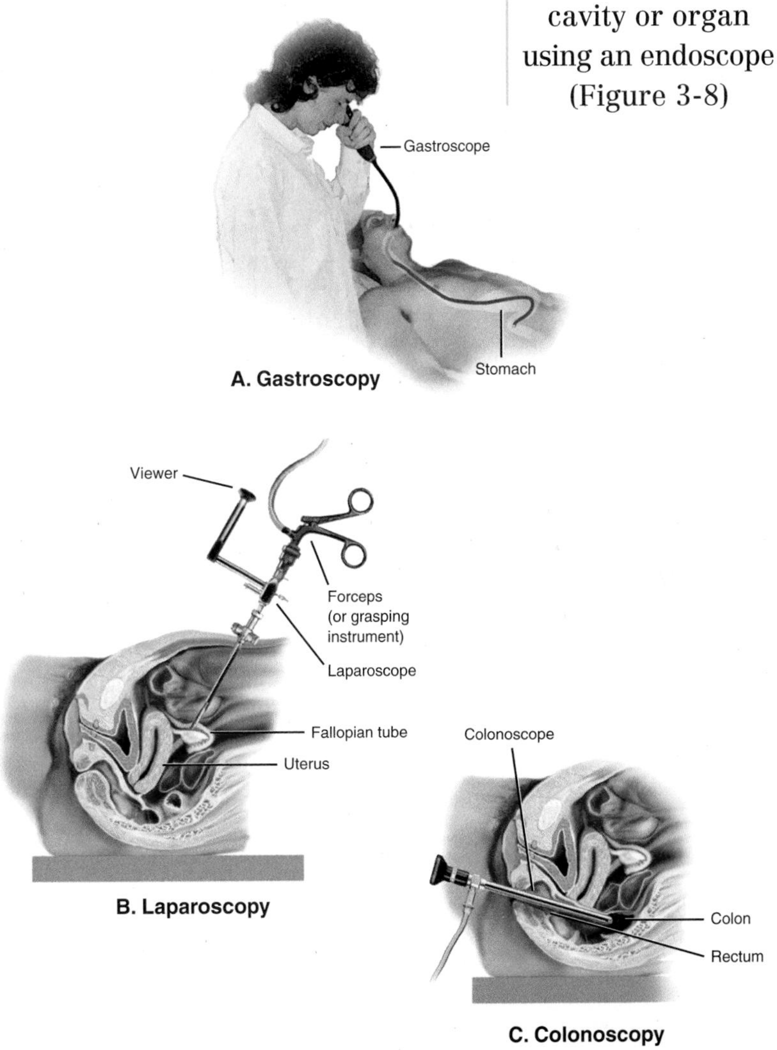

A. Gastroscopy

B. Laparoscopy

C. Colonoscopy

FIGURE 3-8   Endoscopies. A. Gastroscopy. B. Laparoscopy. C. Colonoscopy.

NOTE: Specific endoscopies are named after the organ being studied.		
bronchoscopy (brong-**KOS**-koh-pee)	bronch/o = bronchus	process of viewing inside the bronchus
laparoscopy (lap-ah-**ROS**-koh-pee)	lapar/o = abdomen	process of viewing the abdomen (refer to Figure 3-8B)

IN BRIEF

-scope = instrument used to view inside a body cavity or organ

-scopy = process of viewing inside a body cavity or organ

Suffix	Meaning
-stenosis	narrowing

Term	Term Analysis	Definition
arteriostenosis (ar-**ter**-ee-oh-steh-**NOH**-sis)	arteri/o = artery	narrowing of an artery

Suffix	Meaning
-stomy	surgical creation of a new opening

Term	Term Analysis	Definition
colostomy (koh-**LOSS**-toh-mee)	col/o = colon	surgical creation of a new opening in the colon
tracheostomy (tray-kee-**OS**-toh-mee)	trache/o = trachea; windpipe	surgical creation of a new opening into the trachea

IN BRIEF

-**stomy** = surgical creation of a new opening

-**tomy** = to cut

incision means to cut into

excision means to cut out

Suffix	Meaning
-tomy	to cut; incision

Term	Term Analysis	Definition
tenotomy (teh-**NOT**-oh-mee)	ten/o = tendon	to cut the tendon; incision of the tendon
tracheotomy (tray-kee-**OT**-toh-mee)	trache/o = trachea; windpipe	to cut the trachea; incision of the trachea

NOTE: Incision means to cut into.

Suffix	Meaning	
-trophy	growth; nourishment	
Term	**Term Analysis**	**Definition**
atrophy (**AH**-troh-fee)	a- = no; not	wasting away of the muscle (Figure 3-9A)
hypertrophy (high-**PER**-troh-fee)	hyper- = excessive	excessive growth or enlargement of an organ or part (Figure 3-9B)

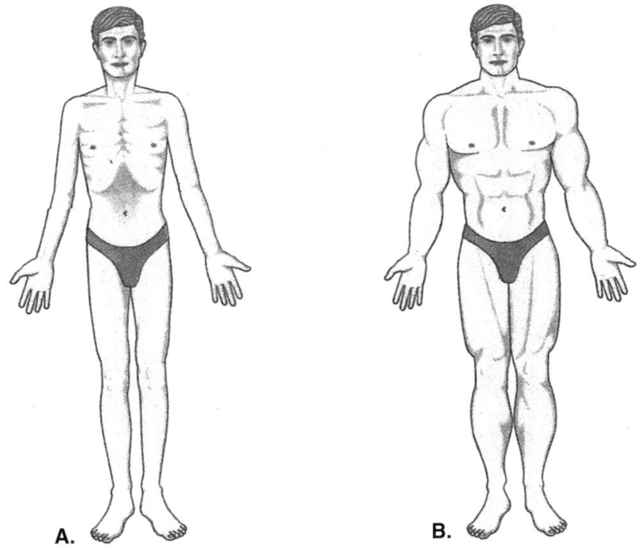

FIGURE 3-9 Differences in muscle size. A. Atrophy. B. Hypertrophy.

Suffixes Used as Adjectives

Suffix	Meaning	
-al; -ar, - ic; -ous	pertaining to	
Term	**Term Analysis**	**Definition**
natal (**NAY**-tal)	nat/o = birth	pertaining to birth
muscular (**MUS**-kyou-lar)	muscul/o = muscle	pertaining to muscle
septic (**SEHP**-tick)	sept/o = infection	pertaining to infection

Suffix	Meaning	
-al; -ar, - ic; -ous	pertaining to	
Term	**Term Analysis**	**Definition**
cutaneous (kyoo-**TAY**-nee-us)	cutane/o = skin	pertaining to the skin

NOTE: Although there are some exceptions, the suffixes meaning "pertaining to" are not interchangeable with a given root. For example, you can say muscul**ar**, but not muscul**al**, muscul**ic**, or muscul**ous**.

3.3 REVIEW EXERCISES

Exercise 3-1 MATCHING WORD PARTS WITH MEANING

Match the word part in Column A *with its meaning in* Column B

Column A	Column B
_____ 1. -algia	A. specialist
_____ 2. -ectomy	B. tumor; mass
_____ 3. -logy	C. nourishment
_____ 4. -logist	D. excision; surgical removal
_____ 5. -ous	E. surgical reconstruction
_____ 6. -scopy	F. pertaining to
_____ 7. -scope	G. pain
_____ 8. -plasty	H. instrument used to view inside an organ
_____ 9. -oma	I. study of
_____ 10. -trophy	J. process of viewing inside an organ

Exercise 3-2 DEFINITIONS

Give the meaning of the following suffixes.

a. **-trophy** _____

b. **-algia** _____

c. **-tomy** _____

d. -ectomy _____

e. -gram _____

f. -logist _____

g. scope _____

h. -itis _____

i. -plasty _____

j. -logy _____

k. -ous _____

l. -oma _____

m. -ic _____

n. -al _____

o. -scopy _____

p. -osis _____

Exercise 3-3   **IDENTIFYING AND DEFINING WORD PARTS**

In the words listed below, separate the medical term into its word parts with a slash (/). Then, define the term in the space provided. The first question is answered for you.

a. **aden/oma** tumor of a gland

b. **otalgia** _____

c. **dermatologist** _____

d. **hysterectomy** _____

e. **cardiology** _____

f. **myelogram** _____

g. **tonsillitis** _____

h. **cutaneous** _____

i. **hypertrophy** _____

j. **rhinoplasty** _____

k. **arthroscopy** _____

l. **arthroscope** _____

m. **tracheotomy** _____

n. **natal** _____

o. **septic** _____

Exercise 3-4

ADJECTIVAL SUFFIX

Match the root with the correct adjectival ending, then complete the sentences below.

Root	Adjectival Suffix
muscul-	-al
nat-	-ic
sept-	-ous
cutane-	-ar

1. I pulled a muscle. I now have _____ pain.

2. I have red marks on my skin. The doctor said it was a _____ rash.

3. I am going to have a baby. I am going to pre-_____ classes.

4. Throw the infectious material away. Put it in the garbage for _____ material.

Exercise 3-5

SPELLING

Circle the word that is correctly spelled in each group below.

1. cephalalga   cefalalgia   cephalgia

2. hysterectomy   histerectomy

3. tonsillitis   tonsilitis

4. cardology   cardiology

5. ophthalmologist   opthalmologist   ophtalmologist

6. nephrosis   nephrosus

7. tracheotomy   traechotomy

8. hypertrophe   hypertrophy

9. enteritis   enteritus

10. mylogram   myelogram

| **Exercise 3-6** | DEFINITIONS |

Define the following terms.

1. **adenoma** _____

2. **arthroplasty** _____

3. **arthroscope** _____

4. **bronchoscopy** _____

5. **cardiology** _____

6. **cephalgia** _____

7. **dermatology** _____

8. **enteritis** _____

9. **gastroscope** _____

10. **laparoscopy** _____

11. **gynecologist** _____

12. **hematoma** _____

13. **hypertrophy** _____

14. **hysterectomy** _____

15. **mastectomy** _____

16. **myelogram** _____

17. **nephropathy** _____

18. **nephrosis** _____

19. **neuropathy** _____

20. **ophthalmologist** _____

21. **osteoma** _____

22. **otalgia** _____

23. **rhinoplasty** _____

24. stomatitis _____

25. tenotomy _____

26. tonsillitis _____

27. tracheotomy _____

28. tracheostomy _____

29. excision _____

30. incision _____

3.4 PRONUNCIATION AND SPELLING

To practice your pronunciation:

1. Listen to each of the following words on the audio CD.

2. Pronounce each word carefully.

3. Spell each word in the space provided.

Word	Pronunciation	Spelling
adenoma	ad-eh-**NOH**-mah	_____
arthroscope	**AR**-throh-skohp	_____
arthroscopy	ar-**THROS**-koh-pee	_____
cardiology	kar-dee-**OL**-oh-jee	_____
colostomy	koh-**LOSS**-toh-mee	_____
dermatology	der-mah-**TOL**-oh-jee	_____
electrocardiograph	ee-**leck**-troh-**KAR**-dee-oh-**graf**	_____
enteritis	en-ter-**EYE**-tis	_____
gastroscopy	gas-**TROS**-koh-pee	_____
gynecologist	guy-neh-**KOL**-oh-jist	_____
hematoma	hem-ah-**TOH**-mah	_____
hypertrophy	high-**PER**-troh-fee	_____
hysterectomy	hiss-ter-**ECK**-toh-mee	_____

Word	Pronunciation	Spelling
mastectomy	mas-**TECK**-toh-mee	
muscular	**MUS**-kyoo-lar	
myelogram	**MY**-eh-loh-gram	
myelography	my-eh-**LOG**-rah-fee	
natal	**NAY**-tal	
nephropathy	nef-**ROP**-pah-thee	
nephrosis	neh-**FROH**-sis	
neuropathy	new-**ROP**-pah-thee	
ophthalmologist	ahf-thal-**MOL**-eh-jist	
osteoma	os-tee-**OH**-mah	
otalgia	oh-**TAL**-gee-ah	
prognosis	prahg-**NOH**-sis	
radiography	ray-dee-**OG**-rah-fee	
stomatitis	sto-mah-**TYE**-tis	
tenotomy	teh-**NOT**-oh-mee	
tomography	toh-**MOG**-rah-fee	
tonsillitis	ton-sih-**LYE**-tis	
tracheotomy	tray-kee-**OT**-toh-mee	

CHAPTER 4

Common Prefixes

LEARNING OBJECTIVES

After studying this chapter and completing the exercises, you should be able to do the following:

1. State the meaning of prefixes found in this chapter.
2. Pronounce, spell, define, and write medical terms that use prefixes in this chapter.
3. Identify prefixes that have the same meaning.
4. Identify prefixes that have the opposite meaning.

INTRODUCTION

This chapter introduces you to the most common prefixes. It starts by listing new roots and suffixes used in this chapter.

The next section displays the prefix and its meaning first, followed by words using the prefix.

4.1 NEW ROOTS AND SUFFIXES

Use these additional roots and suffixes when studying the medical terms in this chapter.

Root	Meaning
cellul/o	cell
cis/o	to cut
cost/o	rib
later/o	side
nat/o	birth
son/o	sound

Suffix	Meaning
-genous	produced by
-ion	process
-mortem	death
-partum	delivery
-plasia; plasm	development; formation
-pnea	breathing
-tic	pertaining to
-um	structure
-uria	urination; urine

4.2 LEARNING THE TERMS

Use the following suggestions for learning medical terms:

1. Pronounce the term repeatedly until it is easy for you.

2. Write it down. Ensure the spelling is correct.

3. Also write the definition. If possible relate the word to a word, thought, or picture that will help you remember it.

4. Analyze the term with the method taught in this text.

Prefix	Meaning
a(n)-	no; not

Term	Term Analysis		Definition
apnea (**AP**-nee-ah)	-pnea = breathing		not breathing
anuria (ah-**NEW**-ree-ah)	-uria = urine; urination		no urine (being formed in the kidney)

NOTE: "a-" is changed to "an-" before suffixes that start with a vowel.

Prefix	Meaning
ante-	before

Term	Term Analysis		Definition
antenatal (**an**-tee-**NAY**-tal)	-al = pertaining to nat/o = birth		pertaining to before birth
antepartum (**an**-tee-**PAR**-tum)	-partum = delivery, labor, childbirth		before childbirth

HELPING YOU REMEMBER

The prefix "anti-" means "against." Note that both the prefix and its meaning contain the letter "i."

The prefix "ante-" means "before." Both the prefix and its meaning contain the letter "e."

Prefix	Meaning
anti-	against

Term	Term Analysis		Definition
antibiotic (**an**-tih-bye-**OT**-ick)	-tic = pertaining to bi/o = life		drugs used against bacteria that have infected the body

HELPING YOU REMEMBER

A bicycle has two wheels.

Prefix	Meaning
bi-	two

Term	Term Analysis		Definition
bilateral (bye-**LAT**-er-al)	-al = pertaining to later/o = side		pertaining to two sides

Prefix	Meaning
dys-	bad; difficult; painful; abnormal

Term	Term Analysis	Definition
dysplasia (dis-**PLAY**-see-ah)	-plasia = development; formation	abnormal development
dyspnea (**DISP**-nee-ah)	-pnea = breathing	difficult breathing
dysuria (dis-**YOO**-ree-ah)	-uria = urine; urination	painful urination
dystrophy (**DIS**-troh-fee)	-trophy = nourishment; growth; development	abnormal development, especially muscular dystrophy

Prefix	Meaning
endo-	within

Term	Term Analysis	Definition
endogenous (en-**DOJ**-eh-nus)	-genous = produced by	produced from within the body; infection that originates from within the body

Prefix	Meaning
epi-	upon; above

Term	Term Analysis	Definition
epicardium (ep-ih-**KAR**-dee-um)	-um = pertaining to cardi/o = heart	pertaining to upon the heart

Prefix	Meaning
ex-	out

Term	Term Analysis	Definition
excision (eck-**SIH**-zhun)	-ion = process cis/o = to cut	process of cutting out; the removal of tissue from the body

Prefix	Meaning
hyper-	above; excessive

Term	Term Analysis	Definition
hyperplasia (high-per-**PLAY**-see-ah)	-plasia = development; formation	excessive formation of cells; abnormal increase in the number of normal cells in normal tissue

Prefix	Meaning
hypo-	below; deficient

Term	Term Analysis	Definition
hypogastric (high-poh-**GAS**-trick)	-ic = pertaining to gastr/o = stomach	pertaining to below the stomach

Prefix	Meaning
in-	in; into

Term	Term Analysis	Definition
incision (in-**SIH**-zhun)	-ion = process cis/o = to cut	process of cutting into

Prefix	Meaning
infra-	below

Term	Term Analysis	Definition
infracostal (in-frah-**KOS**-tal)	-al = pertaining to cost/o = rib	pertaining to below the rib

Prefix	Meaning
inter-	between

Term	Term Analysis	Definition
intercellular (in-ter-**SEL**-yoo-lar)	-ar = pertaining to cellul/o = cell	pertaining to between the cells
intercostal (in-ter-**KOS**-tal)	-al = pertaining to cost/o = rib	pertaining to between the ribs

Prefix	Meaning
intra-	within

Term	Term Analysis	Definition
intracranial (in-trah-**KRAY**-nee-al)	-al = pertaining to crani/o = head	pertaining to within the head
intramuscular (in-trah-**MUS**-kyoo-lar)	-ar = pertaining to muscul/o = muscle	pertaining to within a muscle
intravenous (in-trah-**VEE**-nus)	-ous = pertaining to ven/o = vein	pertaining to within a vein

Prefix	Meaning
neo-	new

Term	Term Analysis	Definition
neoplasm (**NEE**-oh-plazm)	-plasm = development; formation	new growth of tissue; a tumor

Prefix	Meaning
peri-	around

Term	Term Analysis	Definition
perineuritis (**per**-ih-nyoo-**RYE**-tis)	-itis = inflammation neur/o = nerve	inflammation around the nerve

Prefix	Meaning
post-	after

Term	Term Analysis	Definition
postmortem (pohst-**MOR**-tehm)	-mortem = death examination = to look at; to inspect	after death; autopsy
postpartum (pohst-**PAR**-tum)	-partum = delivery; labor; childbirth	after childbirth

Prefix	Meaning
pre-	before

Term	Term Analysis	Definition
prenatal (pre-**NAY**-tal)	-al = pertaining to nat/o = birth	pertaining to before birth

Prefix	Meaning
pro-	before

Term	Term Analysis	Definition
prodrome (**PROH**-drohm)	-drome = run	symptom or symptoms occurring before the onset of disease. *Example: chest pain, tiredness, and shortness of breath are prodromal symptoms of a heart attack.*

Prefix	Meaning
sub-	under; below

Term	Term Analysis	Definition
subcutaneous (sub-kyoo-**TAY**-nee-us)	-ous = pertaining to cutane/o = skin	pertaining to under the skin (Figure 4-1)

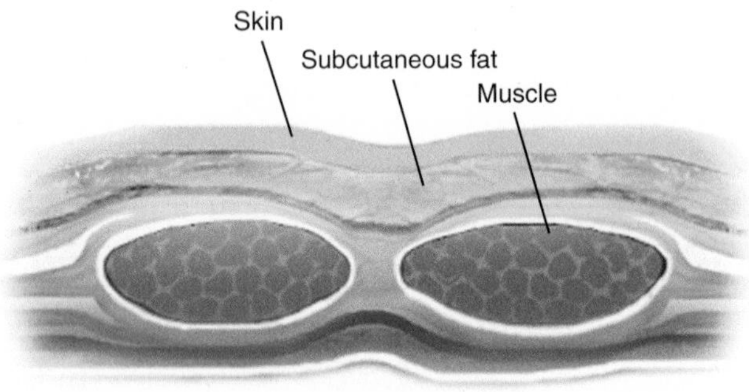

FIGURE 4-1 Skin and subcutaneous fat.

Term	Term Analysis	Definition
sublingual (sub-**LING**-gwal)	-al = pertaining to lingu/o = tongue	pertaining to under the tongue

Prefix	Meaning
trans-	through; across

Term	Term Analysis	Definition
transection (tran-**SECK**-shun)	-ion = process sect/o = cut	process of cutting across (Figure 4-2)

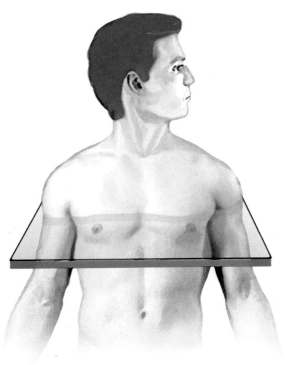

FIGURE 4-2 Transection (the process of cutting across the body or an organ).

Prefix	Meaning
ultra-	beyond

Term	Term Analysis	Definition
ultrasonography (ul-trah-son-**OG**-rah-fee)	-graphy = process of recording son/o = sound	process of recording an image of internal structures by using high frequency sound waves (Figure 4-3). Also known as ultrasound.

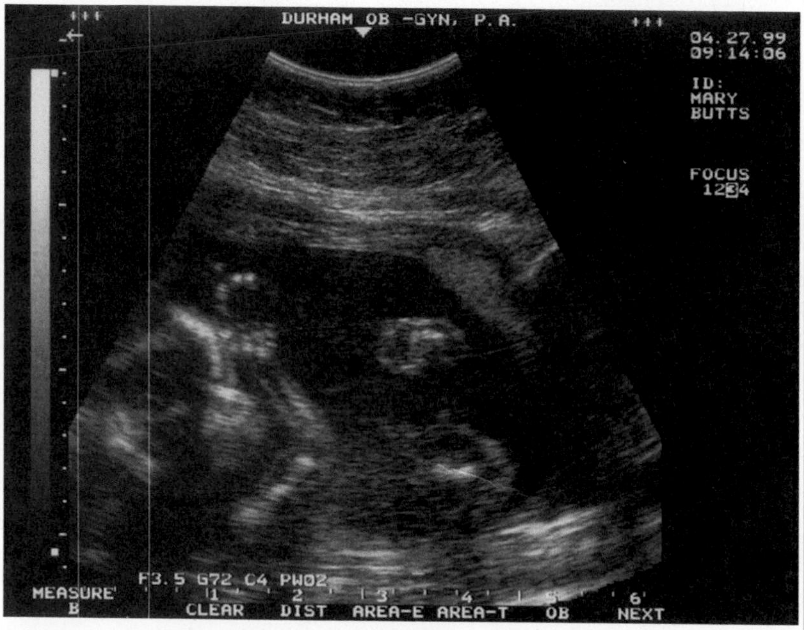

FIGURE 4-3 An image is produced by ultrasonography.

4.3 SUMMARY OF PREFIXES THAT HAVE THE SAME MEANING

Meaning	Prefix
above	epi-; hyper-
before	ante-; pre-; pro-
below	hypo-; infra-; sub-
within	endo-; intra-

4.4 SUMMARY OF PREFIXES THAT HAVE THE OPPOSITE MEANING

Meaning	Prefix
excessive deficient	hyper- hypo-
after before	post- ante-; pre-; pro-
above below	epi-; hyper- hypo-; infra-; sub-
in; into out	in- ex-

4.5 REVIEW EXERCISES

Exercise 4-1   MATCHING WORD PARTS WITH MEANING

Match the word element in Column A *with its meaning in* Column B.

Column A		Column B
_____	1. trans-	A. before
_____	2. anti-	B. difficult
_____	3. endo-	C. below
_____	4. sub-	D. across
_____	5. ante-	E. excessive
_____	6. infra-	F. after
_____	7. hyper-	G. against
_____	8. post-	H. under
_____	9. dys-	I. around
_____	10. peri-	J. within

Exercise 4-2   DEFINITIONS

Write the meaning of the prefix in the space provided.

a. sub- _____

b. dys- _____

    c. ex- _____

    d. bi- _____

    e. post- _____

    f. anti- _____

    g. intra- _____

    h. ante- _____

    i. hypo- _____

    j. a(n)- _____

    k. hyper- _____

    l. endo- _____

    m. pre- _____

    n. peri- _____

Exercise 4-3	IDENTIFYING AND DEFINING WORD PARTS

In the words listed below, separate the medical term into its word parts with a slash. Then, define the term in the space provided. The first question is answered for you.

    a. **pre/nat/al** pertaining to before birth_____

    b. **postmortem**_____

    c. **perineuritis**_____

    d. **apnea**_____

    e. **dysuria**_____

    f. **antenatal**_____

    g. **subcutaneous**_____

    h. **hypogastric**_____

    i. **bilateral**_____

    j. **intramuscular**_____

    k. **dyspnea**_____

    l. **infracostal**_____

    m. **hyperplasia**_____

    n. **endogenous**_____

| Exercise 4-4 | WORD BUILDING AND SENTENCE COMPLETION |

Build a known medical word by matching one of the prefixes from the left-hand column with the correct root or suffix in the right-hand column. Then, complete the following sentences using the correct medical word.

Prefix	Root or Suffix
anti-	-cutaneous
a-	-gnosis
infra-	-pnea
sub-	-biotics
pro-	-costal

1. I have an infection. The doctor gave me a prescription for _____ .

2. Salina broke her arm. The doctor said her bone would repair itself quickly. He said that the _____ was good.

3. Miguel received an injection under his skin. It is called a(n) _____ injection.

4. Sometimes when I am sleeping I stop breathing. The doctor says I have sleep _____ .

5. The pain is located below the ribs. The physician said this was _____ pain.

| Exercise 4-5 | SPELLING |

Circle the word that is correctly spelled in each group below.

1. antenatal   antinatal   antenatul

2. antebiotic   antibyotic   antibiotic

3. bylateral   bilateral   billateral

4. dispnea   dyspnea   dysneea

5. dysuria   dysurea   disuria

6. exsision	eccision	excision
7. intracranal	intracranial	intracraneal
8. perineuritis	perenuritis	perineuritus
9. postmortum	postmortem	postmoretem
10. subqutaneus	subcutaneus	subcutaneous

4.6 PRONUNCIATION AND SPELLING

1. Listen to each word on the audio CD.

2. Pronounce each word carefully.

3. Spell each word in the space provided.

Word	Pronunciation	Spelling
antenatal	an-tee-**NAY**-tal	
antepartum	an-tee-**PAR**-tum	
antibiotic	an-tih-bye-**OT**-ick	
anuria	ah-**NOO**-ree-ah	
apnea	**AP**-nee-ah	
bilateral	bye-**LAT**-er-al	
dysplasia	dis-**PLAY**-see-ah	
dyspnea	**DISP**-nee-ah	
dysuria	dis-**YOO**-ree-ah	
endogenous	en-**DOJ**-eh-nus	
epicardium	ep-ih-**KAR**-dee-um	
excision	eck-**SIH**-zhun	
hyperplasia	high-per-**PLAY**-see-ah	
hypogastric	high-poh-**GAS**-trick	
incision	in-**SIH**-zhun	
infracostal	in-frah-**KOS**-tal	
intracranial	in-trah-**KRAY**-nee-al	

Word	Pronunciation	Spelling
intramuscular	**in**-trah-**MUS**-kyoo-lar	
perineuritis	**per**-ih-nyoo-**RYE**-tis	
postmortem	pohst-**MOR**-tehm	
postpartum	pohst-**PAR**-tum	
prenatal	pre-**NAY**-tal	
subcutaneous	**sub**-kyoo-**TAY**-nee-us	
sublingual	sub-**LING**-gwal	
transection	tran-**SECK**-shun	
ultrasonography	**ul**-trah-son-**OG**-rah-fee	

CHAPTER 5

Body Organization

CHAPTER OUTLINE

LEARNING OBJECTIVES

After studying this chapter and completing the exercises, you should be able to do the following:

1. Name the cavities of the body and their related organs.
2. Define the anatomical position.
3. Define common terms used for directions.
4. Name and locate the abdominopelvic regions.
5. Name and locate the abdominopelvic quadrants.
6. Pronounce, spell, define, and write medical terms common to the body as a whole.
7. Listen, read, and study, so you can speak and write.

INTRODUCTION

This chapter will teach you common terminology relating to the organization of the body. You will also learn the terms used to describe the position of the body and the placement of various body parts.

5.1 BODY CAVITIES

PRACTICE FOR LEARNING: BODY CAVITIES

Write the words below in the correct spaces on Figure 5-1. To help you, the number beside the word tells you where it goes on the figure. Be sure to pronounce each word as you write it. Repeat the pronunciation several times if you find the word hard to say.

1. dorsal cavity (**DOOR**-sal **KAH**-vih-tee)

2. ventral cavity (**VEN**-tral)

3. cranial cavity (**KRAY**-nee-al)

4. vertebral cavity (**VER**-teh-bral)

5. abdominal cavity (ab-**DOM**-ih-nal)

6. pelvic cavity (**PEL**-vick)

7. thoracic cavity (thoh-**RAS**-ick)

When you study the body cavities, think of a backpack. The backpack has empty spaces called pouches. Some are big, some are small. The body has empty spaces inside it as well. But they are not called pouches. They are called cavities.

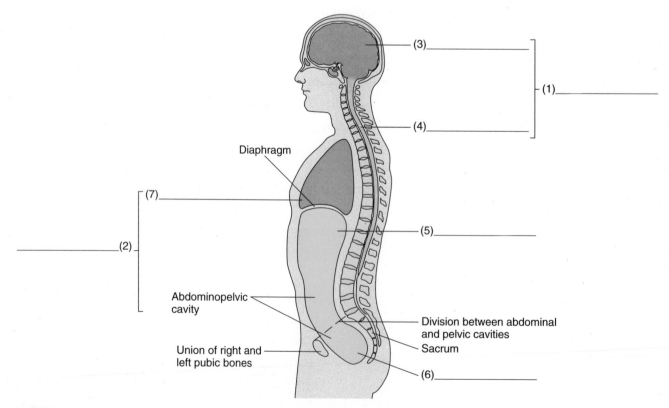

FIGURE 5-1 Major body cavities and subdivisions.

The body has two main cavities: the dorsal and the ventral. The dorsal cavity is also called the posterior cavity, because it is at the back of the body. Posterior refers to the back. The ventral cavity is also called the anterior cavity, because it is at the front of the body. Anterior refers to the front. Each of these cavities has further subdivisions, which are shown in Figure 5-1.

Dorsal Cavity

The dorsal cavity is subdivided into two parts: the cranial cavity and vertebral cavity. The cranial cavity is inside the skull. The brain is contained in the cranial cavity. The vertebral cavity is inside the vertebral column, or spine. The spinal cord (a group of nerves) is contained in the vertebral cavity.

Ventral Cavity

The ventral cavity contains many internal organs including the heart, lungs, kidneys, digestive organs, and others. These internal organs are also called viscera (**VIS**-er-ah). A large muscle called the diaphragm (**DYE**-ah-fram) divides the ventral cavity into upper and lower cavities. The upper cavity is called the thoracic cavity. The lower cavity is the abdominopelvic (ab-**dom**-ih-noh-**PEL**-vick) cavity.

The thoracic cavity contains the heart and lungs. The abdominopelvic cavity is divided into two smaller cavities: the abdominal cavity and the pelvic cavity. The abdominal cavity is above the pelvic cavity. It contains organs such as the liver, intestines, stomach, and kidneys. The pelvic cavity contains some reproductive organs, the urinary bladder, and parts of the intestine.

IN BRIEF

The **dorsal cavity** is subdivided into the cranial and vertebral cavities.

The **ventral cavity** is subdivided into the thoracic and abdominopelvic cavities.

PRACTICE FOR LEARNING: BODY CAVITIES

Fill in the blanks with the most appropriate answer.

1. Write the two major body cavities. _____ and _____

2. What body organ would you find in the cranial cavity? _____ Vertebral cavity? _____

3. Name the two cavities contained in the ventral cavity. _____ and _____

4. The stomach and kidneys are found in which body cavity? _____

5. The urinary bladder is found in which body cavity? _____

Answers: **1.** dorsal and ventral. **2.** brain; spinal cord. **3.** thoracic; abdominopelvic. **4.** abdominal. **5.** pelvic.

5.2 DIRECTIONAL TERMINOLOGY

Anatomical Position

If you are going to tell someone how to get somewhere, you both need to understand what east, west, north, and south mean. These words are called directional terms because they tell direction.

In health care, we need directional terms that will accurately describe where particular body structures are located. The problem is that bodies can move. You can lie on your back, your front, or either side. You can stand or sit. A change in position would change the meaning of the directional terms.

There is a simple solution to this problem. Everyone using directional terminology in health care must think of the body in a standard position. This is known as the anatomical position. It is illustrated in Figure 5-2A. The body is standing erect, arms by the side, with head, palms, and feet facing forward. All directional terms assume that the body is in this position.

> ### IN BRIEF
>
> Anatomical position is standing erect, arms by the side, head, palms, and feet facing forward.

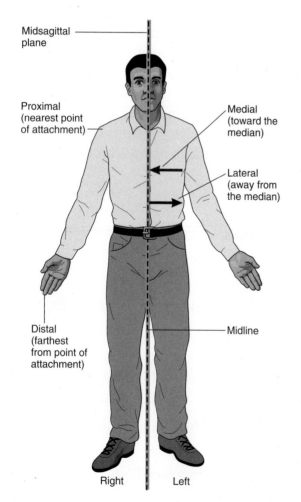

Midsagittal plane

Proximal (nearest point of attachment)

Medial (toward the median)

Lateral (away from the median)

Distal (farthest from point of attachment)

Midline

Right   Left

(A) Anatomical position

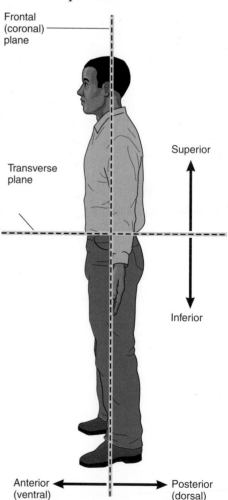

Frontal (coronal) plane

Transverse plane

Superior

Inferior

Anterior (ventral)   Posterior (dorsal)

(B)

FIGURE 5-2 (A–F) Anatomical position and directional terms.

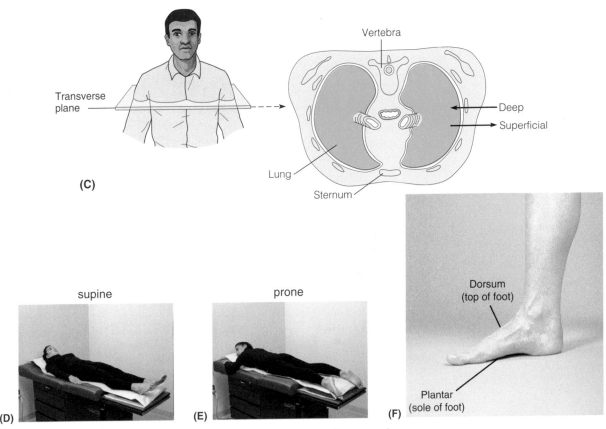

FIGURE 5-2 (A–F) Anatomical position and directional terms (continued).

Directional Terms

As stated above, we need directional terms to describe the position of body parts, particularly in relation to each other. Directional terms are also useful in communicating the location of diseases when they appear in the body.

All of the directional terms are listed in Table 5-1. To help you remember them, they are grouped in opposite pairs. For example, the terms "superior" and "inferior" are grouped because they are opposites: superior means "above," and inferior means "below." Figures 5-2 A–F illustrate the use of the terms.

HELPING YOU REMEMBER

To remember the meaning of supine, notice that supine has "up" as part of the word.

PRACTICE FOR LEARNING: DIRECTIONAL TERMS

    A. Write the opposite meaning of the following directional terms. The first one is done for you.

        1. anterior <u>posterior</u>

        2. lateral _____

(continued on page 79)

TABLE 5-1 Directional Terms

superior	above	The head is superior to the neck.
inferior	below	The neck is inferior to the head.
anterior (ventral)	front	The thoracic cavity is anterior to the vertebral cavity.
posterior (dorsal)	back	The vertebral cavity is posterior to the thoracic cavity.
medial	toward the midline of the body	The big toe is medial to the small toe.
lateral	away from the midline of the body	The small toe is lateral to the big toe.
proximal	1. nearest to the point of attachment to the trunk	The elbow is proximal to the wrist.
	2. nearest the point of origin	The stomach is proximal to the intestine. (In the digestive tract, the mouth is the point of origin.)
distal	1. farthest from the point of attachment to the trunk	The knee is distal to the hip.
	2. farthest from the point of origin	The intestine is distal to the stomach.
superficial	near the surface of the body	The skin is superficial to muscle.

TABLE 5-1 Directional Terms *(continued)*

deep	away from the surface of the body	The muscle is deep to skin.
supine	lying on the back, face up	During an operation on the abdomen, the patient is placed in the supine position.
prone	lying on the abdomen	For a back operation, the patient is placed in the prone position.
plantar	bottom of the foot; sole of the foot	Plantar warts are on the sole of the foot.
dorsum	top of the foot	The dorsum of the foot is the top of the foot.

3. proximal _____

4. deep _____

5. prone _____

6. dorsum _____

B. Underline the correct answer.

1. The neck is (inferior/superior) to the chin.

2. Your mouth is (medial/lateral) to your ear.

3. You have stepped on a sharp object. The bottom of your foot starts to bleed. You have cut the (plantar/dorsum) area of your foot.

4. Jack has a sunburn on the surface of his skin. The sunburn is said to be (superficial/deep).

5. A patient is having an operation on her breast. The patient will be placed on the operating table in the (supine/prone) position.

6. Ed has a rash on his chest and a bruise under is armpit. The bruise is (lateral/medial) to the rash.

Answers: **A. 1.** posterior. **2.** medial. **3.** distal. **4.** superficial. **5.** supine.
6. plantar. **B. 1.** inferior. **2.** medial. **3.** plantar. **4.** superficial. **5.** supine.
6. lateral.

5.3 BODY PLANES

Directional terms help us describe where structures are located in the body. In health care, we also need to describe those structures inside the body. This is called internal anatomy.

When internal anatomy is described, we think of the body or organ as being cut or sectioned (**SECK**-shunned) in a specific way to make a particular structure clearly visible. Once the body or organ is sectioned, an internal flat surface is exposed. This surface is called a plane (**PLAYN**). Because an organ can be cut in different ways, there are different kinds of planes. They are listed in Table 5-2 and illustrated in Figure 5-3.

HELPING YOU REMEMBER

To help you remember that sagittal separates a structure into right and left, think of the astrological sign of Sagittarius. With its bow and arrow, Sagittarius can hit a body structure, slicing it into right and left portions.

TABLE 5-2 Plane of the Body

Plane	Definition
frontal; coronal	separates a structure into anterior and posterior portions
sagittal	separates a structure into right and left portions. If the sagittal section divides the body into equal portions, it is called a **midsagittal** section.
transverse; horizontal	separates a structure into superior and inferior portions

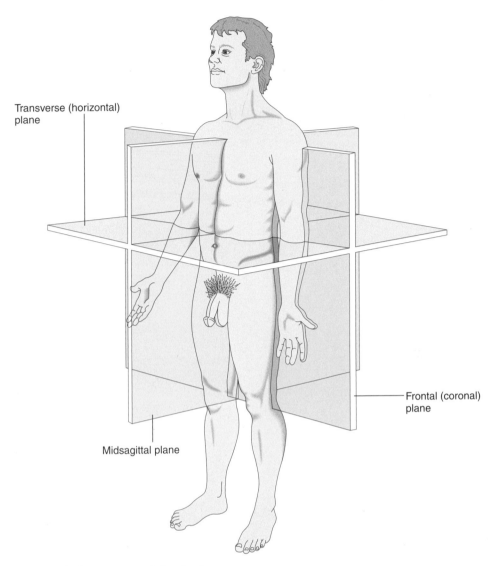

Transverse (horizontal) plane

Frontal (coronal) plane

Midsagittal plane

FIGURE 5-3 Planes of the body.

5.4 ABDOMINOPELVIC REGIONS

PRACTICE FOR LEARNING: ABDOMINOPELVIC REGIONS

Write the words below in the correct spaces on Figure 5-4. To help you, the number beside the word tells you where it goes on the figure. Be sure to pronounce each word as you write it. Repeat the pronunciation several times if you find the word hard to say.

1. right hypochondriac region (**high**-poh-**KON**-dree-ack)

2. epigastric region (**ep**-ih-**GAS**-trick)

3. left hypochondriac region (**high**-poh-**KON**-dree-ack)

4. right lumbar region (**LUM**-bar)

5. umbilical region (**um-BILL-ih-cahl**)

6. left lumbar region (**LUM**-bar)

7. right inguinal or iliac region (**ING**-gwih-nal or **ILL**-ee-ack)

8. hypogastric region (**high-poh-GAS**-trick)

9. left inguinal or iliac region (**ING**-gwih-nal or **ILL**-ee-ack)

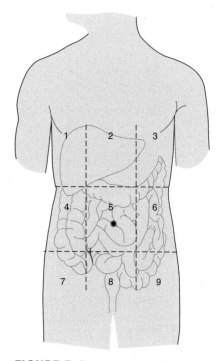

1. _____

2. _____

3. _____

4. _____

5. _____

6. _____

7. _____

8. _____

9. _____

FIGURE 5-4   Abdominopelvic regions.

Looking at the outside of the body, the abdominopelvic area can be divided into nine regions. As you can see in Figure 5-4, it looks like a tic-tac-toe board. Each region is given a name and each region contains specific organs.

When a patient has pain in the abdominopelvic area, the name of the region is used to communicate the exact location of the pain. For example, a doctor may say, "The pain is in the right iliac region." This means the pain is located in the patient's right hip area. When you are looking at illustrations, be careful to remember that the right and left abdominal regions refer to the patient's right or left, not yours.

5.5 ABDOMINOPELVIC QUADRANTS

PRACTICE FOR LEARNING: ABDOMINOPELVIC QUADRANTS

Write the words below in the correct spaces on Figure 5-5. To help you, the number beside the word tells you where it goes on the figure. Be sure to pronounce each word as you write it. Repeat the pronunciation several times if you find the word hard to say.

1. right upper quadrant (RUQ)

2. left upper quadrant (LUQ)

3. right lower quadrant (RLQ)

4. left lower quadrant (LLQ)

The abdominopelvic area can also be divided into four areas called quadrants (Figure 5-5).

1. _____

2. _____

3. _____

4. _____

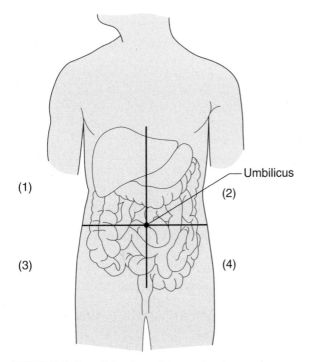

Umbilicus
(1)
(2)
(3)
(4)

FIGURE 5-5 Abdominopelvic quadrants.

5.6 NEW ROOTS

Use these additional roots when studying the medical terms of this chapter.

Root	Meaning
anter/o	front
dors/o	back
ili/o	hip
infer/o	below; downward
inguin/o	groin
medi/o	middle
poster/o	back
proxim/o	near
super/o	above; toward the head
ventr/o	front
vertebr/o	vertebra (any of 33 bones making up the spine)

5.7 LEARNING THE TERMS

Use the following suggestions for learning medical terms:

1. Pronounce the term repeatedly until it is easy for you.

2. Write it down. Ensure the spelling is correct.

3. Also write the definition. If possible, relate the word to a word, thought, or picture that will help you remember it.

4. Analyze the term with the method taught in this text.

Root	Meaning
gastr/o	stomach

Term	Term Analysis	Definition
epigastric (**ep**-ih-**GAS**-**TRICK**)	-ic = pertaining to epi- = above; upon	pertaining to upon the stomach. (Figure 5-4).
hypogastric (**high**-poh-**GAS**-trick)	-ic = pertaining to hypo- = below	pertaining to below the stomach. (Figure 5-4).

Root	Meaning
ili/o	hip

Term	Term Analysis	Definition
iliac (**ILL**-ee-ack)	-ac = pertaining to	pertaining to the hip

Suffix	Meaning
-al	pertaining to

Term	Term Analysis	Definition
abdominal (ab-**DOM**-ih-nal)	abdomin/o = abdomen	pertaining to the abdomen. The abdomen is the portion of the body between the chest and pelvis

HELPING YOU REMEMBER

The combining form is spelled abdomin/o. The word is spelled abdomen.

(continued)

Term	Term Analysis	Definition
cranial (**KRAY**-nee-al)	crani/o = skull	pertaining to the skull
dorsal (**DOOR**-sal)	dors/o = back	pertaining to the back; posterior (Figure 5-2B)
inguinal (**ING**-gwih-nal)	inguin/o = groin (the fold between the thigh and lower abdomen)	pertaining to the groin
medial (**MEE**-dee-al)	medi/o = middle	pertaining to the middle (Figure 5-2A)
proximal (**PROCK**-sih-mal)	proxim/o = near; close to	pertaining to something being near a specific point (Figure 5-2A)
spinal (**SPYE**-nal)	spin/o = spine; vertebral column	pertaining to the spine
ventral (**VEN**-tral)	ventr/o = front	pertaining to the front; anterior (Figure 5-2B)
vertebral (**VER**-teh-bral)	vertebr/o = vertebra (bones making up the spine)	pertaining to any one of the 33 bones making up the spine
visceral (**VIS**-er-al)	viscer/o = internal organs	pertaining to the internal organs

Suffix		Meaning
-ic		pertaining to
Term	**Term Analysis**	**Definition**
pelvic (**PEL**-vick)	pelv/o = pelvis	pertaining to the pelvis
thoracic (thoh-**RAS**-ick)	thorac/o = chest	pertaining to the chest

Suffix	Meaning
-ior	pertaining to

Term	Term Analysis	Definition
anterior (an-**TEER**-ee-or)	anter/o = front	pertaining to the front (Figure 5-2B)
inferior (in-**FEER**-ee-or)	infer/o = below; downward	pertaining to below or in a downward position; a structure below another structure (Figure 5-2B)
posterior (pos-**TEER**-ee-or)	poster/o = back	pertaining to the back of the body or an organ (Figure 5-2B)
superior (soo-**PEER**-ee-or)	super/o = above; toward the head	pertaining to a structure located above another (Figure 5-2B)

5.8 REVIEW EXERCISES

Exercise 5-1   MATCHING WORD PARTS WITH MEANING

Match the meaning in Column A *with the word part in* Column B.

Column A	Column B
_____ 1. hip	A. gastr/o
_____ 2. back	B. thorac/o
_____ 3. near	C. anter/o
_____ 4. above; upon	D. -ic
_____ 5. stomach	E. ili/o
_____ 6. below	F. epi-
_____ 7. front	G. crani/o

(continued)

Column A	Column B
_____ 8. pertaining to	H. dors/o
_____ 9. chest	I. infer/o
_____ 10. skull	J. proxim/o

Exercise 5-2

DIRECTIONAL TERMS

Match each directional term in Column A *with its meaning in* Column B.

Column A	Column B
_____ 1. superior	A. pertaining to the skull
_____ 2. anterior	
_____ 3. thoracic	B. pertaining to the hip
_____ 4. visceral	C. above; toward the head
_____ 5. epigastric	
_____ 6. iliac	D. pertaining to the front
_____ 7. cranial	E. pertaining to below the stomach
_____ 8. hypogastric	
	F. pertaining to upon the stomach
	G. pertaining to the chest
	H. pertaining to internal organs

Exercise 5-3

DEFINING DIRECTIONAL TERMS

Underline the root or combining form, then define the medical word. The first question is answered for you.

1. **hypogastric** pertaining to below the stomach

2. **iliac** _____

3. **dorsal** _____

4. **inguinal** _____

5. visceral _____

6. cranial _____

7. anterior _____

8. superior _____

Exercise 5-4	TRUE/FALSE

Circle True if the statement is true. Circle False if the statement is false.

1. The liver is located in the pelvic cavity.   True   False

2. The abdominal cavity is superior to the thoracic cavity.   True   False

3. The small toe is medial to the big toe.   True   False

4. The wrist is proximal to the elbow.   True   False

5. Prone is lying on the abdomen.   True   False

6. The right iliac region is in the right upper quadrant.   True   False

7. Dorsum may refer to the back of a structure   True   False

8. The right hypochondriac region of the abdomen is in the RUQ.   True   False

Exercise 5-5	SPELLING

Circle the words that are spelled incorrectly in the list below. Then correct the spelling in the space provided.

1. epigastric _____

2. abdomenal _____

3. inquinal _____

4. thorasic _____

5. vicseral _____

6. anterior _____

7. medial _____

5.9 PRONUNCIATION AND SPELLING

1. Listen to each word on the audio CD.
2. Pronounce each word carefully.
3. Spell each word in the space provided.

Word	Pronunciation	Spelling
epigastric	ep-ih-**GAS**-trick	
hypogastric	high-poh-**GAS**-trick	
iliac	**ILL**-ee-ack	
abdominal	ab-**DOM**-ih-nal	
cranial	**KRAY**-nee-al	
dorsal	**DOOR**-sal	
inguinal	**ING**-gwih-nal	
medial	**MEE**-dee-al	
proximal	**PROCK**-sih-mal	
spinal	**SPYE**-nal	
ventral	**VEN**-tral	
visceral	**VIS**-er-al	
pelvic	**PEL**-vick	
thoracic	thoh-**RAS**-ick	
inferior	in-**FEER**-ee-or	
posterior	pos-**TEER**-ee-or	
superior	soo-**PEER**-ee-or	

CHAPTER 6

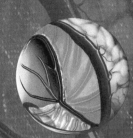

The Skin and Related Structures

LEARNING OBJECTIVES

After studying this chapter and completing the exercises, you should be able to do the following:

1. Identify the cells, tissues, and organs of the system.
2. Identify the layers of the skin and describe the structures found in these layers.
3. List the functions of the skin.
4. Pronounce, spell, define, and write medical terms common to this system.
5. Describe common diseases of the system.
6. Listen, read, and study, so you can speak and write.

INTRODUCTION

The body is covered with skin, nails, and hair. Together, they make up the integumentary (in-**teg**-yoo-**MEN**-tar-ee) system. It gets its name from the Latin word *integumentum* meaning "covering."

The skin is an organ, just like the heart and lungs. It is the largest organ in the body.

The skin has two layers. The outer layer (epidermis) helps prevent harmful substances from entering the body. The inner layer (dermis) contains glands that secrete important substances, nerves that carry electrical impulses, and blood vessels that help to keep the body at the right temperature.

6.1 LAYERS OF THE SKIN

PRACTICE FOR LEARNING: LAYERS OF THE SKIN

Write the words below in the correct spaces on Figure 6-1. To help you, the number beside the word tells you where it goes on the figure. Be sure to pronounce each word as you write it. Repeat the pronunciation several times if you find the word hard to say.

1. epidermis (**ep-ih-DER**-mis).

2. dermis (**DER**-mis).

3. subcutaneous tissue (**sub**-kyoo-**TAY**-nee-us **TISH**-yoo)

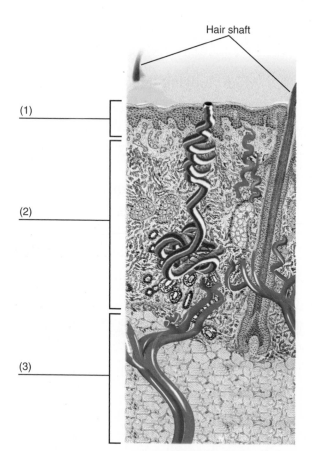

FIGURE 6-1 Layers of the skin and subcutaneous tissue.

IN BRIEF

The **epidermis** is the outer layer of skin.

The **dermis** is under the epidermis.

Subcutaneous tissue is under the dermis.

Figure 6-1 shows you the layers of tissue. The outer layer is part of the skin and is called the epidermis. Underneath it is another layer of skin called the dermis. Underneath the dermis is a layer called subcutaneous tissue. It is not part of the skin. The muscles lie below the subcutaneous layer.

Epidermis

In Chapter 2, you learned that organs are made of tissues and tissues are made of cells. The epidermis is an organ made of tissue called **epithelium** (**ep-ih-THEE-lee-um**). The cells are called **epithelial** (**ep-ih-THEE-lee-al**) cells.

The epidermis protects us from the sun's rays by producing **melanin** (**MEL-ah-nin**). Melanin is produced by cells in the epidermis called **melanocytes** (**meh-LAN-oh-sights**). Darker skin has more melanocytes than lighter skin. Skin with more melanin has better protection from the sun.

Dermis

PRACTICE FOR LEARNING: DERMIS

Write the words below on the correct spaces in Figure 6-2. To help you, the number beside the word tells you where it goes on the figure. Be sure to pronounce each word as you write it. Repeat the pronunciation several times if you find the word hard to say.

1. sebaceous (**seh-BAY-shus**) gland

2. nerve (**NURV**)

3. sweat gland (**SWET GLAND**)

4. vein (**VAYN**)

5. artery (**AR-ter-ee**)

The dermis is made of connective tissue. If you look at Figure 6-2, you can see that the dermis contains blood vessels. If you are cut down to this layer, you will bleed. The blood vessels supply nutrients to the epidermis and dermis. They also help control body temperature.

The dermis also contains nerves. They give us sensations such as touch, pain, temperature, and pressure.

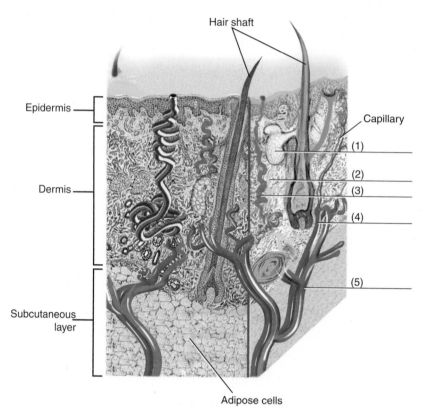

FIGURE 6-2 Structures found in the dermis.

There are glands in the dermis that secrete substances necessary for skin function. Sebaceous glands secrete oil called sebum (**SEE-bum**). It keeps the skin and the hair soft and pliable. Sweat glands regulate temperature by secreting sweat onto the surface of the skin.

There are also hair follicles in the dermis. They grow the hairs that cover our skin in certain places. When hair is lost on top of the head, the person is said to be bald. The medical word for bald is alopecia (**al-oh-PEE-she-ah**).

PRACTICE FOR LEARNING: EPIDERMIS AND DERMIS

Complete the sentence by underlining the correct answer.

1. The function of the epidermis is (protection/sensation).

2. The tissue making up the epidermis is (epithelial/connective) tissue.

3. The substance that gives the skin a darker color is (melanin/sebum).

4. The dermis is made of (epithelial/connective) tissue.

5. A function of the blood vessels in the dermis is (sensation/temperature regulation).

6. Sebaceous glands secrete an (oil/wax).

Answers: **1.** protection. **2.** epithelial. **3.** melanin. **4.** connective. **5.** temperature regulation. **6.** oil.

6.2 NEW ROOTS, SUFFIXES, AND PREFIX

Use these additional roots, suffixes, and prefixes when studying the medical terms in this chapter.

Root	Meaning
chem/o	drug
cry/o	cold
melan/o	black
myc/o	fungus

Suffix	Meaning
-ion	process
-opsy	to view
-ose; -tic	pertaining to
-sis	condition

Prefix	Meaning
ab-	away from

6.3 LEARNING THE TERMS

Use the following suggestions for learning medical terms.

1. Pronounce the term repeatedly until it is easy for you.

2. Write it down. Ensure the spelling is correct.

3. Also write the definition. If possible, relate the word to a word, thought, or picture that will help you remember it.

4. Analyze the term with the method taught in this text.

Root	Meaning
adip/o (see also lip/o)	fat

Term	Term Analysis	Definition
adipose (**AD**-ih-pohs)	-ose = pertaining to	pertaining to fat

Root	Meaning
bi/o	life

Term	Term Analysis	Definition
biopsy (**BYE**-op-see)	-opsy = to view	a procedure involving the removal of a piece of living tissue, which is then examined for any abnormalities

Root	Meaning
cutane/o (see also derm/o and dermat/o)	skin

Term	Term Analysis	Definition
subcutaneous (**sub**-kyoo-**TAY**-nee-us)	sub- = under -ous = pertaining to	pertaining to under the skin

Root	Meaning
cyan/o	blue

Term	Term Analysis	Definition
cyanosis (**sigh**-ah-**NOH**-sis)	-sis = condition	bluish discoloration of skin (Figure 6-3)

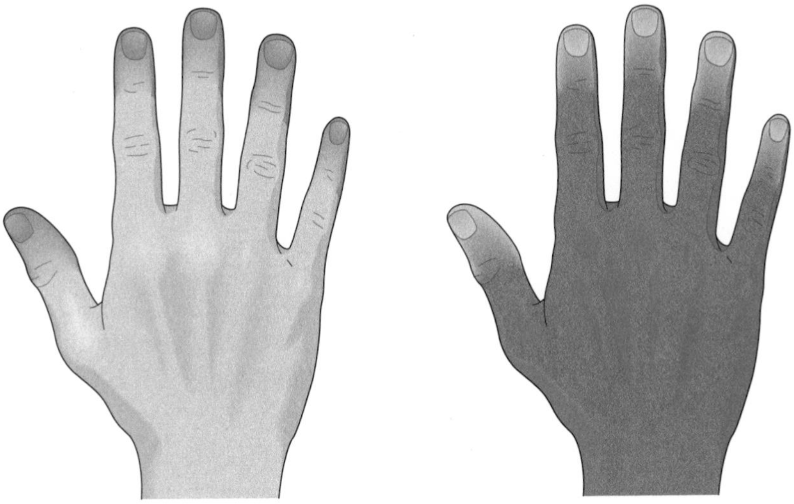

FIGURE 6-3 Cyanosis.

Root	Meaning
derm/o; dermat/o	skin

Term	Term Analysis	Definition
dermatitis (**der**-mah-**TYE**-tis)	-itis = inflammation	inflammation of the skin
dermatologist (**der**-mah-**TOL**-oh-jist)	-logist = one who specializes in the study of	one who specializes in the study of the skin and its diseases
hypodermic (**high**-poh-**DER**-mick)	-ic = pertaining to hypo- = under; below	pertaining to under the skin

NOTE: The prefixes hypo- and sub- cannot be interchanged with the roots meaning skin. Hypo- is used with the root **derm/o,** and sub- is used with the root **cutane/o.**

Root	Meaning
erythem/o	red

Term	Term Analysis	Definition
erythema (er-ih-**THEE**-mah)	"-a" is a noun ending	red discoloration of the skin

Root	Meaning
lip/o	fat

Term	Term Analysis	Definition
lipoma (lih-**POH**-mah)	-oma = tumor; mass	tumor or mass containing fat
liposuction (lip-oh-**SUCK**-shun)	suction = process of aspirating or withdrawing	withdrawal of fat from the subcutaneous tissue

Root	Meaning
necr/o	death

Term	Term Analysis	Definition
necrotic tissue (neh-**KROT**-ick)	-tic = pertaining to	pertaining to the death of tissues (Figure 6-4)

FIGURE 6-4 Decubitus ulcer (pressure sore, bedsore). (Permission to reproduce this copyrighted material has been granted by the owner, Hollister Incorporated.)

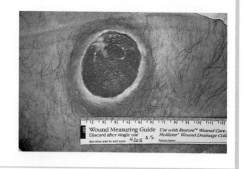

NOTE: A decubitus ulcer is also known as a pressure sore or bedsore. It is caused by constant pressure on the skin, especially over bony areas such as the elbows. The pressure cuts off circulation to the skin. The skin becomes necrotic (dies) because of the lack of oxygen. When necrotic tissue is sloughed (falls off), it leaves an open sore (Figure 6-4). Figure 6-7c illustrates necrotic tissue before it is sloughed. In this case it resulted from a burn.

Root	Meaning
onych/o	nail

Term	Term Analysis	Definition
onychomycosis (**on**-ih-koh-my-**KOH**-sis)	-osis = abnormal condition myc/o = fungus	fungal infection of the skin

Root	Meaning
ras/o	scrape

Term	Term Analysis	Definition
abrasion (ab-**RAY**-zhun)	-ion = process ab- = away from	scraping away of the superficial layers of injured skin; for example, scraping your skin on the cement results in an abrasion. Also known as an excoriation (ecks-**kor**-ee-**AY**-shun)

Suffix	Meaning
-cyte	cell

Term	Term Analysis	Definition
melanocyte (meh-**LAN**-oh-sight)	melan/o = black	cells producing melanin

Suffix	Meaning
-therapy	treatment

Term	Term Analysis	Definition
chemotherapy (**kee**-moh-**THER**-ah-pee)	chem/o = drugs	treatment with drugs. Usually refers to the use of drugs on cancer patients.

(continued)

Term	Term Analysis	Definition
cryotherapy (**krye**-oh-**THER**-ah-pee)	cry/o = cold	destruction of unwanted tissue, such as warts, by freezing with liquid nitrogen. The freezing destroys the tissue (Figure 6-5).

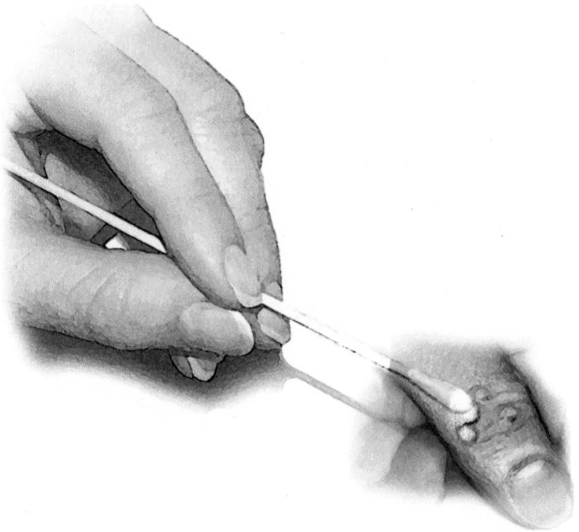

FIGURE 6-5 Cryotherapy.

Term	Term Analysis	Definition
laser therapy (**LAY**-zer **THER**-ah-pee)	laser = intense beam of light	removal of skin lesions such as birthmarks or tattoos using an intense beam of light called a laser. Lasers are also used in cosmetic surgeries.

NOTE: In this example, therapy is used as a word rather than a suffix as in cryotherapy.

Term	Term Analysis	Definition
radiotherapy (ray-dee-oh-**THER**-ah-pee)	radi/o = x-rays	treatment of disease, usually cancer, using radiation (x-rays).

6.4 PATHOLOGY

Burns

An injury to the skin caused by heat, chemicals, electricity, or radiation. Burns can be described by how deep the burn is and by the area of skin burned. Look at Figures 6-6 and 6-7as you read the descriptions below:

first-degree burn (superficial burn) burn to the epidermis only. There is redness but no blisters, for example, a sunburn.

second-degree burn (partial-thickness burn) involves the epidermis and upper portion of the dermis. The skin is red. There are blisters.

third-degree burn (full-thickness burn) involves the epidermis and all of the dermis. The subcutaneous tissue may be damaged.

fourth-degree burn involves the epidermis, dermis, subcutaneous tissue, and muscle

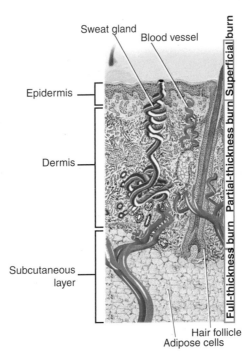

FIGURE 6-6 Superficial, partial-thickness, and full-thickness burn.

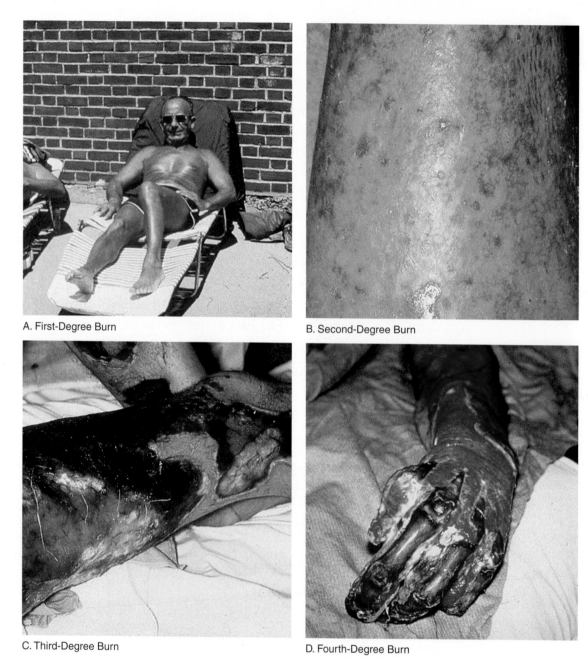

A. First-Degree Burn

B. Second-Degree Burn

C. Third-Degree Burn

D. Fourth-Degree Burn

FIGURE 6-7 Burns. A, First-degree burn. B, Second-degree burn. C, Third-degree burn. D, Fourth-degree burn. (All photographs courtesy of the Phoenix Society for Burn Survivors, Inc.)

Psoriasis (sor-EYE-ah-sis)

A chronic inflammation of the skin (Figure 6-8). The skin appears red with silvery scales. It is not infectious. The cause is unknown.

Tumors, Neoplasms

An abnormal growth of tissue cells. Tumors can be benign (bee-NIGHN) or malignant (mah-LIG-nant). Benign tumors are noncancerous, are usually harmless, and do not spread from one location to another. Malignant tumors are cancerous and harmful and usu-

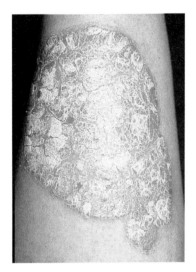

FIGURE 6-8 Psoriasis. (Courtesy of Robert A. Silverman, MD, Pediatric Dermatology, Georgetown University.)

ally spread or metastasize (**meh-TAS-tah-size**). Common benign and malignant tumors are listed below. Treatment involves removal of the tumor by surgery, laser, radiation, and/or chemotherapy.

Benign Tumors

papilloma (**pap-ih-LOH-mah**) benign nipple-like growths projecting from epithelial tissue (papill/o = nipple). Example: a wart.

lipoma (**lih-POH-mah**) benign tumor of fatty tissue

Malignant Tumors

carcinoma (**kar-sih-NOH-mah**) malignant tumor of epithelial cells. Two types include:

basal (**BAY-sal**) cell carcinoma malignant tumor of the epidermis. Unlike other malignant skin cancers, it rarely spreads to other locations (Figure 6-9A).

squamous (**SKWAY-mus**) cell carcinoma also a malignant tumor of the epidermis. It has a tendency to spread to other organs (Figure 6-9B).

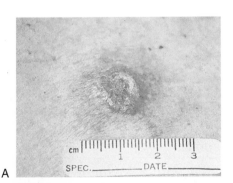

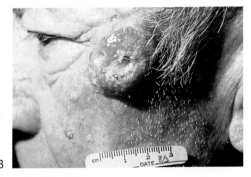

FIGURE 6-9 Carcinoma of the skin. A, Basal cell carcinoma. B, Squamous cell carcinoma. (Courtesy of Robert A. Silverman, MD, Pediatric Dermatology, Georgetown University.)

melanoma (**mel-ah-NOH-mah**) malignant tumor arising from the melanocytes (Figure 6-10).

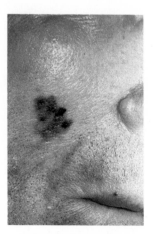

FIGURE 6-10 Melanoma. (Courtesy of Robert A. Silverman, MD, Pediatric Dermatology, Georgetown University.)

REVIEW EXERCISES

| Exercise 6-1 | LOOK-ALIKE AND SOUND-ALIKE |

Below is a list of look-alike and sound-alike words. Study the definitions of each set of words, then read the sentences carefully and circle the word in parentheses that correctly completes the meaning.

glands	organs that secrete chemicals
glans	the tip of the penis (glans penis)
patience	showing self-control
patients	a person under medical care
vesical	pertaining to the bladder (adj)
vesicle	blister (noun)
plantar	the sole of the foot
planter	container for a plant
cirrhosis	yellow discoloration of the skin
psoriasis	skin condition characterized by silvery scales
Mohs'	surgery for melanoma
mows	to mow (cut) the lawn with a lawnmower

1. Genital warts are sexually transmitted. They often appear on the (**glands/glans**) penis.

2. After swallowing the medication, the patient broke out in (**vesicals/vesicles**).

3. Cryotherapy was used to treat the (**plantar/planter**) warts on the bottom of the foot.

4. All of the (**patients/patience**) showed up at the medical clinic at the same time. It took a lot of (**patients/patience**) to look after them.

5. The patient has been given a cream to treat his (**cirrhosis/psoriasis**).

6. After he (**mohs/mows**) the lawn, Juan will travel to the hospital for treatment of his melanoma. (**Mohs'/Mows'**) surgery will be performed.

Exercise 6-2   ## MATCHING WORD PARTS WITH MEANING

Match the word part in Column A *with its meaning in* Column B.

Column A	Column B
_____ 1. adip/o	A. blue
_____ 2. cry/o	B. scrape
_____ 3. bi/o	C. nail
_____ 4. cyan/o	D. life
_____ 5. necr/o	E. tumor
_____ 6. erythem/o	F. fungus
_____ 7. radi/o	G. fat
_____ 8. myc/o	H. pertaining to
_____ 9. ras/o	I. away from
_____ 10. -opsy	J. skin
_____ 11. -tic	K. cold
_____ 12. ab-	L. death
_____ 13. -onych/o	M. x-rays
_____ 14. derm/o	N. red
_____ 15. -oma	O. to view

| Exercise 6-3 | **MATCHING MEDICAL WORDS WITH DEFINITIONS** |

Match the term in Column A *with its definition in* Column B.

Column A	Column B
_____ **1.** epidermis	A. tissue making up the dermis
_____ **2.** sebum	
_____ **3.** alopecia	B. bald
_____ **4.** epithelium	C. pertaining to fat
_____ **5.** adipose	D. treatment with drugs
_____ **6.** erythema	E. top layer of skin
_____ **7.** connective	F. scraping away of skin
_____ **8.** chemotherapy	G. keeps hair soft
_____ **9.** abrasion	H. death of tissue
_____ **10.** necrotic	I. red discoloration
	J. tissue making up the epidermis

| Exercise 6-4 | **WORD COMPLETION** |

Complete the medical word by adding the most appropriate word element. The first question is completed for you.

1. A specialist in the study of the skin is a derma**tologist.**

2. Pertaining to fat is _____ose.

3. Under the skin is _____cutaneous.

4. Under the skin is _____dermic.

5. Pertaining to the death of tissues is _____tic.

6. A tumor or mass containing fat is _____oma.

7. Cell producing melanin is called melan_____ .

8. Treatment with drugs _____therapy.

| **Exercise 6-5** | SPELLING |

Circle any misspelled words in the list below and correctly spell them in the space provided.

1. subqutaneous _____

2. sebaceous _____

3. malanin _____

4. sweet glands _____

5. epithelial _____

6. airythemia _____

7. soriasis _____

8. metastasize _____

6.6 PRONUNCIATION AND SPELLING

Listen, read, and study, so you can speak and write.

1. Listen to each word on the audio CD.

2. Pronounce each word carefully.

3. Spell each word in the space provided.

Word	Pronunciation	Spelling
abrasion	ab-**RAY**-zhun	
adipose	**AD**-ih-pohs	
biopsy	**BYE**-op-see	
carcinoma	kar-sih-**NOH**-mah	
cryotherapy	krye-oh-**THER**-ah-pee	
cyanosis	sigh-ah-**NOH**-sis	
dermatitis	der-mah-**TYE**-tis	
dermatologist	der-mah-**TOL**-oh-jist	
dermis	**DER**-mis	

Word	Pronunciation	Spelling
epidermis	ep-ih-**DER**-mis	
epithelial	ep-ih-**THEE**-lee-al	
epithelium	ep-ih-**THEE**-lee-um	
hypodermic	**high**-poh-**DER**-mick	
laser therapy	**LAY**-zer **THER**-ah-pee	
lipoma	lih-**POH**-mah	
liposuction	**lip**-oh-**SUCK**-shun	
melanin	**MEL**-ah-nin	
melanocytes	meh-**LAN**-oh-sights	
melanoma	**mel**-ah-**NOH**-mah	
necrotic	neh-**KROT**-ick	
onychomycosis	**on**-ih-koh-my-**KOH**-sis	
papilloma	**pap**-ih-**LOH**-mah	
psoriasis	sor-**EYE**-ah-sis	
sebaceous	seh-**BAY**-shus	
subcutaneous	**sub**-kyoo-**TAY**-nee-us	

CHAPTER 7

Skeletal System

CHAPTER OUTLINE

LEARNING OBJECTIVES

After studying this chapter and completing the review exercises, you should be able to do the following:

1. Name and locate the major bones of the body.
2. Pronounce, spell, and define the medical terms related to the skeletal system.
3. Describe the common diseases related to the skeletal system.
4. Listen, read, and study so you can speak and write.

INTRODUCTION

The skeletal system is made up of 206 bones. They are attached to each other at joints.

In this chapter you will learn about the structure of bones, the location of the major bones, and how bones contribute to body function. You will also learn about the structure of joints and how they function to produce movement.

7.1 MAJOR BONES OF THE BODY

PRACTICE FOR LEARNING: MAJOR BONES OF THE BODY

Write the words below in the correct spaces on Figure 7-1. To help you, the number beside the word tells you where it goes on the figure. Be sure to pronounce each word as you write it. Repeat the pronunciation several times if you find the word hard to say. The common names are listed in Table 7-1.

1. cranium (**KRAY**-nee-um)

2. facial bones (**FAY**-shal)

3. thorax (**THOH**-racks)

4. carpals (**KAR**-palz)

5. metacarpals (**met**-ah-**KAR**-palz)

6. phalanges (fah-**LAN**-jeez)

7. tarsals (**TAHR**-salz)

8. metatarsals (**met**-ah-**TAHR**-salz)

9. phalanges (fah-**LAN**-jeez)

10. fibula (**FIB**-yoo-lah)

11. tibia (**TIB**-ee-ah)

12. patella (pah-**TEL**-ah)

13. femur (**FEE**-mur)

14. pelvis (**PEL**-vis)

15. ulna (**ULL**-nah)

16. radius (**RAY**-dee-us)

17. humerus (**HEW**-mer-us)

18. vertebra (**VER**-teh-brah)

19. scapula (**SKAP**-yoo-lah)

20. clavicle (**KLAV**-ih-kul)

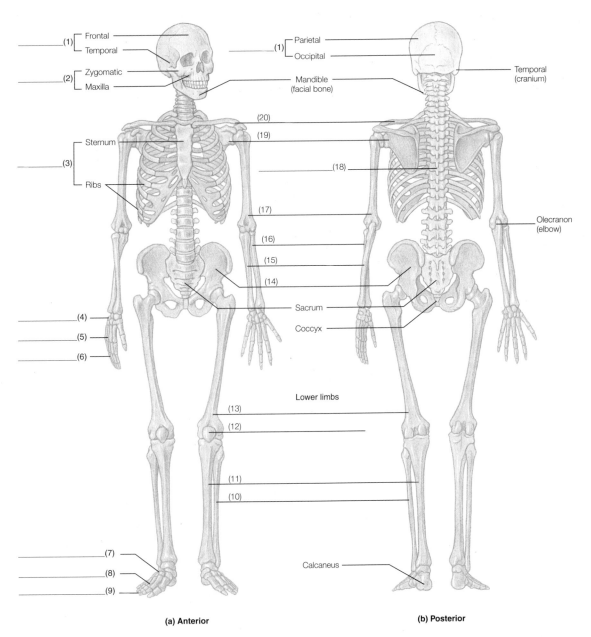

FIGURE 7-1   Major bones of the body. A. Anterior view. B. Posterior view.

BONE STRUCTURE AND FUNCTION

Bone Structure

Cells and Minerals

Just like other organs, bones are made up of cells and tissues.

Bones grow and renew themselves. Immature bone cells are called osteoblasts (**OS-tee-oh-blasts**). They grow into mature cells called osteocytes (**OS-tee-oh-sights**). Osteocytes form bone tissue called osseous (**OS-ee-us**) tissue.

IN BRIEF

Ostoblasts are immature bone cells.

Osteocytes are mature bone cells.

Osteocytes form osseous tissue.

Calcium and phosphorus are minerals that make bone hard.

TABLE 7-1 Bones and their Common Names

Bone	Common Name
carpals	wrist
clavicle	collarbone
coccyx	tailbone
cranium	skull
femur	thigh
humerus	upper arm
ilium	hip or pelvis
mandible	lower jaw
maxilla	upper jaw
metacarpals	hand
olecranon	elbow
patella	kneecap
phalanges	fingers or toes
scapula	shoulder blade
sternum	breastbone
thorax	chest
tibia	shin
zygomatic bone	cheek

For bones to properly form and become hard and strong, we need to eat food that contains two minerals: calcium (**KAL-see-um**) and phosphorus (**FOS-for-us**). We also need plenty of vitamin D to help us absorb the calcium.

Cartilage is similar to bone but it is soft because it lacks the calcium deposits that make bone hard. Cartilage is found in all joints, the spinal column, and the rib cage.

Bone Function

Bones have many functions. They provide protection and support, and allow movement to happen because they provide a rigid structure for the muscles to pull on. They also act as a storehouse for calcium and phosphorus, and release these minerals into the bloodstream when required. The bone marrow produces blood cells that are necessary for life.

PRACTICE FOR LEARNING: BONE STRUCTURE AND FUNCTION

Underline true or false

1.	Calcium is a mineral found in bone.	True or False
2.	Bone marrow produces blood cells.	True or False
3.	Osseous is a type of bone cell.	True or False
4.	Osteoblasts are a type of bone cell.	True or False

Answers: **1.** True. **2.** True. **3.** False. **4.** True.

 # 7.3 VERTEBRAL COLUMN

PRACTICE FOR LEARNING: VERTEBRAL COLUMN

Write the bones of the vertebral column in the correct space on Figure 7-2. To help you, the number beside the bone tells you where it goes on the figure. Be sure to pronounce each word as you write it. Repeat the pronunciation several times if you find the word hard to say.

1. cervical vertebrae (**SER**-vih-kal **VER**-teh-bree)

2. thoracic (thoh-**RAS**-ick)

3. lumbar (**LUM**-bar)

4. sacrum (**SAY**-krum)

5. coccyx (**KOCK**-sicks)

The bones of the vertebral (**VER**-teh-brahl) column are organized into five groups. They are illustrated in Figure 7-2. The vertebral column is usually called the spine or backbone.

The vertebral column consists of 33 bones arranged in a column that extends from the base of the skull to the lower back. Each bone is called a vertebra (**VER**-teh-brah) (plural = vertebrae (**VER**-teh-bree). There are 7 cervical vertebrae (C1 to C7), 12 thoracic vertebrae (T1 to T12), 5 lumbar vertebrae (L1 to L5), 5 fused bones called the sacrum (S1 to S5), and 4 fused bones called the coccyx or tailbone. Each vertebra has a round hole in the middle. The holes line up to form a canal. The spinal cord lies within this

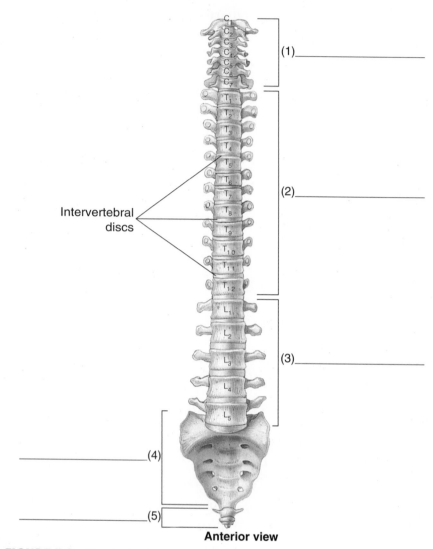

Intervertebral discs

(1)_____

(2)_____

(3)_____

(4)_____

(5)_____

Anterior view

FIGURE 7-2 Vertebral column, anterior view.

IN BRIEF

The **vertebral column** is also known as the spine or backbone.

The **vertebral column** is made up of bone.

The **spinal cord** is made up of nerves.

canal. The vertebrae protect the spinal cord, which is made up of nerves.

In Figure 7-2 there is a diagram of a cushion of cartilage called the **interverte-bral** (**in-ter-VER-teh-bral**) disc, which lies between each vertebrae. These discs allow the vertebrae to glide over each other, making movement smooth and painless.

HELPING YOU REMEMBER

Think of the vertebral column as a stack of doughnuts with the spinal cord passing through the holes. The inter-vertebral discs would be like thick wax paper placed be-tween the doughnuts to prevent sticking.

7.4 JOINTS

A joint is where two bones come together. Movement occurs at joints. A joint is usually named after the bones that it joins. For example, the sacroiliac joint in the pelvis is the union between the sacrum (sacr/o) and iliac (ili/o) bones.

For joints to work properly and without pain, it is important that the two bones glide smoothly over each other (Figure 7-3). This is accomplished by articular (**ar-TIK-yoo-lar**) cartilage and synovial (**sih-NOH-vee-al**) fluid inside the joint. The synovial fluid is produced by synovial membrane lining the joint.

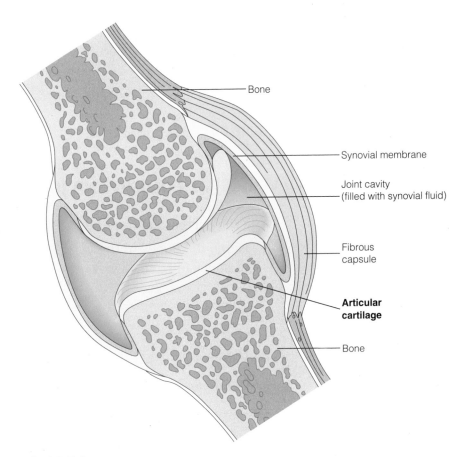

Bone

Synovial membrane

Joint cavity
(filled with synovial fluid)

Fibrous
capsule

**Articular
cartilage**

Bone

FIGURE 7-3 A joint cavity.

Also at joints (but not inside) are tendons (**TEN-donz**), ligaments (**LIG-ah-ments**), and bursae (**BUR-see**) (Figure 7-4). Tendons attach muscle to bone. Ligaments attach bone to bone. Bursae are tiny, purse-like sacs lined with synovial membrane and filled with synovial fluid. Each bursa (**BUR-sah**) prevents friction between two structures that need to glide past each other when they move. The bursa can become inflamed through overuse, resulting in a condition called **bursitis** (bur-**SIGH**-tis). Golfers will sometimes develop bursitis at the shoulder, while tennis players often develop it in the elbow.

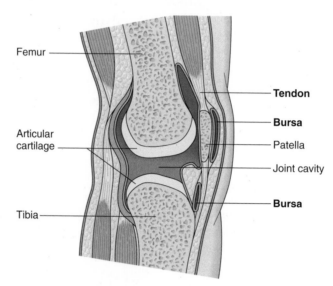

Femur

Tendon

Bursa

Articular cartilage

Patella

Joint cavity

Bursa

Tibia

FIGURE 7-4   Bursae around a joint.

PRACTICE FOR LEARNING: VERTEBRAL COLUMN AND JOINTS

Write the correct answers on the line

1. Name the bones of the vertebral column. Write the number of bones in each segment.

   _____

   _____

2. Define a joint. _____

3. Define articular cartilage. _____

Answers: **1.** 7 cervical, 12 thoracic, 5 lumbar, 5 fused sacral bones, 4 fused coccygeal bones. **2.** A joint is where two bones come together. **3.** Articular cartilage covers the ends of bone and protects the bone.

7.5 NEW SUFFIXES

Use these additional suffixes when studying the medical words in this chapter.

Suffix	Meaning
-centesis	surgical puncture to remove fluid
-immune	immunity; safe (The immune system protects the body against disease.)
-malacia	softening

7.6 LEARNING THE TERMS

Following these steps will make it easier for you to learn medical terms:

1. Pronounce the term repeatedly until it is easy for you.

2. Write it down. Ensure the spelling is correct.

3. Also write the definition. If possible, relate the word to a word, thought, or picture that will help you remember it.

4. Analyze the term with the method taught in this text.

Root		Meaning
arthr/o		joint
Term	**Term Analysis**	**Definition**
arthralgia (ar-**THRAL**-jee-ah)	-algia = pain	joint pain
arthritis (ar-**THRIGH**-tis)	-itis = inflammation	inflammation of a joint. See pathology section for more detail.
arthrocentesis (**ar**-throh-sen-**TEE**-sis)	-centesis = surgical puncture to remove fluid	surgical puncture to remove fluid from the joint cavity
arthropathy (ar-**THROP**-ah-thee)	-pathy = disease	diseased joint

(continued)

Root		Meaning
Term	**Term Analysis**	**Definition**
arthroplasty (**AR**-thro-**plas**-tee)	-plasty = surgical repair or construction	surgical repair of a joint. (Figure 7-5).

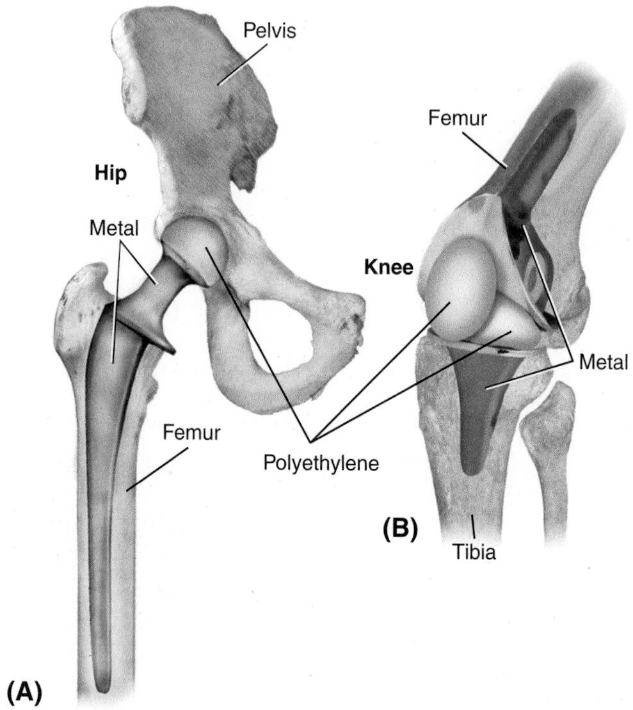

FIGURE 7-5 Arthroplasty. A. Total hip replacement. B. Total knee replacement.

arthroscopy (ar-**THROS**-koh-pee)	-scopy = process of visual examination	process of visually examining the joint cavity by using an arthroscope (Figure 7-6A and B).

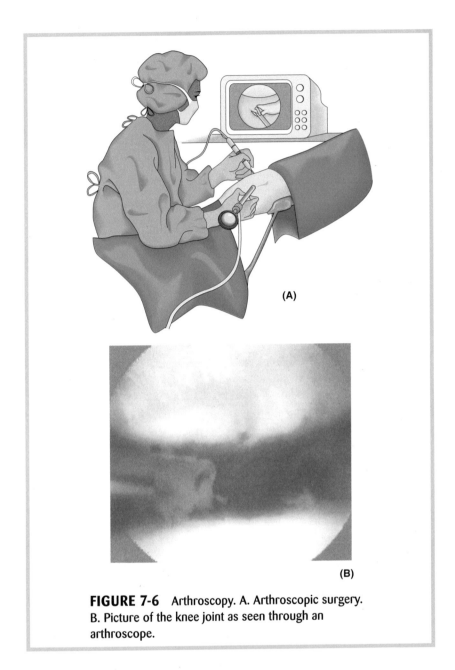

FIGURE 7-6   Arthroscopy. A. Arthroscopic surgery.
B. Picture of the knee joint as seen through an
arthroscope.

Root	Meaning
chondr/o	cartilage

Term	Term Analysis	Definition
chondromalacia (kon-dro-mah-LAY-she-ah)	-malacia = soft	softening of cartilage
chondroma (kon-DROH-mah)	-oma = tumor	tumor of cartilage
chondrocyte (KON-droh-sight)	-cyte = cell	cartilage cell

Root	Meaning
cost/o	rib

costal (KOS-tal)	-al = pertaining to	pertaining to the ribs
subcostal (sub-KOS-tal)	-al = pertaining to sub- = under	pertaining to under the ribs

Root	Meaning
ili/o	hip

iliac (ILL-ee-ack)	-ac = pertaining to	pertaining to the hip

Root	Meaning
myel/o	bone marrow

myelogenous (my-eh-LOJ-en-us)	-genous = produced by	produced by the bone marrow

Root	Meaning
oste/o	bone

Term	Term Analysis	Definition
osteitis (os-tee-**EYE**-tis)	-itis = inflammation	inflammation of the bone
osteoma (os-tee-**OH**-ma)	-oma = tumor	tumor of bone
osteomalacia (**os**-tee-oh-mah-**LAY**-shee-ah)	-malacia = softening	softening of bone
osteomyelitis (**os**-tee-oh-my-eh-**LYE**-tis)	-itis = inflammation myel/o = bone marrow	inflammation of bone and bone marrow
osteosarcoma (**os**-tee-oh-sar-**KOH**-mah)	-sarcoma = malignant tumor of connective tissue	malignant tumor of bone

Prefix	Meaning
auto-	self

Term	Term Analysis	Definition
autoimmune disease (aw-toh-ih-**MYOON**)	-immune = immunity; safe	immune response to one's own body tissue; destruction of one's own cells by one's own immune system.

NOTE: The immune system helps to protect the body against harmful substances.

Prefix	Meaning
ortho-	straight

Term	Term Analysis		Definition
orthopedics (or-thoh-**PEE**-dicks)	-ic = pertaining to ped/o = child		surgical specialty dealing with the correction of deformities and dysfunctions of the skeletal system

7.7 PATHOLOGY

Fractures

A break or crack in a bone (Figure 7-7A and B).

Treatment involves reduction and immobilization. Reduction means placing the bones back together (Figure 7-7C). Immobilization results from placing a cast over the broken bone to prevent movement.

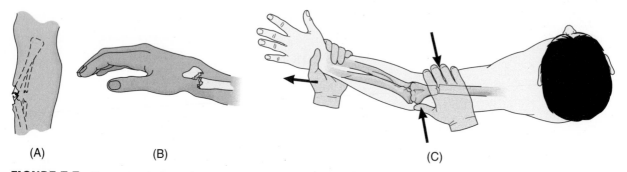

(A)   (B)   (C)

FIGURE 7-7 Fractures. A. Open fracture of the tibia. This is an open fracture because the skin is broken. B. Closed fracture of the wrist. This is a closed fracture because the skin is not broken. C. Reduction of a fracture. Bones are placed back together.

Herniated Intervertebral Disc; Slipped Disc

A portion of the intervertebral disc moves out of place (herniates). The result is that a nerve may be pinched, causing pain (Figure 7-8). Although herniation can occur at any point along the spinal column, the lumbar vertebrae are most often affected because of the weight they bear.

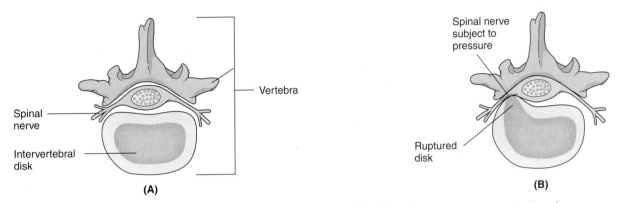

FIGURE 7-8 A. Normal intervertebral disc. B. Herniated intervertebral disc places pressure on spinal cord.

Osteoarthritis (os-tee-oh-ar-THRIGH-tis) (OA)

Chronic progressive degeneration of the articular cartilage. It is the most common form of arthritis (Figure 7-9). The exact cause is unknown, but joint injury and cartilage degeneration may leave the bones unprotected. Movement is painful because bone rubs on bone without protection from the articular cartilage.

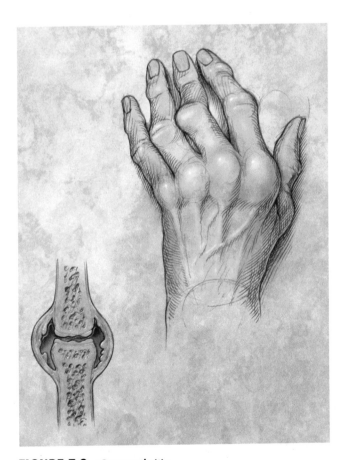

FIGURE 7-9 Osteoarthritis.

Osteoporosis (oss-tee-oh-por-OH-sis)

Loss of bone mass (density of bone), especially in the thoracic vertebrae (Figure 7-10). The bone becomes thin, porous, and weak. Fractures are common because of the weak bone.

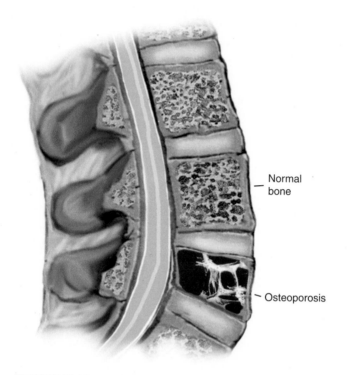

FIGURE 7-10   Osteoporosis.

Rheumatoid Arthritis (ROO-mah-toyd) (RA)

A chronic autoimmune disease that first attacks joints. It can progress to other body organs including skin, blood vessels, and lungs. An autoimmune disease occurs when the body's immune system fails to recognize its own cells as normal and attacks the body's tissues as if they were foreign invaders. In rheumatoid arthritis, the synovial membranes at the joint are attacked, making movement difficult.

 REVIEW EXERCISES

Exercise 7-1   LOOK-ALIKE AND SOUND-ALIKE WORDS

Below is a list of look-alike and sound-alike words. Study the definitions of each set of words, then read the sentences carefully and circle the word in parentheses that correctly completes the meaning.

hypercalcemia	increased amounts of calcium in the blood
hyperkalemia	increased amounts of potassium in the blood
humeral	pertaining to the humerus
humoral	pertaining to body fluids.
humerus	the arm bone
humorous	funny
ilium	hip bone
ileum	third portion of the small intestine
malleolus	bony bump on the distal end of the tibia and fibula
malleus	bone of the middle ear
sprain	stretching or tearing of a ligament
strain	stretching or tearing of a tendon or muscle

1. In (**humoral/humeral**) immunity, antibodies are released into the blood.

2. While bouncing on the bed, Julio fell off and broke his (**humorous/humerus**). This was not (**humorous/humerus**).

3. José slipped on the rocks and broke the distal tibia at the (**malleus/malleolus**).

4. Jack had a difficult time hearing. The MRI showed degeneration of the (**malleolus/malleus**).

5. While skiing, Anastasia tore her shoulder ligaments. The diagnosis was a (**sprain/strain**) of the shoulder.

6. (**Hypercalcemia/hyperkalemia**) is due to kidney dysfunction resulting in abnormal potassium levels.

Exercise 7-2

MATCHING WORD PARTS WITH MEANING

Match the word part in Column A *with its meaning in* Column B.

Column A	Column B
_____ **1.** arthr/o	A. cartilage
_____ **2.** -pathy	B. inflammation
_____ **3.** -plasty	C. softening
_____ **4.** -scopy	D. tumor
_____ **5.** chondr/o	E. under
_____ **6.** cost/o	F. joint
_____ **7.** oste/o	G. rib
_____ **8.** myel/o	H. straight
_____ **9.** -itis	I. malignant tumor of connective tissue
_____ **10.** orth/o	J. self
_____ **11.** -malacia	K. child
_____ **12.** -cyte	L. safe
_____ **13.** -oma	M. disease
_____ **14.** -al	N. bone
_____ **15.** sub-	O. cell
_____ **16.** -sarcoma	P. process of viewing
_____ **17.** -centesis	Q. bone marrow
_____ **18.** auto-	R. surgical puncture
_____ **19.** -immune	S. pertaining to
_____ **20.** ped/o	T. surgical reconstruction

Exercise 7-3

SHORT ANSWER—ANATOMY

Answer the following in the space provided.

    1. Name two cells found in osseous tissue._____

    _____

    2. Bones come together to form _____ .

    3. How are joints named? _____

    4. Name two mineral substances found in bone.

    _____

5. The tailbone is also known as the _____ .

6. The bones of the skull are called the _____ .
The bones of the chest are called the _____ .

7. Tendons attach _____ . Ligaments attach

_____ .

8. What type of tissue is the spinal column made up of?
The spinal cord? _____

9. Name the five divisions of the vertebral column. State
the number of bones in each division.

_____

_____

_____

10. Name five functions of bone. _____

_____

Exercise 7-4 **LOCATION OF BONES**

Match the bones with its location:

arm _____

cranium _____

face _____

foot _____

hand _____

leg _____

pectoral girdle _____

pelvis _____

thoracic cage _____

vertebral column _____

wrist _____

1. calcaneus _____

2. fibula _____

3. carpals _____

4. sternum _____

5. metatarsals _____

6. olecranon _____

7. radius _____

8. occipital _____

9. zygomatic _____

10. maxilla _____

11. parietal _____

12. metacarpals _____

13. coccyx _____

14. ilium _____

15. sacrum _____

16. femur _____

17. humerus _____

18. ulna _____

19. patella _____

20. mandible _____

Exercise 7-5 NAMING BONES

Write the common name of the following bones.

1. cranium _____

2. zygomatic _____

3. mandible _____

4. maxilla _____

5. sternum _____

6. coccyx _____

7. humerus _____

8. olecranon _____

9. carpals _____

10. metacarpals _____

11. phalanges _____

12. ilium _____

13. femur _____

14. tibia _____

15. patella _____

Exercise 7-6 PATHOLOGY

Match the term in Column A *with its description in* Column B.

Column A	Column B
_____ 1. rheumatoid arthritis	A. loss of bone mass
_____ 2. reduction and immobilization	B. treatment for osteoarthritis
_____ 3. osteoarthritis	C. autoimmune disease
_____ 4. osteoporosis	D. treatment for fractures
_____ 5. arthroplasty	E. degeneration of articular cartilage

Exercise 7-7 DEFINITIONS—LEARNING THE TERMS

Give the meanings of the following terms.

1. arthralgia _____

2. chondromalacia_____

3. subcostal _____

4. osteitis _____

5. osteosarcoma_____

6. osteomyelitis_____

7. orthopedics_____

8. myelogenous_____

9. arthropathy_____

10. osteomalacia _____

| Exercise 7-8 | **DEFINITIONS IN CONTEXT** |

Define the bolded terms in context. Use your dictionary if necessary.

1. Severe **arthropathy** in the back involves the **sacroiliac joint**.

    a. arthropathy _____

    b. sacroiliac joint _____

2. **Reduction** and **immobilization** have been performed on a previously noted **fractured radius**.

    c. reduction and immobilization _____

    d. fractured radius _____

3. It was felt he would benefit from **arthroscopy** and repair of the **articular cartilage**.

    e. arthroscopy _____

    f. articular cartilage _____

| Exercise 7-9 | **WORD BUILDING** |

I. Use arthr/o to build medical words for the following definitions:

   a. joint pain _____

   b. inflammation of a joint _____

   c. surgical puncture to remove fluid from the joint cavity
    _____

   d. diseased joint _____

   e. surgical reconstruction of a joint
    _____

   f. process of visually examining a joint cavity
    _____

II. Use chondr/o to build medical words for the following definitions:

   a. softening of cartilage _____

   b. tumor of cartilage _____

   c. cartilaginous cell _____

III. *Use oste/o to build medical words for the following definitions:*

a. inflammation of bone _____

b. tumor of bone _____

c. softening of bone _____

d. inflammation of bone and bone marrow

_____

e. malignant tumor of bone

_____

| **Exercise 7-10** | SPELLING |

Circle any words that are spelled incorrectly in the list below. Then correct the spelling in the space provided.

1. calcaneus _____

2. osseous _____

3. mylogenus _____

4. cocyxx _____

5. humeral _____

6. vertabral _____

7. phalanges _____

8. reumatoid _____

9. imobilization _____

10. cartalage _____

| Exercise 7-11 | LABELING—BONES |

Label Figure 7-11 using the body structures listed on the following page. Space is provided on this page if you prefer to write your answers there. Example: 1. -cranium.

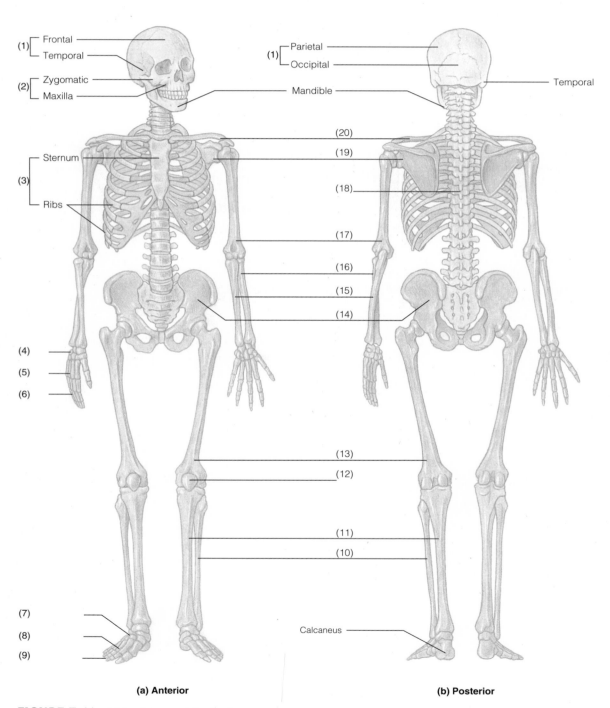

(a) Anterior   (b) Posterior

FIGURE 7-11 Major bones of the body.

carpals

clavicle

cranium

facial bones

femur

fibula

hip bones

humerus

metacarpals

metatarsals

patella

phalanges

radius

scapula

tarsals

thorax

tibia

ulna

vertebra

1. <u>cranium</u>

2. _____

3. _____

4. _____

5. _____

6. _____

7. _____

8. _____

9. _____

10. _____

11. _____

12. _____

13. _____

14. _____

15. _____

16. _____

17. _____

18. _____

19. _____

20. _____

7.9 PRONUNCIATION AND SPELLING

1. Listen to each word on the audio CD.

2. Pronounce each word carefully.

3. Spell each word in the space provided.

Word	Pronunciation	Spelling
arthralgia	ar-**THRAL**-jee-ah	
arthritis	ar-**THRIGH**-tis	
arthrocentesis	ar-throh-sen-**TEE**-sis	
arthroplasty	**AR**-thro-**plas**-tee	
arthroscopy	ar-**THROS**-koh-pee	
carpals	**KAR**-palz	
chondrocyte	**KON**-droh-sight	
chondroma	kon-**DROH**-mah	
chondromalacia	**kon**-droh-mah-**LAY**-she-ah	
clavicle	**KLAV**-ih-kul	
coccyx	**KOCK**-sicks	
cranium	**KRAY**-nee-um	

Word	Pronunciation	Spelling
femur	**FEE**-mur	
fibula	**FIB**-yoo-lah	
frontal	**FRON**-tal	
humerus	**HEW**-mer-us	
metacarpals	**met**-ah-**KAR**-palz	
metatarsals	**met**-ah-**TAHR**-salz	
myelogenous	**my**-eh-**LOJ**-en-us	
occipital	ock-**SIP**-ih-tal	
orthopedics	**or**-thoh-**PEE**-dicks	
osteitis	os-tee-**EYE**-tis	
osteoma	os-tee-**OH**-ma	
osteomalacia	**os**-tee-oh-mah-**LAY**-shee-ah	
osteomyelitis	**os**-tee-oh-**my**-eh-**LYE**-tis	
osteoporosis	**oss**-tee-oh-por-**OH**-sis	
osteosarcoma	**o**-tee-oh-sar-**KOH**-mah	
patella	pah-**TEL**-ah	
phalanges	fah-**LAN**-jeez	
radius	**RAY**-dee-us	
sacrum	**SAY**-krum	
scapula	**SKAP**-yoo-lah	
sternum	**STER**-num	
subcostal	sub-**KOS**-tal	
tarsals	**TAHR**-salz	
thorax	**THOH**-racks	
tibia	**TIB**-ee-ah	
ulna	**ULL**-nah	
vertebral column	**VER**-teh-bral **KOL**-um	
zygomatic	**zye**-goh-**MAT**-ick	

CHAPTER 8

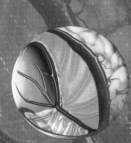

Muscular System

LEARNING OBJECTIVES

After studying this chapter and completing the review exercises, you should be able to:

1. Name three types of muscle tissue and state the location of each.
2. Name and define types of muscular movement.
3. Name and locate common skeletal muscles.
4. Pronounce, spell, define, and write the medical terms related to the muscular system.
5. Describe common diseases related to the muscular system.
6. Describe the diagnostic tests related to the muscular system.
7. Listen, read, and study so you can speak and write.

INTRODUCTION

All bodily movement is performed by muscle. Bend your arm and move your hand toward your shoulder. The muscles in your forearm and upper arm have made this happen. They are called **voluntary** muscles because you can make them move when you want them to. At the same time you were doing this, your heart kept beating even though you weren't thinking about it. The heart is an example of **involuntary** muscle. It does its job without being told.

8.1 MAJOR MUSCLES OF THE BODY

PRACTICE FOR LEARNING: MAJOR MUSCLES OF THE BODY

Write the muscles listed below on the correct spaces in Figure 8-1A and B. To help you, the number beside the muscle tells you where it goes on the figure. Be sure to pronounce each word as you write it. Repeat the pronunciation several times if you find the word hard to say.

Anterior View

1. facial muscles (**FAY**-shul **MUSS**-els)

2. sternocleidomastoid (**stern**-oh-**kleye**-doh-**MASS**-toyd)

3. pectoralis major (**peck**-tor-**AL**-iss **MAY**-jor)

4. serratus anterior (seh-**RAY**-tuss an-**TEER**-ee-or)

5. abdominal muscles (ab-**DOM**-ih-nul)

6. adductors of thigh (ah-**DUCK**-terz)

7. sartorius (sar-**TOR**-ee-us)

8. quadriceps femoris (**KWA**-drih-seps **FEM**-or-iss)

9. biceps brachii (**BYE**-seps **BRAY**-kee)

Posterior View

10. trapezius (trah-**PEE**-zee-us)

11. triceps brachii (**TRIGH**-seps **BRAY**-kee)

12. latissimus dorsi (lah-**TIS**-ih-mus)

13. gluteus maximus (**GLOO**-tee-us **MAX**-ih-muss)

14. gastrocnemius (**gas**-troh-**NEE**-mee-us)

15. Achilles tendon (ah-**KILL**-eez **TEN**-don)

16. hamstrings (**HAM**-stringz)

17. deltoid (**DEL**-toyd)

HELPING YOU REMEMBER

The words biceps and triceps always end in "s," whether they are referring to one muscle or more than one.

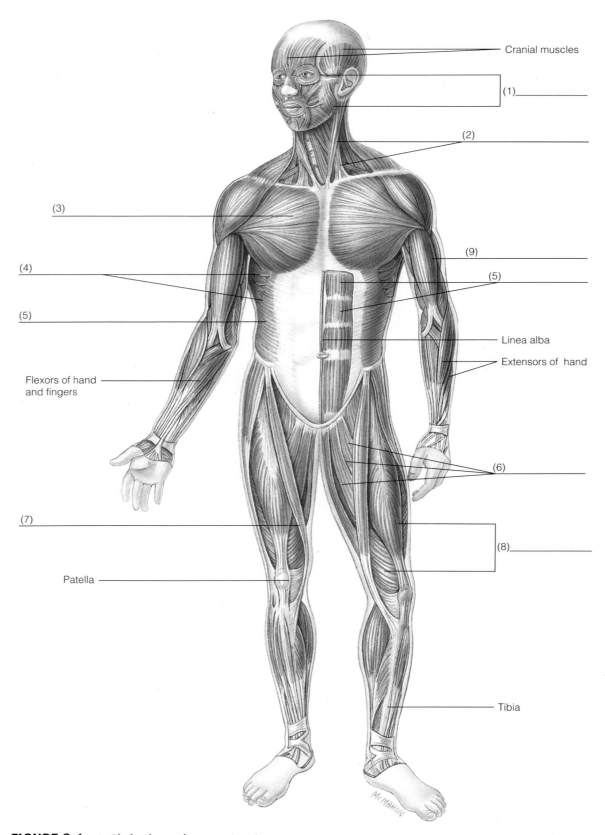

Cranial muscles

(1)

(2)

(3)

(9)

(4)

(5)

(5)

Linea alba

Extensors of hand

Flexors of hand
and fingers

(6)

(7)

(8)

Patella

Tibia

FIGURE 8-1 A. Skeletal muscles, anterior view.

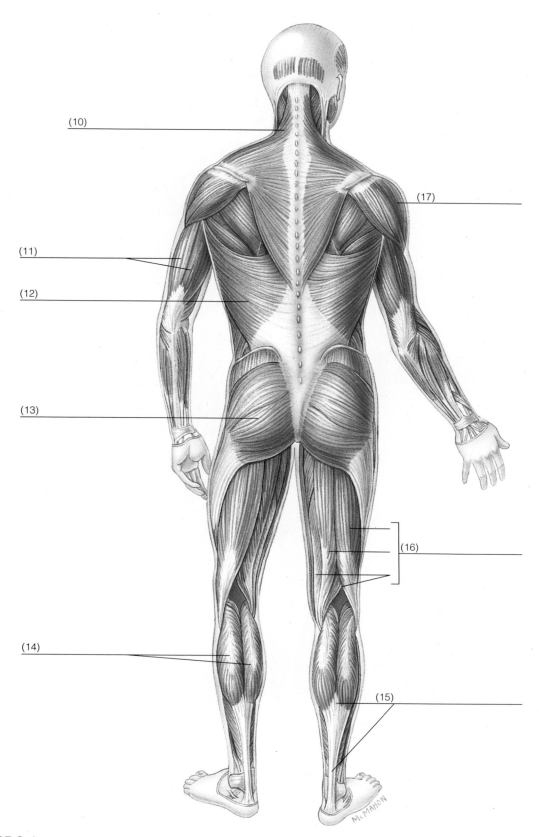

FIGURE 8-1 B. Skeletal muscles, posterior view.

TYPES OF MUSCLE TISSUE

The cells found in muscle are called muscle fibers. They are long, slender, and thread-like. They can **contract (kon-TRAKT)**, which means they can shorten their length. This makes movement possible. These cells form three types of muscle tissue: **cardiac (KAR-dee-ack)**, **visceral (VISS-er-al)**, and **skeletal (SKEL-eh-tal)**. Cardiac muscle is located in the heart and functions to pump blood. Visceral muscles move internal organs (viscer/o = internal organs) such as the respiratory tract, digestive tract, and blood vessels. Skeletal muscles are located on top of bone. They move bone by pulling on it.

All muscle is wrapped in a band of connective tissue called **fascia (FASH-ah)**, as illustrated in Figure 8-2.

In this chapter you will learn only about the skeletal muscles, because the cardiac and visceral muscles are covered in other chapters.

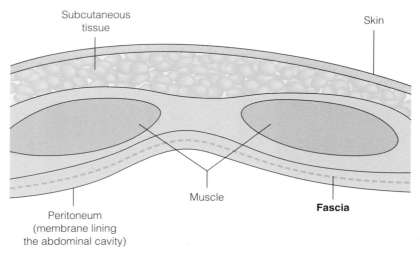

FIGURE 8-2 Fascia wraps around muscle.

PRACTICE FOR LEARNING: MUSCLE TYPES

Fill in the blanks with the correct answer.

1. Muscle cells are also called _____ .

2. Name three types of muscle tissue: _____ , _____ , and _____ .

3. What is the main function of muscle tissue?
_____

4. Where are visceral muscles located? _____

5. Where are skeletal muscles located? _____

6. Define fascia. _____

> *Answers:* **1.** muscle fibers. **2.** cardiac, skeletal, and visceral. **3.** movement.
> **4.** internal organs. **5.** on top of bones. **6.** band of connective tissue around
> the muscle.

8.3 MOVEMENTS OF SKELETAL MUSCLE

All skeletal muscles are connected to two bones. This makes movement possible. When the muscle contracts, one of the two bones it is connected to moves. This is illustrated in Figure 8-3.

The muscles are connected to bones by bands of connective tissue. Some of these tissues are thin and cordlike. They are called tendons (Figure 8-3). Broader connective tissues are called aponeuroses (**ah-poh-new-ROH-**seez).

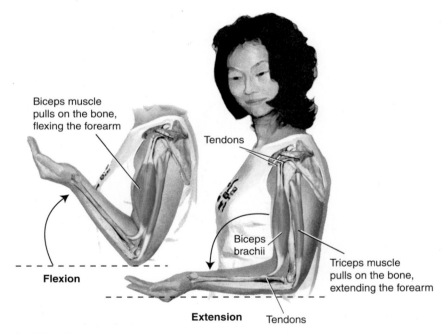

FIGURE 8-3 Movement of the forearm by biceps and triceps muscles. All skeletal muscles are connected to bones by tendons. Bone movement occurs when the muscle pulls on the bone.

Types of Muscle Movements

Muscles move bone in different ways. The common movements are listed below and are illustrated in Figures 8-3 to 8-8.

flexion decreasing the angle between two bones such as bending the neck forward or bending a limb

extension increasing the angle between two bones; return from flexion

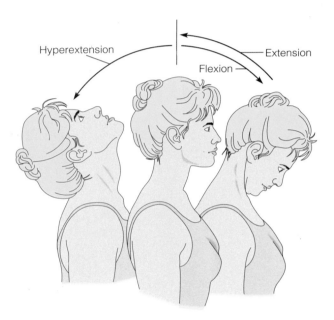

FIGURE 8-4 Muscle movements: flexion, extension, and hyperextension.

hyperextension overextending the joint beyond the anatomical position

abduction movement **away** from the midline of the body, usually involving the upper or lower limbs

adduction movement **toward** the midline of the body, usually involving the upper or lower limbs

pronation turning the palm down or backward

supination turning the palm up or toward the front

HELPING YOU REMEMBER

Notice that **adduction** *has the word "add" in it, meaning "to bring things together."*

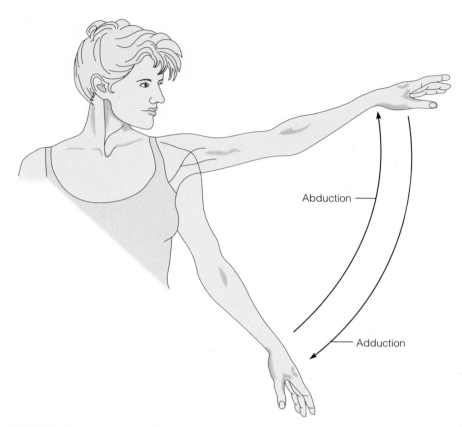

FIGURE 8-5   Muscle movements: abduction and adduction.

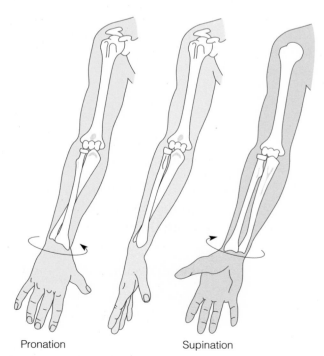

Pronation   Supination

FIGURE 8-6   Muscle movements: pronation and supination.

eversion movement of the sole of the foot outward, away from the midline

inversion movement of the sole of the foot inward, toward the midline

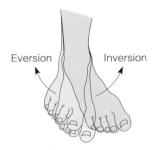

FIGURE 8-7 Muscle movements: eversion and inversion.

dorsiflexion flexion at the ankle moving the foot upward

plantar flexion flexion at the ankle pointing the toes toward the ground

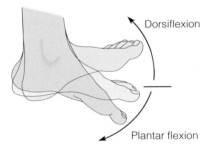

FIGURE 8-8 Muscle movements: dorsiflexion, plantar flexion.

PRACTICE FOR LEARNING: MUSCLE MOVEMENTS

Fill in the blanks with the correct muscle movement

1. Overextending the joint beyond the anatomical position.

   _____

2. Movement of the sole inward toward the midline.

   _____

3. Turning the palm down or backward.

   _____

4. Movement toward the midline of the body.

   _____

5. Decreasing the angle between two bones.

   _____

6. Turning the palm up or toward the front.

   _____

7. Flexion at the ankle pointing the toes toward the ground.

   _____

8. Movement away from the midline of the body.

   _____

Answers: **1.** hyperextension. **2.** inversion. **3.** pronation. **4.** adduction. **5.** flexion. **6.** supination. **7.** plantar flexion. **8.** abduction.

8.4 NEW ROOTS

Use these additional roots when studying the terms in this chapter.

Root	Meaning
fibr/o	fiber
skelet/o	skeleton

8.5 LEARNING THE TERMS

Following these steps will make it easier for you to learn medical terms:

1. Pronounce the term repeatedly until it is easy for you.

2. Write it down. Ensure the spelling is correct.

3. Also write the definition. If possible, relate the word to a word, thought or picture that will help you remember it.

4. Analyze the term with the method taught in this text.

Root	Meaning
fasci/o	fascia (band of tissue surrounding the muscle)

Term	Term Analysis	Definition
fascial (**FASH**-ee-al)	-al = pertaining to	pertaining to fascia
fasciitis; fascitis (**fas**-ee-**EYE**-tis); (fah-**SIGH**-tis)	-itis = inflammation	inflammation of the fascia

Root	Meaning
kinesi/o	movement

Term	Term Analysis	Definition
kinesiology (kih-**nee**-see-**OL**-oh-jee)	-logy = study of	study of movement

Root	Meaning
muscul/o (see also my/o)	muscle

Term	Term Analysis	Definition
muscular (**MUS**-kyoo-lar)	-ar = pertaining to	pertaining to muscle
musculoskeletal (**mus**-kyoo-loh-**SKEL**-eh-tal)	-al = pertaining to skelet/o = skeleton	pertaining to the muscles and skeleton

Root	Meaning
my/o	muscle

Term	Term Analysis	Definition
fibromyalgia (**figh**-broh-my-**AL**-jee-ah)	-algia = pain fibr/o = fiber	chronic muscle pain
myopathy (my-**OP**-ah-thee)	-pathy = disease	any muscular disease

Root	Meaning
tendin/o; ten/o	tendon

Term	Term Analysis	Definition
tendinitis (ten-dih-**NIGH**-tis)	-itis = inflammation	inflammation of a tendon
tendinous (**TEN**-dih-nus)	-ous = pertaining to	pertaining to a tendon
tenotomy (teh-**NOT**-oh-me)	-tomy = to cut	cutting of a tendon

Root	Meaning
ton/o	tone; tension

Term	Term Analysis	Definition
atonic (a-**TON**-ick)	-ic = pertaining to a- = no; not; lack of	pertaining to no tone or tension
dystonia (dis-**TOH**-nee-ah)	-ia = condition dys- = bad; difficult; painful	abnormal muscle tone
myotonia (**my**-oh-**TOH**-nee-ah)	-ia = condition my/o = muscle	muscle is unable to relax; a type of dystonia
tonic (**TON**-ick)	-ic = pertaining to	pertaining to tone

Suffix	Meaning
-kinesia; kinesis	movement

Term	Term Analysis	Definition
bradykinesia (**brad**-ee-kih-**NEE**-zee-ah)	brady-	slow movement
dyskinesia (dis-kih-**NEE**-zee-ah)	dys- = bad; difficult; painful; poor	poor muscle movement
hyperkinesis (**high**-per-kih-**NEE**-sis)	hyper- = excessive; above normal	excessive movement; hyperactivity

Suffix		Meaning
-taxia		order

Term	Term Analysis	Definition
ataxia (ah-**TACKS**-ee-ah)	a- = no; not; lack of	no muscular coordination

8.6 PATHOLOGY

Muscular Dystrophy (MD)

Muscular dystrophy is a broad term that includes a number of inherited disorders of the skeletal muscles. The main features are muscular weakness and degeneration of muscle tissue. The most common type is Duchenne's (**doo-SHENZ**) muscular dystrophy. There is no cure for the disease.

Rotator Cuff Tendinitis

The rotator cuff refers to a group of tendons that holds the shoulder joint in place (Figure 8-9A). Rotator cuff tendinitis is the inflammation of these tendons (Figure 8-9B). Overuse of the tendons in such sports as swimming, tennis, and pitching in baseball is the major cause.

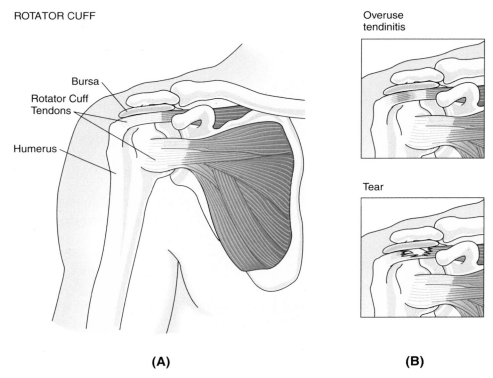

ROTATOR CUFF

Bursa

Rotator Cuff
Tendons

Humerus

Overuse
tendinitis

Tear

(A) (B)

FIGURE 8-9 Rotator cuff. A. Healthy rotator cuff. B. Injured rotator cuff (overuse tendinitis and tear).

Strain

A strain is overstretching or tearing a muscle. It is commonly called a pulled muscle.

 8.7 REVIEW EXERCISES

Exercise 8-1 LOOK-ALIKE AND SOUND-ALIKE WORDS

Below is a list of look-alike and sound-alike words. Study the definitions of each set of words, then read the sentences carefully and circle the word in parentheses that correctly completes the meaning.

abduction	to draw away from the midline of the body
adduction	to draw toward the midline of the body
myelography	process of recording the spinal cord
myography	process of recording a muscle
fascial	pertaining to the fascia
facial	pertaining to the face
flexor	a muscle that flexes a joint
flexure	a portion of a structure that is bent
peroneal	pertaining to the muscles over the fibula
peritoneal	pertaining to the peritoneum. The peritoneum is a membrane lining the abdominopelvic cavity.
perineal	pertaining to the perineum. The perineum is the area between the vagina and anus in the female. In the male, it is the area between the scrotum and anus.

1. Move your leg away from the midline of your body. This motion is (**abduction/adduction**).

2. Muscle disease may be assessed by (**myelography/myography**).

3. Plantar (**fascial/facial**) pain can be caused by flatfeet.

4. The (**fascial/facial**) muscles can wrinkle the forehead and pucker the lips.

5. Bob cannot bend his wrist because the (**flexor/flexure**) muscles were damaged in a motorcycle accident.

6. Debra tore the (**peroneal/peritoneal/perineal**) area when she delivered her baby.

7. The (**peroneal/peritoneal/perineal**) cavity in the abdomen was filled with fluid.

8. The (**peroneal/peritoneal/perineal**) muscle is responsible for abduction of the foot.

Exercise 8-2   MATCHING WORD PARTS WITH MEANING

Match the word part in Column A *with its meaning in* Column B

Column A	Column B
_____ 1. fasci/o	A. order
_____ 2. -ia	B. pertaining to
_____ 3. kinesi/o	C. pain
_____ 4. my/o	D. to cut
_____ 5. -taxia	E. tendon
_____ 6. -ous	F. muscle
_____ 7. -tomy	G. band of tissue surrounding muscle
_____ 8. -algia	H. tension
_____ 9. ton/o	I. movement
_____ 10. ten/o	J. condition

Exercise 8-3   SHORT ANSWER

Answer the following in the space provided.

1. Name three types of muscle tissue.

   _____

   _____

2. What is the primary function of muscle?

   _____

3. State the difference between:

   a. pronation and supination _____

   b. dorsiflexion and plantar flexion _____

   c. hyperextension and extension _____

| **Exercise 8-4** | **LOCATION OF MUSCLES** |

Name the muscle with its location:

arm _____

back _____

chest _____

leg _____

neck _____

shoulder _____

trunk (area between the chest and legs) _____

1. quadriceps _____

2. serratus anterior _____

3. pectoralis major _____

4. adductors _____

5. gastrocnemius _____

6. triceps brachii _____

7. hamstrings _____

8. Achilles tendon _____

9. biceps brachii _____

10. trapezius _____

11. latissimus dorsi _____

12. deltoid _____

13. sartorius _____

14. sternocleidomastoid _____

| **Exercise 8-5** | **DEFINITIONS** |

Give the meaning of the following:

1. muscle fibers _____

2. tendons _____

3. fascia _____

4. adduction _____

5. eversion _____

6. ataxia _____

7. rotator cuff tendinitis _____

8. fibromyalgia _____

9. dystonia _____

10. tenotomy _____

Exercise 8-6   MEDICAL TERMS IN CONTEXT

Define the bolded terms in context in the space below. Use your dictionary if necessary.

DISCHARGE SUMMARY

HISTORY OF PRESENT ILLNESS: The patient is a seven-year-old boy who showed signs of muscular weakness at age three to four years. The diagnosis of muscular dystrophy was made when the muscle biopsy confirmed degeneration of muscle fibers. He is still walking and was started on drug therapy four months ago.

PHYSICAL EXAMINATION: On examination, the patient is a pleasant young fellow. He has proximal muscle weakness. He has hypertrophy and some shortening of the Achilles tendons. General physical examination is within normal limits.

COURSE IN HOSPITAL: While in the hospital, an intravenous line was started, and blood samples were taken for tests during a 24-hour period. The course in hospital was uneventful.

MOST RESPONSIBLE DIAGNOSIS: MUSCULAR DYSTROPHY

1. muscular dystrophy _____

2. biopsy _____

3. degeneration _____

4. therapy _____

5. proximal _____

6. hypertrophy _____

7. Achilles tendons _____

8. intravenous _____

Exercise 8-7 WORD BUILDING

    I. Use the root ton/o to build terms for the following definitions.

      a. pertaining to no tone or tension _____

      b. abnormal muscle tone _____

      c. muscle is unable to relax _____

      d. pertaining to tone _____

    II. Use the suffix -kinesia to build terms for the following definitions.

      a. slow movement _____

      b. impaired movement _____

      c. excessive movement _____

Exercise 8-8 SPELLING

Circle any misspelled words in the list below and correctly spell them in the space provided.

    1. quadraceps _____

    2. sternocliedomastoid _____

    3. serratus _____

    4. adducter muscles _____

    5. plantar _____

    6. trapezious _____

    7. latisimus dorsi _____

    8. gastrocnemius _____

    9. Achilles _____

    10. biceps brachii _____

| Exercise 8-9 | LABELING |

I. Skeletal Muscles, Anterior View
Using the body structures listed below, write the name of each numbered structure in Figure 8-10 on the corresponding lines below.

abdominal muscles _____

adductors _____

biceps brachii _____

facial muscles _____

pectoralis major _____

quadriceps femoris _____

sartorius _____

serratus anterior _____

sternocleidomastoid _____

1. _____

2. _____

3. _____

4. _____

5. _____

6. _____

7. _____

8. _____

9. _____

II. Skeletal Muscles, Posterior View
Using the body structures listed below and on page 158, write the name of each numbered structure in Figure 8-11 on the corresponding line on page 158.

Achilles tendon _____

deltoid _____

gastrocnemius _____

gluteus maximus _____

hamstrings _____

latissimus dorsi _____

(continued on page 158)

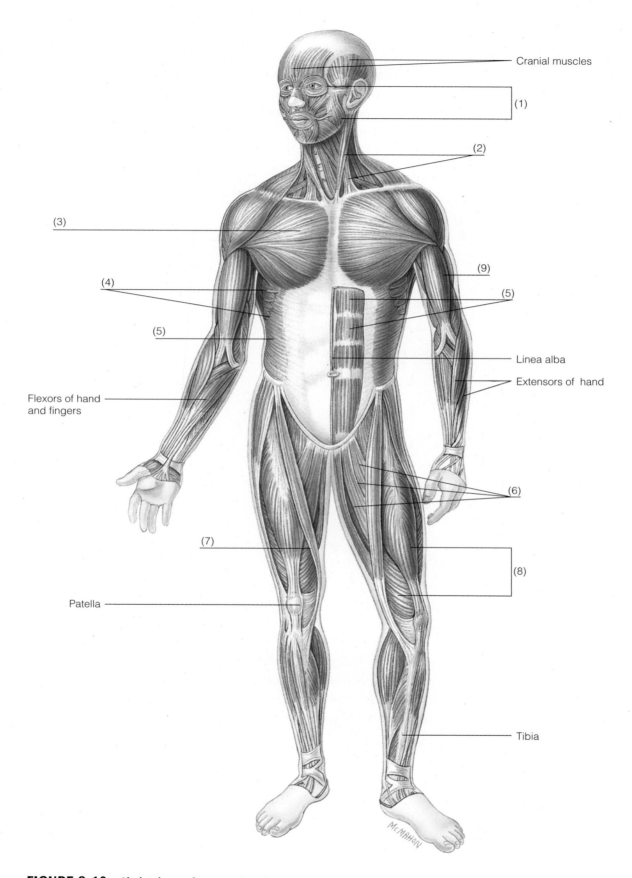

Cranial muscles

(1)

(2)

(3)

(9)

(4)

(5)

(5)

Linea alba

Extensors of hand

Flexors of hand
and fingers

(6)

(7)

(8)

Patella

Tibia

McMAHON

FIGURE 8-10   Skeletal muscles, anterior view.

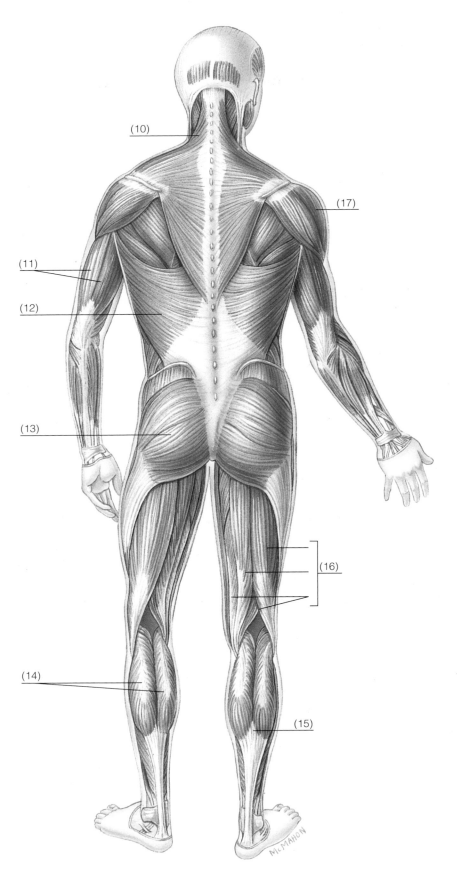

FIGURE 8-11 Skeletal muscle, posterior view.

(continued from page 155)

trapezius

triceps brachii

10. _____

11. _____

12. _____

13. _____

14. _____

15. _____

16. _____

17. _____

8.8 PRONUNCIATION AND SPELLING

Listen, read, and study, so you can speak and write effectively.

1. Listen to each word on the audio CD.

2. Pronounce each word carefully.

3. Spell each word in the space provided.

Word	Pronunciation	Spelling
atonic	a-**TON**-ick	
biceps brachii	**bye**-seps **BRAY**-kee	
deltoid	**DEL**-toyd	
dorsiflexion	dor-sih-**FLECK**-shun	
dyskinesia	dis-kih-**NEE**-zee-ah	
dystonia	dis-**TOH**-nee-ah	
fascia	**FASH**-ah	
fasciitis	fas-ee-**EYE**-tis	
fibromyalgia	figh-broh-my-**AL**-jee-ah	
gastrocnemius	gas-troh-**NEE**-mee-us	
inversion	in-**VER**-zhun	

Word	Pronunciation	Spelling
kinesiology	kih-**nee**-see-**OL**-oh-jee	
latissimus dorsi	lah-**TISS**-ih-mus **DOR**-see	
muscular	**MUS**-kyoo-lar	
muscular dystrophy	**MUS**-kyoo-lar **DISS**-troh-fee	
musculoskeletal	**mus**-kyoo-loh-**SKEL**-eh-tal	
myopathy	my-**OP**-ah-thee	
plantar flexion	**PLAN**-tar **FLECK**-shun	
pronation	proh-**NAY**-shun	
supination	**soo**-pih-**NAY**-shun	
tendinous	**TEN**-dih-nus	
tenotomy	teh-**NOT**-oh-me	
trapezius	trah-**PEE**-zee-us	
triceps brachii	**TRIGH**-seps **BRAY**-kee	

CHAPTER 9

Nervous System

LEARNING OBJECTIVES

After studying this chapter and completing the review exercises, you should be able to:

1. Name and describe the divisions of the nervous system.
2. State the functions of nerve cells.
3. Name and describe the structures of the brain and spinal cord.
4. Describe the peripheral nervous system.
5. Pronounce, spell, define, and write the medical terms related to the nervous system.
6. Describe common diseases related to the nervous system.
7. Listen, read, and study so you can speak and write.

INTRODUCTION

The nervous system helps your body adjust to what is happening to it. If you touch something hot, the nervous system sends signals to the brain that make you quickly pull away. If the light around you grows stronger, the nervous system tells your eyes to adjust. If your body needs water, the nervous system makes you thirsty. The organs that carry the messages are called nerves (**NERVZ**). This chapter will teach you the terms you need to know about this very complicated system.

9.1 MAJOR ORGANS OF THE NERVOUS SYSTEM

PRACTICE FOR LEARNING: MAJOR ORGANS AND DIVISIONS

Write the words below on the correct space in Figure 9-1. To help you, the number beside the word tells you where it goes on the figure. Be sure to pronounce each word as you write it. Repeat the pronunciation several times if you find the word hard to say.

1. brain (**BRAYN**)

2. spinal cord (**SPYE**-nal **KORD**)

3. central nervous system (CNS) (**SEN**-tral **NERV**-us **SIS**-tem)

4. peripheral nerves (per-**IF**-er-al **NERVZ**)

5. peripheral nervous system (PNS)

9.2 DIVISIONS OF THE NERVOUS SYSTEM

Figure 9-1 shows you the two main divisions of the nervous system. They are the central nervous system (CNS) and the peripheral nervous system (PNS).

The CNS consists of the brain and the spinal cord.

The PNS consists mostly of nerves. The cranial (**KRAY**-nee-ul) nerves extend from the brain. The spinal nerves extend from the spinal cord. These nerves branch out into different parts of the body.

9.3 NERVE CELLS AND NERVES

IN BRIEF

Neurons are nerve cells.

Some neurons are myelinated; some neurons are unmyelinated.

Neurons (**NOO**-ronz) are nerve cells. They are very tiny, long, and slender (Figure 9-2). They make up organs called nerves. Neurons carry electrical impulses (messages) to and from the brain and spinal cord. They vary in size (some are as long as 3 feet or 90 centimeters).

Some neurons are covered with a white fatty substance called a myelin sheath (**MY**-eh-lin **SHEETH**). The myelin sheath acts as an insulator, keeping the impulse traveling from

HELPING YOU REMEMBER

Neurons are like electrical wires. The myelin sheath is like the wrapping on an electric wire. Electric impulses move through an electrical wire, and nerve impulses travel from neuron to neuron. If the electric wire is broken, the impulses won't travel. Similarly, if the neuron is torn, the nerve impulses will not be transmitted.

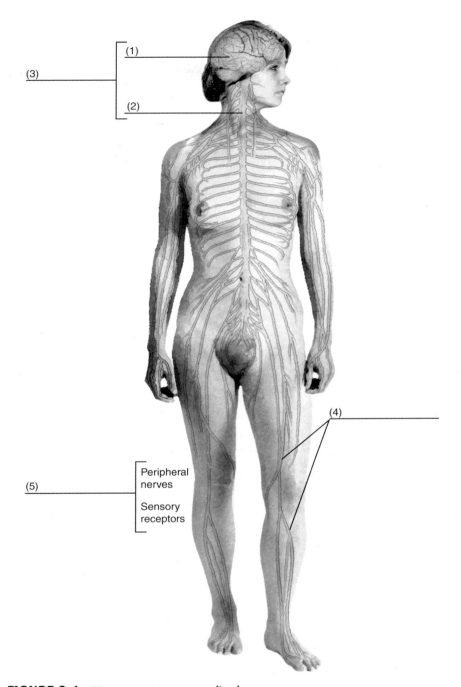

(3)

(1)

(2)

(4)

(5)

Peripheral
nerves

Sensory
receptors

FIGURE 9-1 Nervous system generalized.

neuron to neuron until its destination is reached (Figure 9-2). Neurons wrapped with myelin sheath are called myelinated (**MY-eh-lih-nay-ted**). They are also called white matter. Neurons that are not covered with myelin are called unmyelinated (**UN-my-eh-lih-nay-ted**). They are called gray matter.

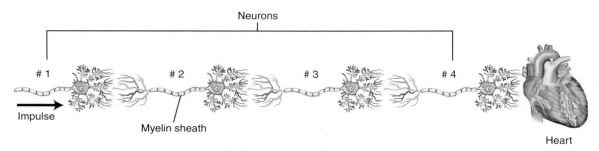

FIGURE 9-2 Neurons placed end-to-end. An electrical impulse travels from one neuron to the next until it reaches its destination, which in this case is the heart.

Nerves

Nerves are made up of neurons bunched together. They can be seen with the naked eye. There are two kinds of nerves. One kind carries impulses **to** the brain and spinal cord. For example, when the skin of your back is itchy, a message travels from the skin through a nerve to the spinal cord and then to the brain. When the message about the itch reaches the brain, the information is analyzed. An appropriate message is sent back from the brain through a second kind of nerve, which carries messages **from** the brain and spinal cord. This messages travels down the spinal cord and stimulates the muscles of the arms and hands. The muscles then respond to the message by scratching the skin.

PRACTICE FOR LEARNING: NERVE CELLS AND NERVES

Circle true if the statement is correct. Circle false if the statement is not correct.

1. The myelin sheath acts an insulator, keeping the nerve impulse on track.   True   False

2. Neurons carry electrical impulses.   True   False

3. Neurons wrapped with myelin sheath are said to be myelinated.   True   False

4. Myelinated neurons are also called white matter.   True   False

5. Electrical impulses travel to and away from the brain and spinal cord.   True   False

6. Neurons are organs made up of nerves.   True   False

Answers: **1.** True. **2.** True. **3.** True. **4.** True. **5.** True. **6.** False.

9.4 CENTRAL NERVOUS SYSTEM

The Brain

PRACTICE FOR LEARNING: **PARTS OF THE BRAIN**

Write the different parts of the brain, listed below, on the correct spaces in Figure 9-3. To help you, the number beside the word tells you where it goes on the figure. Be sure to pronounce each word as you write it. Repeat the pronunciation several times if you find the word hard to say.

1. cerebrum (**seh-REE-brum**)

2. thalamus (**THAL-ah-mus**)

3. hypothalamus (**high-poh-THAL-ah-mus**)

4. midbrain (**MID-brayn**)

5. pons (**PONZ**)

6. medulla oblongata (**meh-DULL-ah ob-long-GAH-tah**)

7. cerebellum (**ser-eh-BELL-um**)

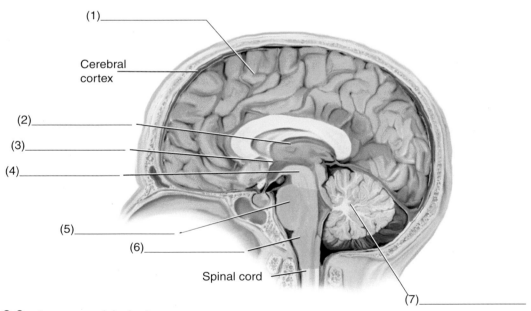

FIGURE 9-3   Structures of the brain.

The brain is protected by the skull, which is also called the cranium.

The brain is made up of billions of neurons and is divided into several parts. Each part has its own function.

Parts of the Brain

The cerebrum is the largest part of the brain. It is covered by gray matter called the cerebral cortex (seh-**REE**-bral **KOR**-tecks). The cerebrum is involved in movement, sensation, as well as thought, reasoning, and judgment.

The thalamus and hypothalamus are two other important structures of the brain.

The thalamus, deep inside the brain, receives stimuli such as pain, touch, and temperature. It sends this information to the cerebral cortex for analysis and interpretation. In the example above under the heading "Nerves," it is the thalamus that first makes the body aware of the hot temperature. However, the sensation must be sent to the cerebral cortex before a proper response to the abnormal temperature can be made.

The hypothalamus is located below the thalamus. It regulates appetite, thirst, and temperature. It is also associated with emotions and behavior.

The midbrain, pons, and medulla oblongata are together called the brainstem. It regulates basic life functions such as waking, respiration, heart rate, and blood pressure. It also serves as a pathway for impulses traveling to and from the brain and spinal cord.

The cerebellum lies under the cerebrum. It is important in maintaining balance and muscle coordination.

IN BRIEF

Parts of the Brain
cerebrum,
cerebral cortex,
thalamus,
hypothalamus,
cerebellum,
brainstem
(midbrain, pons,
medulla oblongata)

PRACTICE FOR LEARNING: BRAIN

Name the part of the brain described below.

1. outer gray matter covering the cerebrum

   _____

2. sends information to the cerebral cortex for analysis and interpretation _____

3. maintains balance and muscle coordination

   _____

4. includes pons, midbrain, and medulla _____

5. regulates appetite and thirst _____

Answers: **1.** cerebral cortex. **2.** thalamus. **3.** cerebellum. **4.** brainstem.
5. hypothalamus.

IN BRIEF

Spinal cord
is made up
of nerves.
Nerves branch
from the spinal
cord to the
rest of the body.

Spinal Cord

The spinal cord is shown in Figure 9-1 on page 163. It is a half-inch–thick cable made up of nerves bunched together. The nerves are soft tissue. They are protected by the bones of the vertebral column. Nerves branch out from both sides of the spinal cord, extending to most parts of the body.

HELPING YOU REMEMBER

The spinal cord and spinal column are not the same structures. The spinal cord is made up of nerves; the vertebral column is made up of bone.

9.5 PERIPHERAL NERVOUS SYSTEM

IN BRIEF

PNS includes
nerves extending
from the brain and
spinal cord to
body organs.

Nerves leave the brain and spinal cord and extend to almost all body structures. This includes structures that are away from the center, which are called peripheral structures. In this case, peripheral means away from the brain and spinal cord. Figure 9-4 illustrates some spinal nerves as they extend from the spinal cord to peripheral sites. The names given to these nerves relate to the organ or structure the nerve serves. For example, the ulnar nerve stimulates the muscles attaching to the ulnar bone of the arm. The tibial nerve stimulates the muscles over the tibia or shin bone.

9.6 NEW ROOTS, SUFFIXES, AND PREFIXES

Use these new roots, suffixes, and prefixes when studying the terms in this chapter.

Root	Meaning
mening/o	membrane; meninges
ment/o	mind
myelin/o	myelin sheath
poli/o	gray matter
spin/o	spinal cord; spine; spinal column; vertebral column
vascul/o	vessel

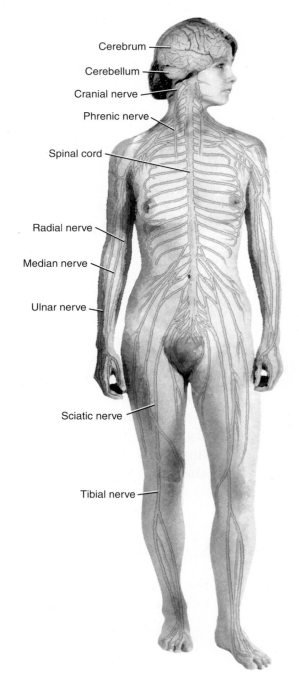

Cerebrum

Cerebellum

Cranial nerve

Phrenic nerve

Spinal cord

Radial nerve

Median nerve

Ulnar nerve

Sciatic nerve

Tibial nerve

FIGURE 9-4 Peripheral nerves branch from the spinal cord.

Suffix	Meaning
-ia	condition
-us	condition; thing

Prefix	Meaning
hemi-	half
para-	beside; near; abnormal
quadri-	four
tetra-	four

9.7 LEARNING THE TERMS

Following these steps will make it easier for you to learn medical terms:

1. Pronounce the term repeatedly until it is easy for you.

2. Write it down. Ensure the spelling is correct.

3. Also write the definition. If possible, relate the word to a word, thought, or picture that will help you remember it.

4. Analyze the term with the method taught in this text.

Root	Meaning
cerebr/o (see also encephal/o)	brain

Term	Term Analysis	Definition
cerebral angiography (seh-**REE**-bral AN-jee-**OG**-rah-fee)	-al = pertaining to -graphy = process of recording; process of producing images angi/o = vessel	process of producing an image of the blood vessels of the brain
cerebrovascular (ser-eh-broh-**VAS**-kyoo-lar)	-ar = pertaining to vascul/o = vessel	pertaining to the brain and blood vessels
cerebrospinal fluid (CSF) (ser-eh-broh-**SPYE**-nal)	-al = pertaining to spin/o = spinal cord fluid = a liquid that can flow	fluid in the brain and spinal cord

Root	Meaning
encephal/o	brain

Term	Term Analysis	Definition
encephalitis (en-**sef**-ah-**LYE**-tis)	-itis = inflammation	inflammation of the brain
encephalopathy (en-**sef**-ah-**LOP**-ah-thee)	-pathy = disease	any disease of the brain

Root	Meaning
hydr/o	water

Term	Term Analysis	Definition
hydrocephalus (**high**-droh-**SEF**-ah-lus)	-us = condition; thing cephal/o = head	accumulation of cerebrospinal fluid in the brain (Figure 9-5)

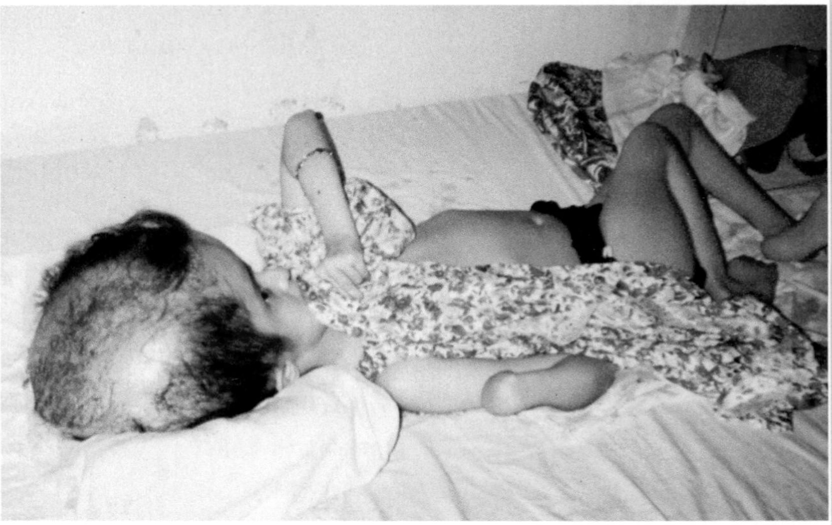

FIGURE 9-5 Hydrocephalus. (Courtesy of Dr. Russell Cox.)

Root	Meaning
magnet/o	magnet

Term	Term Analysis	Definition
magnetic resonance imaging (MRI) (mag-**NET**-ik **RES**-oh-nance **IM**-ah-jing)	-ic = pertaining to resonance = magnification imaging = picture	a picture of the brain produced by using magnetic waves (Figure 9-6)

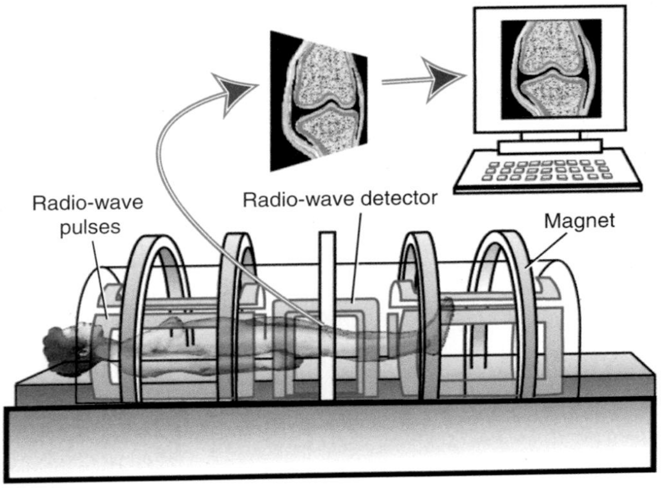

Radio-wave pulses

Radio-wave detector

Magnet

FIGURE 9-6 Magnetic resonance imaging.

Root	Meaning
mening/o	membrane; meninges (membranes around the brain and spinal cord)

Term	Term Analysis	Definition
meningitis (**men**-in-**JIGH**-tis)	-itis = inflammation	inflammation of the membranes surrounding the brain and spinal cord

Root	Meaning
myel/o	spinal cord

NOTE: In the skeletal system, myel/o means bone marrow.

Term	Term Analysis	Definition
poliomyelitis **poh**-lee-oh-**my**-eh-**LYE**-tis	-itis = inflammation poli/o = gray matter	inflammation of the gray matter of the spinal cord. Also known as polio.

NOTE: Poliomyelitis or polio is an infection caused by a virus. It is highly contagious. It attacks the nervous system and may cause paralysis. There is no cure. Polio can only be prevented by immunization with a weakened polio vaccine. Widespread use of the vaccine has eliminated the disease in most of the world.

Postpoliomyelitis has been identified in people who have had polio. The condition is characterized by muscle fatigue and weakness 15 years or more after they have recovered from polio.

Root	Meaning
neur/o	nerve

Term	Term Analysis	Definition
neuromuscular (noo-row-**MUS**-kyoo-lar)	-ar = pertaining to muscul/o = muscle	pertaining to the nerve and muscle; myoneural
neurology (noo-**ROL**-oh-jee)	-logy = study of	the study of the nervous system including diseases and treatment

Suffix	Meaning
-cele	hernia (protrusion or displacement of an organ through a structure that normally contains it)

Term	Term Analysis	Definition
meningocele (meh-**NIN**-goh-**seel**)	mening/o = meninges; membrane	displacement of the meninges from its normal position through an abnormal opening in the skull or vertebra (Refer to Figure 9-9A in Section 9.8 Pathology.)

Suffix	Meaning
-esthesia	sensation

Term	Term Analysis	Definition
anesthesia (an-es-**THEE**-zee-ah)	an- = no; not	loss of sensation
dysesthesia (dis-es-**THEE**-zee-ah)	dys- = bad; painful; difficult; poor	painful sensation in response to normal stimulation
paresthesia (par-es-**THEE**-zee-ah)	para- = abnormal	abnormal sensation such as numbness and tingling

Suffix	Meaning	
-phasia	speech	
Term	**Term Analysis**	**Definition**
aphasia (ah-**FAY**-zee-ah)	a- = no; not; lack of	no speech
dysphasia (dis-**FAY**-zee-ah)	dys- = bad; poor; difficult; painful	poor speech

Suffix	Meaning	
-plegia	paralysis	
Term	**Term Analysis**	**Definition**
hemiplegia (**hem**-ee-**PLEE**-jee-ah)	hemi- = half	paralysis affecting one side of the body, either the right or left
paraplegia (**par**-ah-**PLEE**-jee-ah)	para- = beside; near; abnormal	paralysis of the lower part of the body and legs
tetraplegia (**TET**-rah-**PLEE**-jee-ah)	tetra- = four	paralysis of all four limbs; quadriplegia (**kwad**-rih-**PLEE**-jee-ah)

Prefix	Meaning	
de-	lack of; removal	
Term	**Term Analysis**	**Definition**
dementia (deh-**MEN**-she-ah)	-ia = condition ment/o = mind	mental deterioration; lack of brain function including memory, judgment, reasoning, and personality changes

9.8 **PATHOLOGY**

Alzheimer's Disease (ALZ-high-merz)

A type of dementia. It is caused by the degeneration of brain cells. The disease results in the loss of memory, judgment, and reasoning. The disease gets worse over time, which means it is progressive. There are personality and behavior disorders.

Brain Tumors; Intracranial Tumors

There are two types of intracranial (within the skull) tumors: gliomas (gligh-**OH**-mahz) and meningiomas (meh-**nin**-jee-**OH**-mahz).

Gliomas are malignant tumors of brain tissue (Figure 9-7). They can be fast or slow growing.

Meningiomas are benign tumors. They are located outside the brain tissue but still within the cranium. They are slow growing.

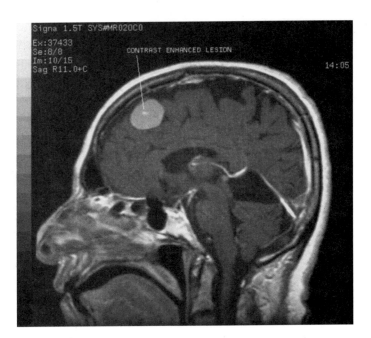

FIGURE 9-7 Brain tumor. Magnetic resonance imaging shows up a brain tumor in the frontal lobe.

Multiple Sclerosis (MS) (MUL-tih-pul skler-OH-sis)

A condition in which the myelin sheath covering the neurons of the brain and spinal cord are destroyed. This is called demyelination ("lack of myelin sheath"). The lack of myelin sheath prevents impulses from being transmitted through the axon. This results in muscle weakness, paralysis, and other physical disabilities.

Parkinson's Disease (PD)

A disease that results in slow movement (bradykinesia), muscular rigidity, and resting tremors (shaking). Parkinson's is a chronic, progressive condition.

The cause is unknown. However, the abnormal movements are due to a decrease in levels of a chemical, named dopamine, in the brain.

Seizure Disorder; Epilepsy

A condition which causes the electrical impulses in the brain to become disorganized, uncoordinated, and excessive. The result is cerebral dysfunction, which causes abnormal movement and sensations. Each attack is called an epileptic seizure.

Electroencephalography (**ee-leck-troh-en-sef-ah-LOG-rah-fee**) can detect the electrical impulses in the brain and register them as brain waves. It is commonly known as an **EEG**. Figure 9-8 illustrates normal and abnormal brain waves. Normal brain waves are the same in height and width. Abnormal brain waves, as seen in seizure disorder, are not the same in height and width.

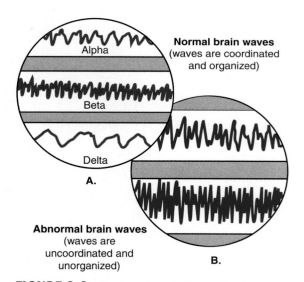

FIGURE 9-8 Brain waves. A. Normal brain waves are usually consistent in height and width. Alpha waves are typical of a normal person who is awake and in a resting state. Beta waves are typical of a brain experiencing intense activity. Delta waves are typical of a normal person in deep sleep. B. Abnormal brain waves. Note the inconsistent height and width of the brain waves as seen in patients with seizure disorders.

Spina Bifida (SPYE-nah-BIF-ih-da)

A defect in fetal development. The vertebrae do not form a complete circle around the spinal cord. It is a congenital (kon-JEN-ih-tal) condition, which means that it is present at birth.

In cases where the opening in the vertebrae is severe, the meninges and/or the spinal cord may protrude outside the vertebrae. They form a sac-like structure. If the sac contains only meninges, the condition is called meningocele (meh-NIN-goh-seel) (Figure 9-9A). If the sac contains meninges and spinal cord, the condition is called meningomyelocele (meh-nin-goh-MY-eh-loh-seel) (Figure 9-9B).

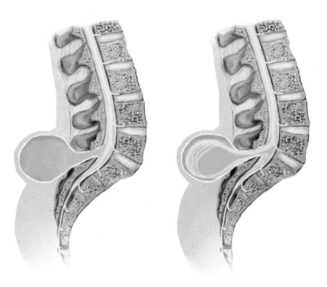

A. Meningocele   B. Meningomyelocele

FIGURE 9-9   Meningocele and meningomyelocele due to spina bifida.

9.9 REVIEW EXERCISES

Exercise 9-1

LOOK-ALIKE AND SOUND-ALIKE WORDS

Below is a list of look-alike and sound-alike words followed by sentences using the words. Study the definitions of each set of words. Then read the sentences carefully. Circle the word in parentheses that correctly completes the meaning.

aphasia	no speech
aphagia	no eating
aphakia	no lens (anatomical structure of the eye)

ataxia	no coordination
attacks	to become sick
clonus	twitching of a muscle
conus	resembling a cone shape
CNS	central nervous system
C&S	culture and sensitivity (a laboratory test)
elicit	to bring on; to elicit a response
illicit	illegal
gait	walking, running
gate	(1) Entrance or opening. (2) Gated cardiac blood-pooling imaging (a diagnostic test)

1. Jacob was admitted to the hospital with loss of blood to the speech centers in the brain due to a motor vehicle accident. On physical examination, at the time of admission, there was noted (**aphakia/aphagia/aphasia**).

2. Expect (**attacks/ataxia**) of delirium tremens following alcohol withdrawal. If there is cerebellar dysfunction, expect (**attacks/ataxia**).

3. The (**clonus/conus**) medullaris is the end portion of the spinal cord.

4. Continual (**clonus/conus**) indicates disruption of nerve impulses to the muscle.

5. To confirm inflammation of the (**CNS/C&S**), Dr. Lorenco withdrew CSF for (**CNS/C&S**).

6. To (**elicit/illicit**) a Babinski reflex on a newborn, stimulate the sole of the foot. The big toe should fan out.

7. Maria was caught with (**elicit/illicit**) drugs in the hospital.

8. Observe the patient carefully. Abnormal (**gate/gait**) may be the result of cerebellar damage.

9. Dr. Rollins ordered a multiple (**gaited/gated**) acquisition following Mr. Mah's abnormal stress test.

| Exercise 9-2 | **MATCHING WORD PARTS WITH MEANING** |

Match the word part in Column A *with its meaning in* Column B.

Column A	Column B
_____ 1. poli/o	A. brain
_____ 2. para-	B. hernia
_____ 3. tetra-	C. painful
_____ 4. cerebr/o	D. mind
_____ 5. ment/o	E. gray matter
_____ 6. -cele	F. vessel
_____ 7. -ar	G. four
_____ 8. dys-	H. membrane
_____ 9. -esthesia	I. abnormal
_____ 10. mening/o	J. pertaining to
_____ 11. hemi-	K. speech
_____ 12. -phasia	L. half
_____ 13. vascul/o	M. sensation
_____ 14. de-	N. condition
_____ 15. -ia	O. lack of

| Exercise 9-3 | **SHORT ANSWER—ANATOMY** |

Answer the following questions on the space provided.

1. (A) Name the organs that make up the central nervous system. (B) The peripheral nervous system.

_____

_____

2. Write one function for the following structures:

   a. cerebrum _____

   b. thalamus _____

   c. hypothalamus _____

   d. brainstem _____

3. What type of tissue makes up the spinal cord?

_____

4. What type of tissue protects the spinal cord?

_____

5. Name three portions of the brainstem.

_____

Exercise 9-4 **LABELING—STRUCTURES OF THE BRAIN**

Using the body structures listed below, write the name of each numbered structure in Figure 9-10 on the corresponding line on page 181.

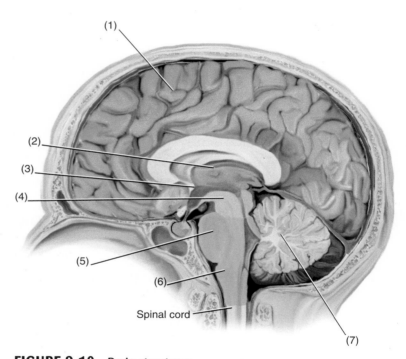

FIGURE 9-10 Brain structures.

cerebellum
cerebrum
hypothalamus
medulla oblongata
midbrain
pons
thalamus

1. _____

2. _____

3. _____

4. _____

5. _____

6. _____

7. _____

Exercise 9-5 | DEFINITIONS—ANATOMY

Define the following terms. Use your dictionary if necessary.

1. **neurons**

_____

2. **nerves**

_____

3. **myelin sheath**

_____

4. **gray matter**

_____

5. **pons**

_____

6. **cerebral cortex**

_____

7. **cerebellum**

_____

8. **spinal cord**

_____

9. **vertebral column**

_____

10. **peripheral nerves**

_____

Exercise 9-6   PATHOLOGY

Match the disease in Column A *with its meaning in* Column B.

Column A	Column B
_____ **1.** Alzheimer's disease	**A.** may result in displaced meninges and/or spinal cord
_____ **2.** multiple sclerosis	
_____ **3.** Parkinson's disease	**B.** characterized by resting tremors and muscle rigidity
_____ **4.** spina bifida	**C.** disorganized, uncoordinated, and excessive electrical impulses in the brain
_____ **5.** seizure disorder	
_____ **6.** meningomyelocele	
_____ **7.** hydrocephalus	**D.** type of dementia
	E. a complication of spina bifida
	F. characterized by demyelination of brain and spinal cord
	G. accumulation of cerebrospinal fluid in the brain

Exercise 9-7   DEFINITIONS—LEARNING THE TERMS

Define the following terms:

1. **cerebrovascular**

   _____

2. **poliomyelitis**

   _____

3. **neurology**

   _____

4. **anesthesia**

   _____

5. **dysesthesia**

   _____

6. paresthesia

_____

7. dysphasia

_____

8. tetraplegia

_____

9. paraplegia

_____

10. cerebrospinal fluid

_____

Exercise 9-8   BUILDING MEDICAL WORDS

I. Use encephal/o to build medical words for the following definitions.

a. inflammation of the brain _____

b. any disease of the brain _____

II. Use neur/o to build medical words for the following definitions.

a. pertaining to the nerve and muscle

_____

b. study of the nervous system _____

III. Use -esthesia to build medical words for the following definitions.

a. loss of sensation _____

b. painful sensations in response to normal stimulation

_____

c. abnormal sensations such as numbness and tingling

_____

IV. Use -plegia to build medical words for the following definitions.

a. paralysis affecting either the right or left side of the body _____

b. paralysis of the lower part of the body and legs

_____

c. paralysis of all four limbs _____

Exercise 9-9 DEFINITIONS IN CONTEXT

Define the bold terms in context. Use your dictionary if necessary.

Alita Lopez is a 62-year-old woman who was diagnosed with a brain tumor two months prior to admission. She suffered from **dysphasia**, abnormal **gait**, and **migraines** prior to admission. **MRI** showed increased **cerebrospinal fluid** in the left ventricle. Ms. Lopez underwent **neurosurgery** to relieve the **intracranial** pressure caused by the tumor. She was then treated with **chemotherapy** and **radiotherapy**.

1. **dysphasia** _____

2. **gait** _____

3. **migraines** _____

4. **MRI** _____

5. **cerebrospinal fluid** _____

6. **neurosurgery** _____

7. **intracranial** _____

8. **chemotherapy** _____

9. **radiotherapy** _____

Exercise 9-10 SPELLING

Circle any words that are spelled incorrectly in the list below. Then correct the spelling in the space provided.

1. disesthesia _____

2. myelin sheath _____

3. siezure _____

4. Parkinsin's diease _____

5. resonence _____

6. thalmus _____

7. cerebellum _____

8. conjenital _____

9. medulla oblongata _____

10. Alzheimer's disease _____

9.10 PRONUNCIATION AND SPELLING

Listen, read, and study, so you can speak and write.

1. Listen to each word on the audio CD.

2. Pronounce each word carefully.

3. Spell each word in the space provided.

Word	Pronunciation	Spelling
anesthesia	an-es-**THEE**-zee-ah	
aphasia	ah-**FAY**-zee-ah	
cerebellum	ser-eh-**BELL**-um	
cerebrospinal	ser-eh-broh-**SPYE**-nal	
cerebrovascular	ser-eh-broh-**VAS**-kyoo-lar	
cerebrum	seh-**REE**-brum	
dementia	deh-**MEN**-she-ah	
demyelination	dee-**my**-eh-lih-**NAY**-shun	
dysesthesia	dis-es-**THEE**-zee-ah	
dysphasia	dis-**FAY**-zee-ah	
electroencephalography	ee-**leck**-troh-en-**sef**-ah-**LOG**-rah-fee	
encephalitis	en-**sef**-ah-**LYE**-tis	
encephalopathy	en-**sef**-ah-**LOP**-ah-thee	
hemiplegia	hem-ee-**PLEE**-jee-ah	
hypothalamus	**high**-poh-**THAL**-ah-mus	
medulla oblongata	meh-**DULL**-ah **OB**-long-**GAH**-tah	
meninges	meh-**NIN**-jeez	
meningocele	meh-**NIN**-goh-**seel**	

Word	Pronunciation	Spelling
meningoencephalitis	meh-**NIN**-goh-en-**sef**-ah-**LYE**-tis	
myelin sheath	**MY**-eh-lin **SHEETH**	
neurology	noo-**ROL**-oh-jee	
neurons	**NOO**-ronz	
paraplegia	**par**-ah-**PLEE**-jee-ah	
paresthesia	**par**-es-**THEE**-zee-ah	
poliomyelitis	**poh**-lee-oh-**my**-eh-**LYE**-tis	
pons	**PONZ**	
thalamus	**THAL**-ah-mus	

CHAPTER 10

The Eyes and Ears

LEARNING OBJECTIVES

After studying this chapter and completing the review exercises, you should be able to:

1. Name and describe the structures and functions of the eyeball.
2. Describe the pathway of vision to the brain.
3. Pronounce, spell, define, and write the medical terms related to the eyes.
4. Describe common diseases related to the eyes.
5. Name and describe the structures and functions of the ear.
6. Describe the pathway of hearing to the brain.
7. Pronounce, spell, define, and write the medical terms related to the ears.
8. Describe common diseases related to the ear.
9. Listen, read, and study so you can speak and write.

INTRODUCTION

Our eyes and ears connect us with the world. The eyes send signals to one part of the brain, and we see. The ears send signals to another part of the brain, and we hear. This chapter explains these amazing organs.

10.1 MAJOR STRUCTURES OF THE EYEBALL

PRACTICE FOR LEARNING: **EYEBALL**

Write the words below on the correct spaces in Figure 10-1. To help you, the number beside the word tells you where it goes on the figure. Be sure to pronounce each word as you write it. Repeat the pronunciation several times if you find the word hard to say.

1. Ciliary body (**SIL**-ee-ahr-ee)
2. Conjunctiva (kon-**JUNK**-tih-vah)
3. Iris (**EYE**-ris)
4. Pupil (**PYOO**-pil)
5. Cornea (**KOR**-nee-ah)
6. Lens (**LENZ**)
7. Optic nerve (**OP**-tick **NERV**)
8. Macula lutea (**MACK**-yoo-lah **LOO**-tee-ah)

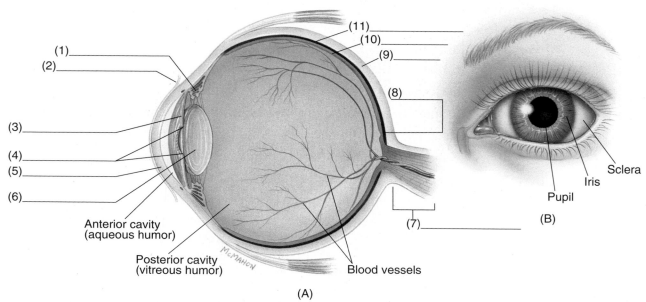

(A)

FIGURE 10-1 Major structures of the eye. A, Sagittal view. B, Anterior view.

9. Sclera (**SKLEHR**-ah)

10. Retina (**RET**-ih-nah)

11. Choroid (**KOH**-roid)

LAYERS OF THE EYEBALL

The eyeball has three layers: outer, middle, and inner. They are described below.

Outer Layer

The outer layer of the eye is made up of the cornea and the sclera. The cornea is transparent. This means that it is clear and lets light into the eye. The sclera is the white of the eye. It is not transparent, and therefore light does not pass through it.

Find the sclera on Figure 10-1A. Using your finger, make a circle by following the sclera. Notice how the sclera joins the cornea at the front of the eye and then becomes the sclera again as the circle is completed.

Middle Layer

Figure 10-1A also illustrates the middle layer of the eyeball. It is called the **uvea** (**YOO**-vee-ah). The uvea has three parts: the choroid, the iris, and the ciliary body.

Find the choroid on Figure 10-1A. Again, using your finger, follow the outline of the middle layer.

The iris is the colored portion of the eye. There is an opening in the middle of the iris called the pupil. It regulates the amount of light that enters the eye. In bright light, the pupil constricts (narrows) to protect the eye from bright light. In dimmer light, the pupil dilates (widens).

Inner Layer

The inner layer of the eye is called the retina. Once again use your finger and trace the outline of the retina on the diagram. The retina contains cells called **rods** (**RODZ**) and **cones** (**KOHNZ**). These structures are named for their shape. They receive light rays and transform them into electrical impulses that travel to the brain along the optic nerve. This allows vision to occur.

The cones are located in the macula lutea. The rods are located peripheral to the macula lutea.

IN BRIEF

Outer layer
Sclera, cornea
Middle layer, or uvea
Choroid, ciliary body, iris
Inner layer
Retina (rods and cones)

PRACTICE FOR LEARNING: OUTER LAYER, MIDDLE LAYER, INNER LAYER

Complete the following statements:

1. Write the structures that make up the following layers of the eye:

   a. outer layer_____

   b. middle layer _____

   c. inner layer_____

2. The middle layer is also known as the _____.

3. Name the location of the cones. _____

4. Write one function of rods and cones. _____

Answers: **1.** A. cornea, sclera. B. choroid, ciliary body, iris. C. retina containing rods and cones. **2.** uvea. **3.** macula lutea. **4.** changes light rays into electrical impulses.

Lens, Anterior Cavity, Posterior Cavity

IN BRIEF

The **lens** is behind the iris.

The **anterior cavity** is in front of the lens and contains aqueous humor.

The **posterior cavity** is behind the lens and contains vitreous humor.

There are structures that are not considered to be part of any one layer of the eye. They are the lens, anterior cavity, and posterior cavity. You can see these in Figure 10-1. The lens is located behind the iris. It bends light rays.

There is a cavity in front of the lens and one behind it. The one in front is the anterior cavity. It is filled with a watery fluid called aqueous humor (**AY-kwee-us HYOO-mer**). The aqueous humor maintains the proper pressure within the eye. This is called intraocular pressure (IOP). As new aqueous humor is produced, the old is drained into the bloodstream.

The posterior cavity (**pos-TEER-ee-or KAV-ih-tee**) is behind the lens. It is filled with gel called vitreous (**VIT-ree-us**) humor. It maintains the round shape of the eyeball and holds the retina in place, firmly against the choroid.

10.3 REFRACTION

IN BRIEF

Refraction means bending

The eye bends light rays so that they come together at the retina at the same time. This is illustrated in Figure 10-2. This bending of light is called refraction (**ree-FRACK-shun**). Without the proper amount of refraction, vision will be blurred.

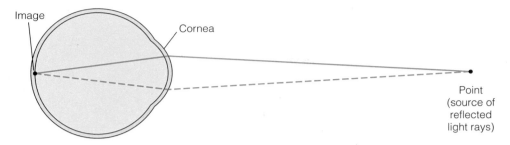

FIGURE 10-2   Refraction: bending of light rays.

PRACTICE FOR LEARNING: **LENS, ANTERIOR AND POSTERIOR CAVITIES**

Write one function for the following:

1. lens _____

2. vitreous humor _____

3. aqueous humor _____

Answers: **1.** A. refraction.   **2.** maintains round shape of the eyeball; holds the retina against the choroid.   **3.** maintains intraocular pressure.

10.4 VISUAL PATHWAY

Sight is possible because various structures work together. Light rays must travel unobstructed through the cornea, aqueous humor, pupil, lens, and vitreous humor. The light rays then focus on the retina. The light rays must focus precisely on the same point on the retina to produce a clear, sharp image. The rods and cones then change the image into electrical impulses. These impulses travel the optic nerve to the brain. The brain then makes us aware of the object we are looking at. Figure 10-3 illustrates light traveling through this visual pathway.

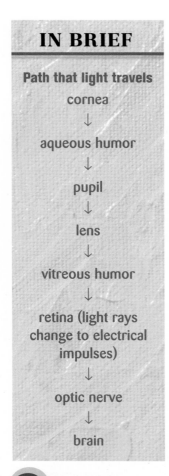

IN BRIEF

Path that light travels

cornea

↓

aqueous humor

↓

pupil

↓

lens

↓

vitreous humor

↓

retina (light rays
change to electrical
impulses)

↓

optic nerve

↓

brain

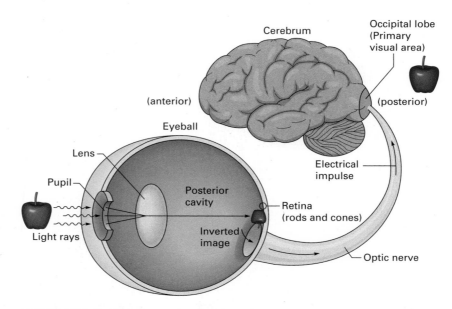

FIGURE 10-3   Visual pathway. Notice the image of the apple is upside down on the retina. The brain turns the image right side up and clear vision is obtained.

10.5 NEW ROOTS, SUFFIXES, AND PREFIXES

Use these additional roots, suffixes, and prefixes when studying the terms in this chapter.

Root	Meaning
ambly/o	dull; dim
dipl/o	double

Suffix	Meaning
-metrist	specialist in the measure of
-pexy	surgical fixation
-phobia	fear

Prefix	Meaning
eso-	inward
exo-	outside
extra-	outside
presby-	old age

10.6 LEARNING THE TERMS

Following these steps will make it easier for you to learn medical terms:

1. Pronounce the term repeatedly until it is easy for you.

2. Write it down. Ensure the spelling is correct.

3. Also write the definition. If possible, relate the word to a word, thought, or picture that will help you remember it.

4. Analyze the term with the method taught in this text.

Root	Meaning
blephar/o (see also palpebr/o)	eyelid

Term	Term Analysis	Definition
blepharoptosis (**blef**-ah-rop-**TOH**-sis)	-ptosis = drooping; sagging	drooping eyelid

Root	Meaning
conjunctiv/o	conjunctiva (membrane lining the eyelids and anterior part of eye)

Term	Term Analysis	Definition
conjunctivitis (kon-**junk**-tih-**VYE**-tis)	-itis = inflammation	inflammation of the conjunctiva

Root	Meaning
corne/o (see also kerat/o)	cornea

Term	Term Analysis	Definition
corneal abrasion (**KOR**-nee-al ab-**RAY**-zhun)	-eal = pertaining to -ion = process ab- = away from ras/o = scrape	scraping of the superficial layers of the cornea

Root	Meaning
irid/o; ir/o	iris

Term	Term Analysis	Definition
iridectomy (ir-ih-**DECK**-toh-mee)	-ectomy = excision; surgical removal	excision of the iris
iritis (eye-**RYE**-tis)	-itis = inflammation	inflammation of the iris

Root	Meaning
kerat/o	cornea

Term	Term Analysis	Definition
keratoplasty (ker-**AT**-oh-plas-tee)	-plasty = surgical reconstruction; surgical repair	surgical reconstruction of the cornea; corneal transplant

Root	Meaning
ocul/o (see also ophthalm/o)	eye

Term	Term Analysis		Definition
extraocular muscles (**ecks**-trah-**OCK**-yoo-lar)	-ar = pertaining to extra- = outside		muscles located outside the eyeball

Root	Meaning
ophthalm/o	eye

Term	Term Analysis	Definition
exophthalmia (**eck**-sof-**THAL**-mee-ah)	-ia = condition ex- = outward	outward protrusion of the eyeball
ophthalmologist (**ahf**-thal-**MOL**-eh-jist)	-logist = specialist	a specialist in the study of the diagnosis and medical and surgical treatment of eye disorders

NOTE: An ophthalmologist is a medical doctor.

Term	Term Analysis	Definition
ophthalmoscopy (**ahf**-thal-**MOS**-koh-pee)	-scopy = process of visually examining	process of visually examining the eye. Also known as a funduscopy.

NOTE: The fundus is the back portion of the eye. It includes the retina and macula lutea.

Root	Meaning
opt/o	vision; sight

Term	Term Analysis	Definition
optician (op-**TISH**-an)	-ician = specialist; one who specializes; expert	expert who fills prescriptions for eyeglasses and contact lenses

NOTE: Opticians are not physicians and do not carry out medical and surgical treatments of eye conditions.

Term	Term Analysis	Definition
optometrist (op-**TOM**-eh-trist)	-metrist = specialist in the measurement of	specialist in the testing of visual function and in the diagnosis and nonsurgical treatment of eye conditions

NOTE: Optometrists prescribe eyeglasses and contact lenses and are licensed in some areas to prescribe medication. They do not have a degree in medicine.

Root	Meaning
palpebr/o	eyelid

Term	Term Analysis	Definition
palpebral (**PAL**-peh-bral)	-al = pertaining to	pertaining to the eyelid

Root	Meaning
phac/o; phak/o	lens

Term	Term Analysis	Definition
aphakia (ah-**FAY**-kee-ah)	a- = no; not; lack of; absence	absence of a lens

Root	Meaning
phot/o	light

Term	Term Analysis	Definition
photophobia (**foh**-toh-**FOH**-bee-ah)	-phobia = fear	intolerance or sensitivity to light

Root	Meaning
retin/o	retina

Term	Term Analysis	Definition
retinopathy (**ret**-ih-**NOP**-ah-thee)	-pathy = disease	any disease of the retina
retinopexy (**RET**-ih-noh-**peck**-see)	-pexy = surgical fixation	surgical fixation of the retina

Suffix	Meaning
-opia	visual condition; vision

Term	Term Analysis	Definition
amblyopia (**am**-blee-**OH**-pee-ah)	ambly/o = dull; dim	dimness of vision
diplopia (dih-**PLOH**-pee-ah)	dipl/o = double	double vision
presbyopia (**pres**-bee-**OH**-pee-ah)	presby- = old age	impaired vision due to advanced age

Suffix	Meaning
-tropia	turning

NOTE: Esotropia and exotropia are also known as **strabismus**.

Term	Term Analysis	Definition
esotropia (**es**-oh-**TROH**-pee-ah)	eso- = inward	turning inward of the eyeball (Figure 10-4B)
exotropia (**eck**-soh-**TROH**-pee-ah)	exo- = outward	outward turning of the eyeball (Figure 10-4C)

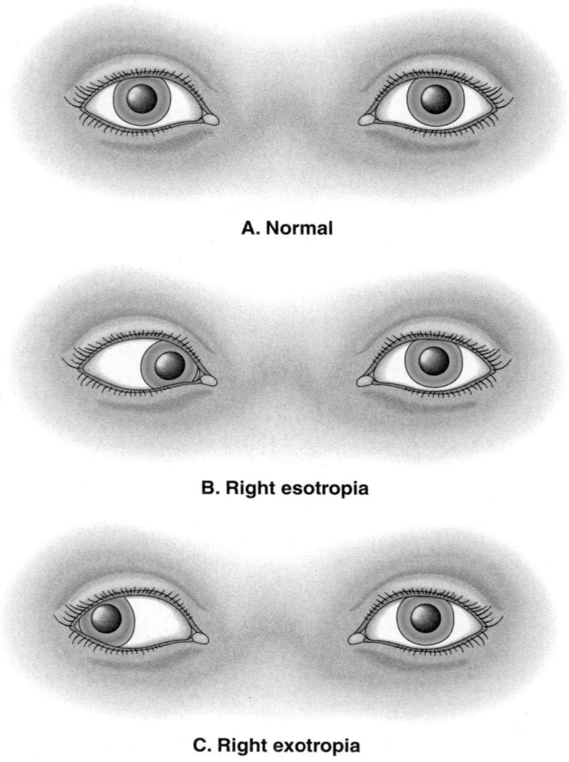

A. Normal

B. Right esotropia

C. Right exotropia

FIGURE 10-4 Normal vision compared with types of strabismus. A, Normal vision. B, Right esotropia. C, Right exotropia.

10.7 PATHOLOGY OF THE EYE

Cataracts (**KAT**-a-rakts)

Fogging of the lens (Figure 10-5). Normally, the lens is clear. When it is foggy, the light rays cannot focus on the retina. As a result, vision becomes blurred. Cataracts can be treated by destroying the diseased lens. This can be done by using ultrasound (high frequency sound waves). The removed lens is replaced with an artificial (prosthetic) intraocular lens (IOL).

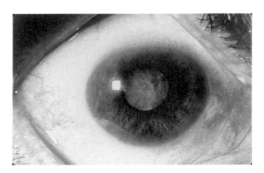

FIGURE 10-5   **Cataract.** Courtesy of the National Eye Institute.

Errors of Refraction

Errors in the bending of light rays in the eye, resulting in blurred vision. Types are myopia, hyperopia, and astigmatism.

*Myopia (*my-**OH**-pee-ah*)*

Nearsightedness. Only near objects can be seen clearly. Light rays focus in front of the retina because they are bent too quickly or because the eyeball is too long. Illustrated in Figure 10-6A.

*Hyperopia (*high-per-**OH**-pee-ah*)*

Farsightedness. Only far-away objects can be seen clearly. Light rays focus behind the retina because they are bent too slowly or because the eyeball is too short. Illustrated in Figure 10-6B.

*Astigmatism (*ah-**STIG**-mah-tiz-um*)*

Blurred vision, both near and far. The curve of the cornea is uneven. Thus, light rays do not reach a point of focus. Illustrated in Figure 10-6C.

All errors of refraction can be treated in a non-surgical or surgical manner. Non-surgical treatment is the prescription of eyeglasses with the appropriate lens to correct the visual distortion (Figure 10-6). Surgical treatment involves using a laser to reshape the curvature of the cornea so that the light rays will focus on the retina.

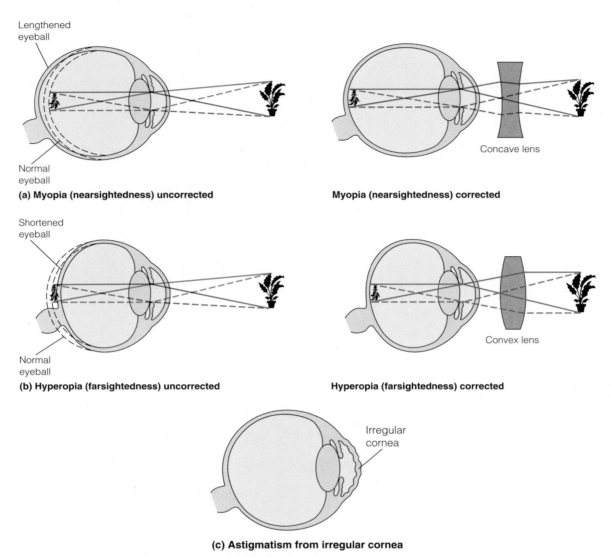

Lengthened eyeball

Normal eyeball

(a) Myopia (nearsightedness) uncorrected

Concave lens

Myopia (nearsightedness) corrected

Shortened eyeball

Normal eyeball

(b) Hyperopia (farsightedness) uncorrected

Convex lens

Hyperopia (farsightedness) corrected

Irregular cornea

(c) Astigmatism from irregular cornea

FIGURE 10-6 Errors of refraction. A, Myopia (nearsightedness). B, Hyperopia (farsightedness). C, Astigmatism.

Glaucoma (glaw-KOH-mah)

Damage to the retina and optic nerve due to increased intraocular pressure. The intraocular pressure increases because the aqueous humor produced is greater than the amount that flows out of the eye. Thus, aqueous humor builds up inside the anterior cavity. This distorts the shape of the eye and impairs vision. The first level of treatment is eyedrops. If this is unsuccessful, surgery is done to increase the outflow of aqueous humor.

Macular Degeneration (MAK-yoo-ler)

Deterioration of the macula lutea. Also known as age-related macular degeneration (AMD) because in some people, deterioration of the macula comes with the aging process. There is loss of central vision. It progresses to blindness.

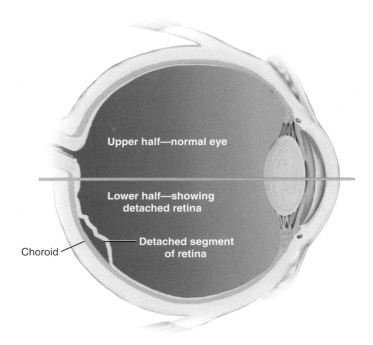

FIGURE 10-7 Retinal detachment.

Retinal Tears (TAYRZ) (do not confuse with TEERZ)

Holes that develop on the retina. With age, the vitreous humor shrinks. As it shrinks, the humor pulls tightly on the retina and results in the creation of holes along the retinal wall. If not treated, they will result in the detachment (separation) of the retina from the layers underneath (Figure 10-7). If not treated, this will lead to blindness.

HELPING YOU REMEMBER

Tears (TEERZ) refer to the droplets of fluid that fall from the eye. Tears (TAYRZ) are holes that develop due to a pulling force.

10.8 MAJOR STRUCTURES OF THE EAR

PRACTICE FOR LEARNING: EAR

Write the words below on the correct spaces in Figure 10-8. To help you, the number beside the word tells you where it goes on the figure. Be sure to pronounce each word as you write it. Repeat the pronunciation several times if you find the word hard to say.

1. external ear

2. middle ear

3. inner ear

4. auricle (**AW-rick-ul**) or pinna (**PIN-ah**)

5. external auditory meatus (**AW-dih-tor-ee mee-AY-tus**)

6. tympanic (**tim-PAN-ik**) membrane or eardrum

7. ossicles (**OSS-ick-les**)

8. cochlea (**KOCK-lee-ah**)

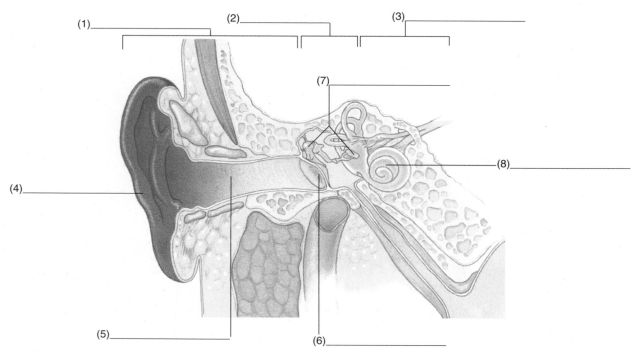

FIGURE 10-8   Major structures of the ear.

External Ear

IN BRIEF
External Ear
Includes: auricle
external auditory
meatus,
tympanic membrane

The external ear can be seen in Figure 10-8. It includes the auricle or pinna, the external auditory meatus, and the tympanic membrane (TM) or eardrum.

The auricle or earflap gathers the sounds. Sound travels down the external auditory meatus to the eardrum. The sound makes the eardrum vibrate. The sound waves from this vibration travel to the middle ear.

Glands in the external auditory meatus secrete a wax called cerumen (**seh-ROO-men**). It protects the ear from infection by trapping microorganisms.

Middle and Inner Ears

PRACTICE FOR LEARNING: MIDDLE EAR AND INNER EARS

Write the words below on the correct spaces in Figure 10-9. To help you, the number beside the word tells you where it goes on the figure. Be sure to pronounce each word as you write it. Repeat the pronunciation several times if you find the word hard to say.

1. malleus (**MAL**-ee-us)

2. incus (**ING**-kus)

3. stapes (**STAY**-peez)

4. oval window

5. eustachian tube (yoo-**STAY**-shun)

6. cochlea (**KOCK**-lee-ah)

7. vestibule (**VES**-tib-yool)

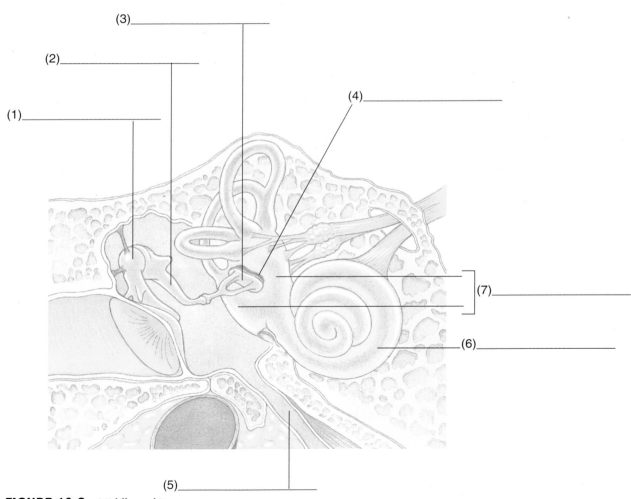

FIGURE 10-9 Middle and inner ear.

The middle ear consists of three tiny bones called ossicles (**OSS-ick-les**). They are the malleus, the incus, and the stapes. The stapes is connected to the oval window. The eustachian tube connects the middle ear to the throat.

The inner ear consists of the cochlea and vestibule. These structures look like winding passageways that resemble a maze, so the inner ear is also called the labyrinth (**LAB-ih-rinth**). The inner ear is responsible for balance and hearing. Balance is maintained through the action of fluid in the inner ear. When we are off balance, the fluid is disturbed, and messages are sent to the brain telling it that the body is not in the right position. The brain then corrects the body's position to get back into balance.

PRACTICE FOR LEARNING: **STRUCTURES OF THE EAR**

1. Circle the structure that does not fit into a given category.

   a. external ear: pinna, malleus, tympanic membrane

   b. middle ear: ossicles, malleus, external auditory meatus, stapes

   c. inner ear: vestibule, cochlea, auricle

2. Name the three ossicles found in the middle ear.

   _____

3. Name the structure that connects the middle ear to the throat.

   _____

4. What is the other name for the inner ear?

   _____

Answers: **1.** a. malleus; b. external auditory meatus; c. auricle.
2. malleus, incus, stapes. **3.** eustachian tube. **4.** labyrinth.

10.9 AUDITORY PATHWAY

Hearing is possible because sound waves travel through the external auditory meatus and hit the tympanic membrane. The sound is transmitted through the middle ear to the inner ear,

IN BRIEF

Path that sound travels

pinna or auricle

↓

external auditory
meatus

↓

tympanic membrane

↓

ossicles (malleus,
incus, stapes)

↓

cochlea

↓

auditory nerve

↓

brain

where it reaches the cochlea. Fluid inside the cochlea is set in motion, which disturbs tiny hair cells inside the cochlea. These hair cells react to the vibration by moving, much as tall grass sways in the wind. The movement of the hair cells stimulates the underlying nerve cells, which create nerve impulses that travel the auditory nerve to the brain for interpretation (Figure 10-10).

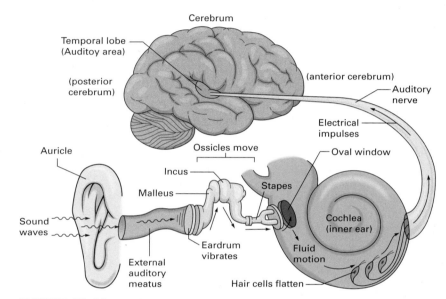

FIGURE 10-10 Auditory pathway.

10.10 NEW SUFFIXES

Use these additional suffixes when studying the terms in this chapter.

Suffix	Meaning
-metry	process of measuring
-ory	pertaining to

10.11 LEARNING THE TERMS

Root	Meaning
audi/o (see also audit/o)	hearing

Term	Term Analysis	Definition
audiometry (**aw-dee-OM-eh-tree**)	-metry = process of measuring	process of measuring a patient's hearing ability

Root	Meaning
audit/o	hearing

Term	Term Analysis	Definition
auditory (**AW-dih-tor-ee**)	-ory = pertaining to	pertaining to hearing

Root	Meaning
aur/o	ear

Term	Term Analysis	Definition
aural (**AW-ral**)	-al = pertaining to	pertaining to the ear

NOTE: Do not confuse with "oral" meaning "pertaining to the mouth."

Root	Meaning
labyrinth/o	inner ear; labyrinth

Term	Term Analysis	Definition
labyrinthitis (**lab-ih-rin-THIGH-tis**)	-itis = inflammation	inflammation of the inner ear

Root	Meaning
myring/o (see also tympan/o)	tympanic membrane; eardrum

Term	Term Analysis	Definition
myringotomy (**mir-ing-GOT-oh-me**)	-tomy = process of cutting; to cut	process of cutting into the eardrum to remove fluid from the middle ear

Root	Meaning
ot/o	ear

Term	Term Analysis	Definition
otalgia (oh-**TAL**-jee-ah)	-algia = pain	earache
otitis media (oh-**TYE**-tis **ME**-dee-ah)	-itis = inflammation media = middle	inflammation of the middle ear
otorrhea (**oh**-toh-**REE**-ah)	-rrhea = discharge; flow	discharge from the ear

Root	Meaning
tympan/o	tympanic membrane

Term	Term Analysis	Definition
tympanoplasty (**tim**-pah-no-**PLAS**-tee)	-plasty = surgical repair; surgical reconstruction	surgical reconstruction of the eardrum; myringoplasty

Suffix	Meaning
-cusis	hearing

Term	Term Analysis	Definition
presbycusis (**pres**-beh-**KOO**-sis)	presby- = old age	diminished hearing due to old age

 10.12 PATHOLOGY OF THE EAR

Hearing Impairment

Loss of hearing with impaired ability to distinguish between speech sounds.

Meniérè's Disease (men-ee-**AYRZ**)

A condition of the inner ear. It includes hearing loss, a feeling of pressure in the ear, dizziness or vertigo (**VER**-tih-goh), and ringing in the ears or tinnitus (**TIN**-ih-tus).

Perforated Tympanic Membrane

Rupture of the tympanic membrane. It often results in hearing loss (Figure 10-11). If surgery is necessary to restore hearing loss, the procedure is called tympanoplasty.

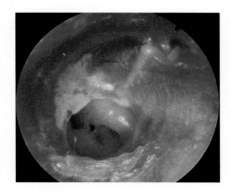

FIGURE 10-11   Perforated **tympanic membrane.** (Courtesy Dr. Andrew B. Silva, Pediatric Otolaryngology).

 REVIEW EXERCISES

| **Exercise 10-1** | **LOOK-ALIKE AND SOUND-ALIKE WORDS** |

Below is a list of look-alike and sound-alike words. Study the definitions of each set of words, then read the sentences carefully and circle the word in parentheses that correctly completes the meaning.

aura	warning signs to the patient that a seizure is starting
aural	pertaining to the ear
oral	pertaining to the mouth
here	the place you are in
hear	to hear sound
malleus	bone of middle ear
malleolus	bony bumps on the lower leg, commonly called the ankle
palpable	to feel
palpebral	pertaining to the eyelid
serious	not joking; causing great harm
serous	watery fluid

| tendinitis | inflammation of the tendon |
| tinnitus | ringing in the ears |

1. On (**aural/oral**) examination, the tympanic membrane was red and inflamed.

2. When the tuning fork is placed (**hear/here**), the patient cannot (**hear/here**) the sound.

3. The swelling over the (**malleus/malleolus**) was caused by a sprained ankle.

4. The (**malleus/malleolus**), incus, and stapes are bones in the middle ear.

5. No (**palpable/palpebral**) neck masses; no (**serious/serous**) abnormalities. However, he did have a discharge from his right ear and was admitted with a diagnosis of (**serious/serous**) otitis media.

6. The patient thinks his (**tendonitis/tinnitus**) is caused by loud noises.

Exercise 10-2   MATCHING WORD PARTS WITH MEANING

Match the word part in Column A *with its meaning in* Column B.

Column A	Column B
_____ 1. aur/o	A. cornea
_____ 2. ophthalm/o	B. lens
_____ 3. phot/o	C. light
_____ 4. audi/o	D. tympanic membrane
_____ 5. kerat/o	E. double
_____ 6. opt/o	F. hearing
_____ 7. myring/o	G. fear
_____ 8. dipl/o	H. eye
_____ 9. -phobia	I. vision
_____ 10. phac/o	J. ear

| Exercise 10-3 | MATCHING—STRUCTURE AND FUNCTION |

Match the structures listed below with its function.

aqueous humor _____

cochlea _____

cornea _____

macula _____

pupil _____

tympanic membrane _____

vestibule _____

vitreous humor _____

   1. maintains intraocular pressure _____

   2. location of cones on the retina _____

   3. regulates amount of light entering the eye

     _____

   4. maintains shape of eyeball _____

   5. entry point of light into the eye _____

   6. vibrates sound _____

   7. function is balance _____

   8. function is hearing _____

| Exercise 10-4 | SHORT ANSWER—ANATOMY AND PHYSIOLOGY |

   I. Arrange the following structures of the ear so that they in-
   dicate the correct sequence in the transmission of sound
   waves to the brain from the external ear.

auditory nerve
brain
cochlea
external auditory meatus
ossicles
pinna or auricle
tympanic membrane

   1. _____

   2. _____

   3. _____

4. _____

5. _____

6. _____

7. _____

II. *Arrange the following structures of the eye so that they indicate the correct sequence in the transmission of light rays to the brain from the external eye.*

aqueous humor
brain
cornea
lens
optic nerve
pupil
retina
vitreous humor

1. _____

2. _____

3. _____

4. _____

5. _____

6. _____

7. _____

8. _____

Exercise 10-5   LABELING—EYE

Write the name of each numbered structure on the corresponding line below the diagram (Figure 10-12). Use the body structures listed below and on page 212.

choroid _____

ciliary body _____

conjunctiva _____

cornea _____

iris _____

lens _____

macula lutea _____

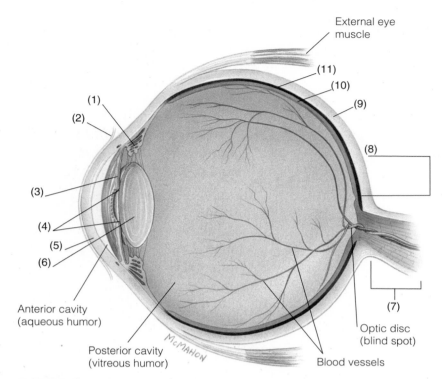

External eye
muscle

(11)

(10)

(9)

(1)

(2)

(8)

(3)

(4)

(5)

(6)

Anterior cavity
(aqueous humor)

Posterior cavity
(vitreous humor)

McMAHON

(7)

Optic disc
(blind spot)

Blood vessels

FIGURE 10-12 Labeling the major structures of the eye.

optic nerve _____

pupil _____

retina _____

sclera _____

1. _____

2. _____

3. _____

4. _____

5. _____

6. _____

7. _____

8. _____

9. _____

10. _____

11. _____

| Exercise 10-6 | LABELING—EAR |

Write the name of each numbered structure on the corresponding line below the diagram (Figure 10-13). Use the body structures listed below.

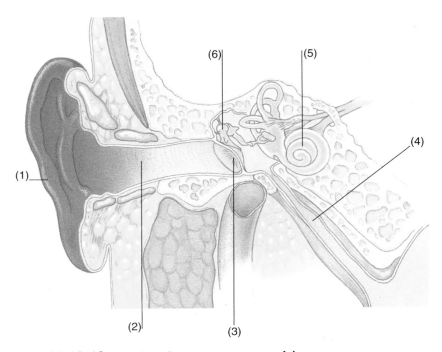

FIGURE 10-13 Labeling the major structures of the ear.

auricle
_____

cochlea
_____

eustachian tube
_____

external auditory meatus
_____

ossicles
_____

tympanic membrane
_____

      1. _____

      2. _____

      3. _____

      4. _____

      5. _____

      6. _____

| **Exercise 10-7** | DEFINITIONS—PATHOLOGY |

Define the following.

1. retinal detachment

_____

_____

_____

2. otitis media

_____

_____

_____

3. perforated tympanic membrane

_____

_____

_____

4. Meniérè's disease

_____

_____

_____

5. myopia

_____

_____

_____

6. astigmatism

_____

_____

_____

7. cataracts

_____

_____

_____

8. glaucoma

_____

_____

_____

| Exercise 10-8 | **DEFINITIONS—LEARNING THE TERMS** |

Define the following terms.

1. blepharoptosis _____

2. ophthalmoscopy _____

3. ophthalmologist _____

4. optician _____

5. optometrist _____

6. aphakia _____

7. photophobia_____

8. retinopathy _____

9. diplopia _____

10. presbyopia _____

11. esotropia_____

12. auditory _____

13. aural _____

14. audiometry_____

15. myringotomy_____

16. otorrhea_____

17. presbycusis _____

18. otalgia_____

| Exercise 10-9 | **BUILDING MEDICAL WORDS** |

I. Using the suffix -opia, build the medical word meaning:

   a. double vision _____

   b. nearsightedness _____

   c. dimness of vision _____

   d. impaired vision due to old age _____

II. Using the suffix -tropia, build the medical word meaning:

    a. turning inward of the eyeball _____

    b. outward turning of the eyeball _____

III. Using the root ot/o, build the medical word meaning:

    a. pain in the ear _____

    b. discharge from the ear _____

Exercise 10-10   DEFINITIONS IN CONTEXT

Define the bolded terms in context. Use your medical dictionary if necessary.

Report #1 Discharge Summary

ADMISSION DIAGNOSIS: LEFT CATARACT FOR EXTRACTION.

HISTORY: Mrs. Serowan had noted progressive deteriorating vision in the right eye over a number of years. Remainder of medical history is unremarkable.

PHYSICAL EXAMINATION: Best corrected visual acuity was 20/70 in the right eye.

COURSE IN HOSPITAL: On June 21, ultrasound was used to destroy the cataract. A prosthetic intraocular lens was inserted. On the first postoperative day, she was discharged home.

    a. cataract _____

    b. deteriorating _____

    c. visual acuity _____

    d. ultrasound _____

    e. prosthetic intraocular lens _____

Report #2 Operative Report

PREOPERATIVE DIAGNOSIS: OTITIS MEDIA.

OPERATION PROPOSED: BILATERAL MYRINGOTOMY AND
TUBE INSERTION.

POSTOPERATIVE DIAGNOSIS: RECURRENT OTITIS MEDIA.

OPERATION PERFORMED: BILATERAL MYRINGOTOMY WITH
TUBE INSERTION.

OPERATIVE NOTE: The patient was brought to the operating room, placed in the supine position, and given a general anesthetic. Using the operative microscope, the right external auditory meatus was cleaned of a small amount of cerumen revealing an abnormal tympanic membrane with a buildup of pus-filled material. A myringotomy was performed and the infectious material was suctioned out. A tube was inserted to drain any further fluid buildup. The procedure was then performed on the left side with a similar technique. A buildup of watery fluid was noted. The patient was then taken to the recovery room in good condition._____

    a. **otitis media**_____

    b. **myringotomy** _____

    c. **recurrent**_____

    d. **bilateral** _____

    e. **supine** _____

    f. **microscope** _____

    g. **external auditory meatus** _____

    h. **cerumen** _____

    i. **tympanic membrane**_____

Exercise 10-11   SPELLING

Circle any words that are spelled incorrectly in the list below. Then correct the spelling in the space provided

    1. tinnitis _____

    2. maleus _____

    3. aqueus _____

    4. glaucoma _____

    5. vitreus _____

    6. otorhea _____

    7. conjunctiva _____

    8. palpebra _____

    9. kornea _____

   10. serumen _____

10.14 PRONUNCIATION AND SPELLING

Listen, read, and study, so you can speak and write.

1. Listen to each word on the audio CD.

2. Pronounce each word carefully.

3. Spell each word in the space provided.

Word	Pronunciation	Spelling
amblyopia	**am**-blee-**OH**-pee-ah	
aphakia	ah-**FAY**-kee-ah	
aqueous humor	**AY**-kwee-us **HYOO**-mer	
audiometry	aw-dee-**OM**-eh-tree	
auditory	**AW**-dih-tor-ee	
aural	**AW**-ral	
auricle	**AW**-rih-kel	
blepharoptosis	blef-ah-roh-**TOH**-sis	
cochlea	**KOCK**-lee-ah	
conjunctivitis	kon-**junk**-tih-**VYE**-tis	
corneal abrasion	**COR**-nee-al ab-**RAY**-zhun	
diplopia	dih-**PLOH**-pee-ah	
esotropia	es-oh-**TROH**-pee-ah	
eustachian tube	yoo-**STAY**-shun	

Word	Pronunciation	Spelling
exotropia	**eck**-soh-**TROH**-pee-ah	
incus	**INK**-us	
iridectomy	ir-ih-**DECK**-toh-mee	
iritis	eye-**RYE**-tis	
labyrinthitis	lab-ih-rin-**THIGH**-tis	
malleus	**MAL**-ee-us	
myopia	my-**OH**-pee-ah	
ophthalmologist	**ahf**-thal-**MOL**-eh-jist	
ophthalmoscopy	**ahf**-thal-**MOS**-koh-pee	
optician	op-**TISH**-an	
optometrist	op-**TOM**-eh-trist	
otalgia	oh-**TAL**-jee-ah	
otitis media	oh-**TYE**-tis **ME**-dee-ah	
otorrhea	**oh**-toh-**REE**-ah	
palpebral	**PAL**-peh-bral	
photophobia	**foh**-toh-**FOH**-bee-ah	
presbycusis	**pres**-beh-**KOO**-sis	
presbyopia	**pres**-bee-**OH**-pee-ah	
retinopathy	**ret**-ih-**NOP**-ah-thee	
retinopexy	**RET**-ih-noh-**peck**-see	
stapes	**STAY**-peez	
tympanic	tim-**PAN**-ik	
tympanoplasty	tim-pah-no-**PLAS**-tee	
vestibule	**VESS**-tih-byool	

CHAPTER 11

Digestive System

LEARNING OBJECTIVES

After studying this chapter and completing the review exercises, you should be able to:

1. Name and locate the major organs of the digestive system.
2. Name and locate the liver, gallbladder, biliary ducts, and pancreas.
3. Describe the peritoneum.
4. Pronounce, spell, define, and write the medical terms related to the digestive system.
5. Describe common diseases related to the digestive system.
6. Listen, read, and study so you can speak and write.

INTRODUCTION

Figure 11-1 shows you the digestive system. The main part is a long tube called the **digestive tract**. It is also known as the **gastrointestinal tract**. It is about 16 feet (5 m) long. It starts at the mouth and ends at the anus. The inside wall is lined with mucous membrane.

The digestive tract takes in food. It then breaks it down so that the body can use it. This is called *digestion*. The food molecules then go into the blood and lymph systems. This is called the process of *absorption*. The waste materials that are left continue to the end of the digestive tract and are eliminated.

 11.1 MAJOR ORGANS OF THE DIGESTIVE SYSTEM

PRACTICE FOR LEARNING: MAJOR ORGANS OF THE DIGESTIVE SYSTEM

Write the words below in the correct spaces on Figure 11-1. To help you, the number beside the word tells you where it goes on the figure. Be sure to pronounce each word as you write it. Repeat the pronunciation several times if you find the word hard to say.

1. oral cavity (**OR**-al)

2. pharynx (**FAR**-inks)

3. esophagus (en-**SOF**-ah-gus)

4. stomach (**STUM**-ick)

5. small intestine (in-**TESS**-tine)

6. large intestine (in-**TESS**-tine)

7. rectum (**RECK**-tum)

8. appendix (ah-**PEN**-dicks)

9. pancreas (**PAN**-kree-as)

10. gallbladder (**GALL**-blad-er)

11. liver (**LIV**-er)

12. salivary gland (**SAL**-ih-vehr-ee)

Figure 11-1 shows you the six regions of the digestive tract. They are the oral cavity (mouth), the pharynx, the esophagus, the stomach, the small intestine, and the large intestine.

Four organs connected to the digestive system help out in the process of digestion. They are the salivary glands, the pancreas, the liver, and the gallbladder. Identify them on Figure 11-1.

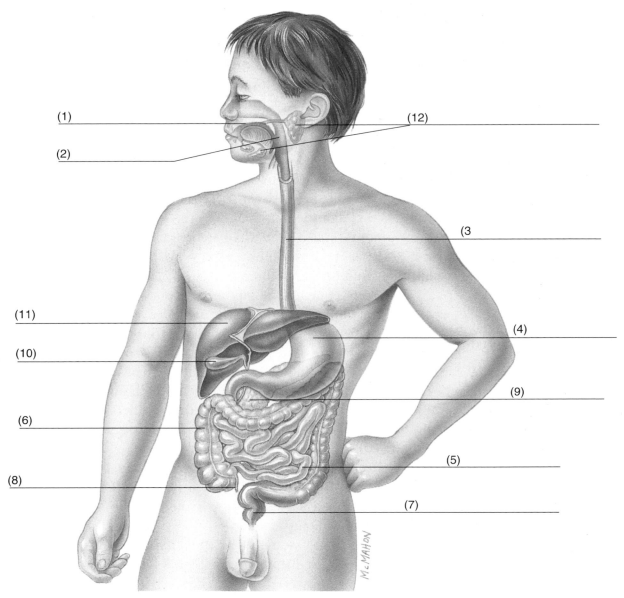

FIGURE 11-1 Major organs of the digestive system.

11.2 ORAL CAVITY

IN BRIEF

Oral cavity is the mouth

Uvula closes of the nasal passage during swallowing

Tongue is for speech, taste and swallowing

The oral (**OR-al**) cavity is the mouth. The roof of the mouth is the palate (**PAL-at**). It separates the mouth from the nasal cavity. At the back of the palate is the uvula (**YOO-vyoo-lah**). It looks like a sack hanging from the soft palate. It closes off the nasal passage during swallowing.

The tongue is the most versatile muscle in the body. Its primary functions are to provide a sense of taste and to assist in swallowing. It is also very important in the production of speech.

PHARYNX, ESOPHAGUS, AND STOMACH

IN BRIEF

Pharynx is also known as the throat

Peristalsis pushes the bolus through the esophagus

Esophagus is located between the pharynx and stomach

Sphincters are circular muscles that keep food moving in one direction

Stomach regions cardia, antrum, body, fundus

Bolus wet ball of food

Chyme partially digested food

Rugae folds in stomach

During chewing, the food is mixed with saliva, producing a softened ball of food called a bolus (**BO-lus**). The bolus is pushed by the tongue into the throat, or pharynx, which is a 5-inch (12.5 cm) tube. This pushing commences the process of swallowing, which moves the bolus into the esophagus.

The esophagus is a 10-inch (25-cm) tube. It begins at the pharynx and passes through an opening in the diaphragm called the esophageal hiatus (**eh-sof-ah-JEE-ul high-AYE-tus**). The esophagus continues through the diaphragm to the stomach. The muscles of the esophagus cause wave-like contractions called peristaltic (**per-ih-STAL-tick**) waves. These waves push the bolus down the esophagus and into the stomach.

As the bolus nears the stomach, it encounters a closed area caused by a tight circular muscle called a sphincter (**SFINK-ter**). The sphincter opens to allow the bolus into the stomach and then closes again to prevent stomach contents from re-entering the esophagus. The sphincter is called the gastroesophageal sphincter because it is located between the stomach and esophagus.

Once the bolus passes through the sphincter into the stomach, the food is broken down, by enzymes, into a semiliquid called chyme (**KYM**).

The stomach is J-shaped, with four regions: the cardia (**KAR-dee-ah**), fundus (**FUN-dus**), body, and antrum (**AN-trum**). The inner lining consists of a series of folds called rugae (**ROO-jee**), which stretch to accommodate food.

Food leaves the stomach for the small intestine through another sphincter called the pyloric (**pie-LOR-ick**) sphincter.

PRACTICE FOR LEARNING: ORAL CAVITY

Underline the correct answer in the following sentences.

1. The sac-like structure at the back of the mouth is the uvea/uvula).

2. The roof of the mouth is the (fundus/cardia/palate).

3. Food enters the small intestine as a semiliquid substance called (bolus/chyme).

4. The esophageal hiatus is located in the (stomach/esophagus/diaphragm).

5. The (fundus/hiatus/antrum/sphincter) is defined as a tight circular muscle.

6. Which of the following is not a part of the stomach? (body/hiatus/rugae/cardia)

Answers: **1.** uvula. **2.** palate. **3.** chyme. **4.** diaphragm. **5.** sphincter. **6.** hiatus.

11.4 SMALL INTESTINE

PRACTICE FOR LEARNING: SMALL INTESTINE

Write the words below on the correct spaces in Figure 11-2. To help you, the number beside the word tells you where it goes on the figure. Be sure to pronounce each word as you write it. Repeat the pronunciation several times if you find the word hard to say.

1. duodenum (**doo-oh-DEE-num**)

2. jejunum (**jeh-JOO-num**)

3. ileum (**ILL-ee-um**)

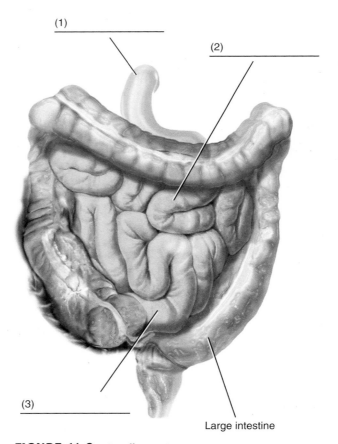

(1) _____

(2) _____

(3) _____

Large intestine

FIGURE 11-2 Small intestine.

Figure 11-2 illustrates the small intestine coiled within the abdominopelvic cavity. It is also called the small bowel. It is 11 feet (3.35 m) long and has three regions: the duodenum, the jejunum, and the ileum. Although the diameter is only about 1 inch (2.54 cm), the small intestine expands to accommodate food as it passes through.

The function of the small intestine is to absorb nutrients from digested food and pass them into the bloodstream. The remaining waste products enter the large intestine.

11.5 LARGE INTESTINE

PRACTICE FOR LEARNING: LARGE INTESTINE

Write the words below on the correct spaces in Figure 11-3. To help you, the number beside the word tells you where it goes on the figure. Be sure to pronounce each word as you write it. Repeat the pronunciation several times if you find the word hard to say.

1. appendix (ah-**PEN**-dicks)

2. cecum (**SEE**-kum)

3. ascending colon (ah-**SEN**-ding **KOH**-lon)

4. transverse colon (tranz-**VERS**)

5. descending colon (dee-**SEN**-ding)

6. sigmoid colon (**SIG**-moid)

7. rectum (**RECK**-tum)

8. anal canal (**AY**-nul)

9. anus (**AY**-nus)

The large intestine is about 5 feet (1.8 m) long. It is also called the large bowel. As illustrated in Figure 11-3, the large intestine has three regions. First is a pouch called the cecum. The appendix, which has no known function, hangs down from the cecum. The next region is the colon. It forms a long, square arch consisting of four areas: the ascending colon, transverse colon, descending colon, and sigmoid colon. The last region of the large intestine is the rectum. It is about 8 inches long and is lined with mucous folds.

The final segment of the rectum is the anal canal.

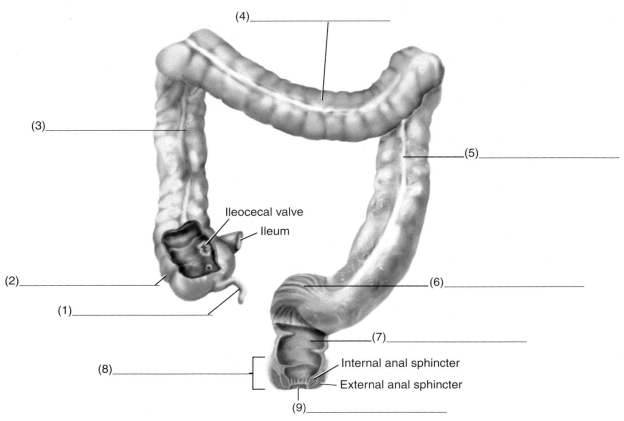

Ileocecal valve

Ileum

Internal anal sphincter

External anal sphincter

FIGURE 11-3   Large intestine.

PRACTICE FOR LEARNING: MAJOR ORGANS OF THE DIGESTIVE SYSTEM

Write the correct term on the line.

1. The organ located between the oral cavity and esophagus is the _____ .

2. The organ that empties food into the stomach is the _____ .

3. Food leaves the stomach and enters the _____ .

4. The transverse colon is part of the _____ .

5. The duodenum is part of the _____ .

6. The function of the small intestine is the _____ of nutrients.

7. The appendix is located on the _____ side of the abdomen.

Answers: **1.** pharynx. **2.** esophagus. **3.** duodenum. **4.** large intestine. **5.** small intestine. **6.** absorption. **7.** right.

11.6 LIVER, GALLBLADDER, BILIARY DUCTS, AND PANCREAS

The liver weighs about 4 pounds (1.75 kg). It is located below the diaphragm in the right upper quadrant (RUQ) of the abdomen (Figure 11-4). The liver has many functions including the production of bile, elimination of toxic substances; and break-down of proteins, fats, and carbohydrates.

The biliary tract includes the liver, the gallbladder (GB), and the biliary ducts. The biliary ducts include the hepatic ducts, the common hepatic duct, the cystic duct, and the common bile duct (CBD) (Figure 11-4).

Bile is a greenish-yellow fluid produced in the liver. Look at the bile ducts in Figure 11-4. Bile goes from the hepatic cells through the right and left hepatic ducts, through the common hepatic duct, and into the cystic duct. It is stored in the gallbladder. The function of bile is to break down fats in the duodenum. When bile is required, it travels through the cystic duct and into the CBD (where the common hepatic and cystic ducts meet). The CBD drains into the duodenum.

The liver is essential to life. However, the gallbladder may be surgically removed without too much disruption to body function.

IN BRIEF

Liver

Location: RUQ

Function: produces bile

Gallbladder

Location: Under the liver

Function: Stores bile

Pancreas

Location: Lies behind the stomach

Function: Secretes enzymes and hormones

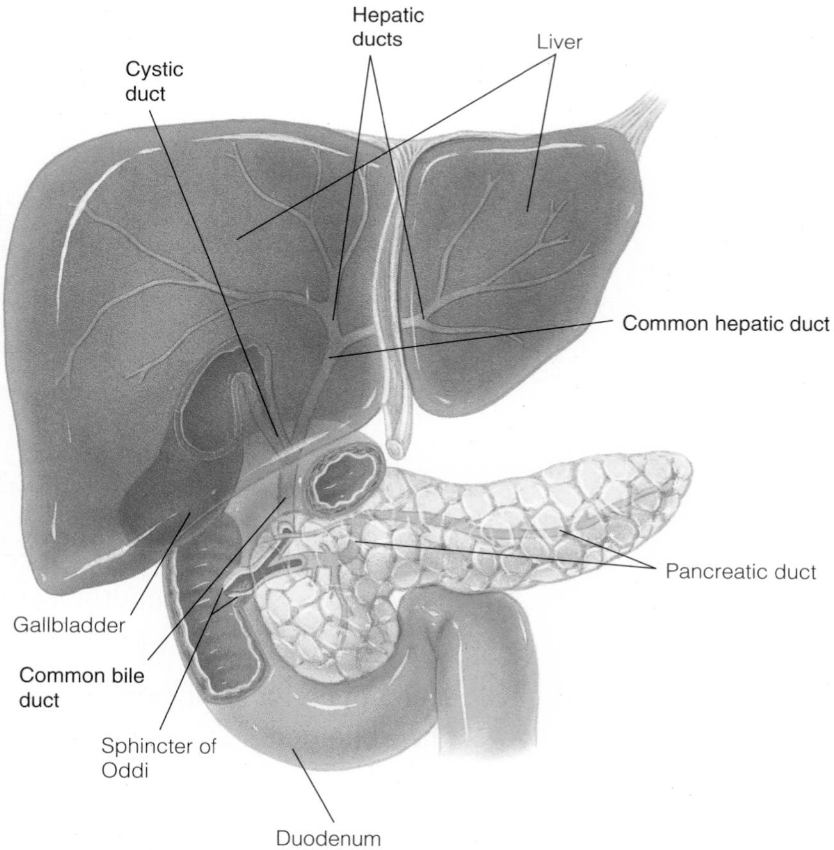

FIGURE 11-4   Liver, gallbladder, pancreas, and biliary tract.

After removal of the gallbladder, the bile may be stored in the biliary ducts, and biliary processes proceed normally.

The pancreas is illustrated in Figure 11-4. It is a long, fish-shaped organ lying behind the stomach. It secretes pancreatic juice, which contains enzymes to break down food in the duodenum.

The pancreas also secretes the hormones **insulin** (**IN-suh-lin**) and **glucagon** (**GLOO-kah-gon**). These hormones work together to regulate the amount of sugar in the bloodstream. See Chapter 19, under Pancreas, for details of sugar regulation.

11.7 PERITONEUM

Figure 11-5 illustrates the **peritoneum** (**per-ih-toh-NEE-um**). It is a membrane lining the abdominopelvic cavity and covering the abdominopelvic organs. It has two layers. The space between the two layers is called the **peritoneal** (**per-ih-toh-NEE-al**) **cavity.** It is filled with peritoneal fluid, a watery substance that prevents friction between the two layers.

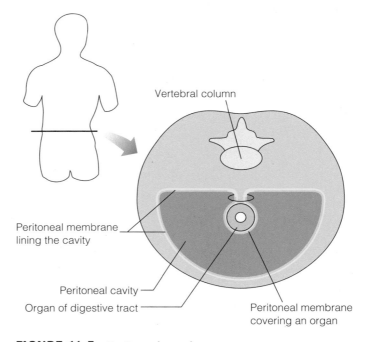

IN BRIEF

Peritoneum

Membrane lining the abdominal and pelvic cavities and covering its organs

Vertebral column

Peritoneal membrane lining the cavity

Peritoneal cavity

Organ of digestive tract

Peritoneal membrane covering an organ

FIGURE 11-5 Peritoneal membrane.

PRACTICE FOR LEARNING: BILIARY TRACT AND THE PERITONEUM

Underline the correct answer in each sentence.

1. The hepatic ducts carry bile from the (gallbladder/liver).

2. A greenish-yellow fluid stored in the gallbladder is (glucagon/bile).

3. The (pancreas/liver) regulates blood sugar.

4. The peritoneum lines the (thoracic/abdominal) cavity.

Answers: **1.** liver. **2.** bile. **3.** pancreas. **4.** abdominal.

11.8 NEW ROOTS, SUFFIXES, AND PREFIX

Use these additional roots, suffixes, and prefix when studying the medical terms in this chapter.

Root	Meaning
intestin/o	intestine

Suffix	Meaning
-aise	ease
-flux	flow
-tripsy	crushing

Prefix	Meaning
re-	back

11.9 LEARNING THE TERMS

Following these steps will make it easier for you to learn medical terms:

1. Pronounce the term repeatedly until it is easy for you.

2. Write it down. Ensure the spelling is correct.

3. Also write the definition. If possible, relate the word to a word, thought, or picture that will help you remember it.

4. Analyze the term with the method taught in this text.

Root	Meaning
append/o; appendic/o	appendix

Term	Term Analysis	Definition
appendicitis (ah-**pen**-dih-**SIGH**-tis)	-itis = inflammation	inflammation of the appendix

Root	Meaning
cholangi/o	bile duct; bile vessel

Term	Term Analysis	Definition
cholangiogram (koh-**LAN**-jee-oh-gram)	-gram = record	record (image) of the bile ducts produced by x-rays

Root	Meaning
cholecyst/o	gallbladder (GB)

Term	Term Analysis	Definition
cholecystectomy (**koh**-lee-sis-**TECK**-toh-mee)	-ectomy = excision; surgical removal	excision of the gallbladder
cholecystitis (**koh**-lee-sis-**TYE**-tis)	-itis = inflammation	inflammation of the gallbladder

Root	Meaning
choledoch/o	common bile duct

Term	Term Analysis	Definition
choledochotomy (**koh**-led-oh-**KOT**-oh-mee)	-tomy = to cut into; incision; process of cutting	incision into the common bile duct

HELPING YOU REMEMBER

The roots chol/e and col/o are often confused. They are pronounced the same, but have entirely different meanings: chol/e means gall and col/o means colon. Therefore, the term for inflammation of the gallbladder is cholecystitis, not colecystitis.

Root		Meaning	
col/o		colon	
Term	**Term Analysis**		**Definition**
colitis (koh-**LYE**-tis)	-itis = inflammation		inflammation of the colon
colic (**KOLL**-ick)	-ic = pertaining to		severe abdominal pain; pertaining to the colon

Root		Meaning	
enter/o		small intestine; intestine	
Term	**Term Analysis**		**Definition**
gastroenteritis (**gas**-troh-**en**-ter-**EYE**-tis)	-itis = inflammation gastr/o = stomach		inflammation of the stomach and intestines often accompanied by nausea (a sick feeling) and vomiting

Root		Meaning	
gastr/o		stomach	
Term	**Term Analysis**		**Definition**
gastroesophageal reflux (GER) (**gas**-troh-eh-**sof**-ah-**JEE**-ul **REE**-flucks)	-eal = pertaining to esophag/o = esophagus -flux = flow re- = back		backward flow of stomach contents into the esophagus

Root	Meaning
gingiv/o	gums; gingiva

Term	Term Analysis	Definition
gingivitis (**jin**-jih-**VYE**-tis)	-itis = inflammation	inflamed gums

Root	Meaning
gloss/o (see also lingu/o)	tongue

Term	Term Analysis	Definition
glossitis (**glos**-EYE-tis)	-itis = inflammation	inflammation of the tongue

Root	Meaning
hepat/o	liver

Term	Term Analysis	Definition
hepatitis (**hep**-ah-**TYE**-tis)	-itis = inflammation	inflammation of the liver

Root	Meaning
ile/o	ileum (first part of the small intestine)

Term	Term Analysis	Definition
ileectomy (**ill**-ee-**ECK**-toh-mee)	-ectomy = excision; surgical removal	excision of the ileum

HELPING YOU REMEMBER

Do not confuse ile/o, which means "intestine," with ili/o, which means "hip." To remember, think of the "e" in ile/o corresponding to the "e" in intestine and the "i" in ili/o corresponding to the "i" in hip.

Root	Meaning
labi/o	lips

Term	Term Analysis	Definition
labial (**LAY**-bee-al)	-al = pertaining to	pertaining to the lips

Root	Meaning
lapar/o	abdomen

Term	Term Analysis	Definition
laparoscope (**LAP**-ah-roh-skohp)	-scope = instrument used to visually examine	instrument used to visually examine the inside of the abdomen

Root	Meaning
lingu/o	tongue

Term	Term Analysis	Definition
sublingual (sub-**LING**-gwal)	-al = pertaining to sub- = under	pertaining to under the tongue

Root	Meaning
lith/o	stone; calculus

Term	Term Analysis	Definition
cholecystoli-thiasis (koh-lee-**sis**-toh-lih-**THIGH**-ah-sis)	-iasis = abnormal condition cholecyst/o = gallbladder	condition of stones in the gallbladder; cholelithiasis
NOTE: For further details, see Section 11.10 Pathology under "cholecystolithiasis."		
lithotripsy (**LITH**-oh-**trip**-see)	-tripsy = crushing	crushing of gallstones into pebbles tiny enough to be eliminated without surgical removal

Root	Meaning
orex/o	appetite

Term	Term Analysis		Definition
anorexia (an-oh-RECK-see-ah)	-ia = condition an - no; not; lack of		loss of appetite

NOTE: Do not confuse anorexia with anorexia nervosa. Anorexia is a loss of appetite due to an underlying condition. Anorexia nervosa is an eating disorder of self-starvation.

Root	Meaning
or/o (see also stomat/o)	mouth

Term	Term Analysis	Definition
oral (OR-al)	-al = pertaining to	pertaining to the mouth

Root	Meaning
stomat/o	mouth

Term	Term Analysis	Definition
stomatitis (sto-mah-TYE-tis)	-itis = inflammation	inflammation of the mouth

HELPING YOU REMEMBER

stomat/o, is usually used in reference to pathology of the mouth.

Suffix	Meaning
-emesis	vomiting

NOTE: -emesis can be used as a suffix, as evident in the following examples; or it can stand alone as a word, as in "There was no emesis."

Term	Term Analysis	Definition
hyperemesis (**high**-per-**EM**-eh-sis)	hyper- = excessive; above normal	excessive vomiting
hematemesis (**hem**-ah-**TEM**-eh-sis)	hemat/o = blood	vomiting of blood
melanemesis (**mel**-ah-**NEM**-eh-sis)	melan/o = black	black vomit caused by the mixing of blood with intestinal contents

NOTE: Melanemesis may be due to bleeding ulcers.

Suffix	Meaning
-phagia	eating; swallowing

Term	Term Analysis	Definition
aphagia (ah-**FAY**-jee-ah)	a- = no; not; lack of	inability to swallow
dysphagia (dis-**FAY**-jee-ah)	dys- = difficult; painful; bad	difficulty in swallowing
polyphagia (**pol**-ee-**FAY**-jee-ah)	poly- = many	excessive eating

Suffix	Meaning
-pepsia	digestion

Term	Term Analysis	Definition
dyspepsia (dis-**PEP**-see-ah)	dys- = difficult; painful; bad	indigestion

Suffix	Meaning
-stomy	new opening

Term	Term Analysis	Definition
colostomy (koh-**LOSS**-toh-mee)	col/o = colon	creation of a new opening between the colon and the abdominal wall. Wastes are then eliminated through this opening (Figure 11-6).

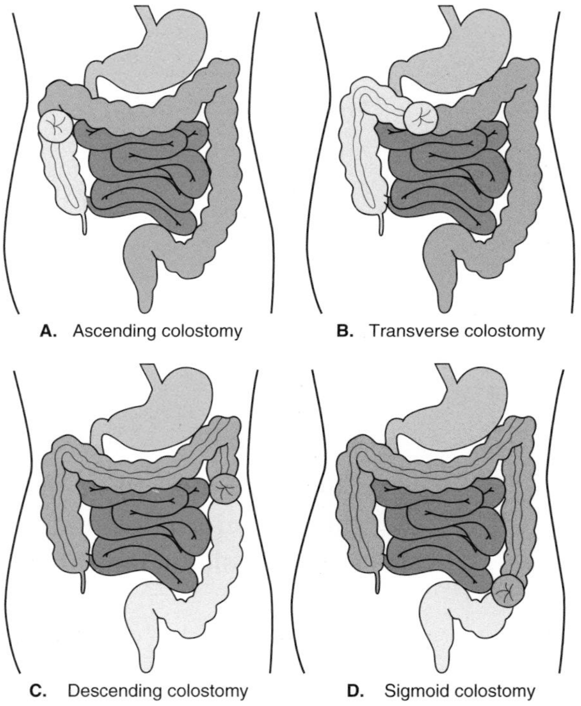

A. Ascending colostomy   B. Transverse colostomy

C. Descending colostomy   D. Sigmoid colostomy

FIGURE 11-6 Colostomies: A colostomy is named for the part of the colon that is removed. In this diagram, the areas of intestine that are removed are shown in **blue**.

Prefix	Meaning	
dia-	through; complete	
Term	**Term Analysis**	**Definition**
diarrhea (**dye-ah-REE-ah**)	-rrhea = flow; discharge	frequent and watery excretion of stool

Prefix	Meaning	
mal-	bad	
Term	**Term Analysis**	**Definition**
malaise (**mah-LAYZ**)	-aise = ease	a feeling of uneasiness or discomfort. A sign of illness.

11.10 PATHOLOGY

Cholecystolithiasis or Cholelithiasis

Calculi (stones) in the gallbladder. Commonly called gallstones. If the calculi are located in the common bile duct, the condition is called choledocholithiasis (Figure 11-7).

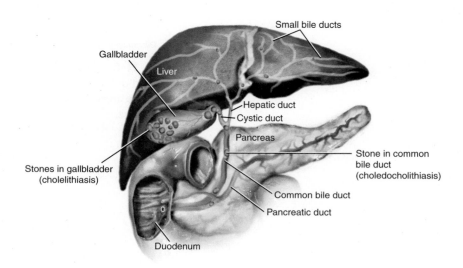

FIGURE 11-7 Stones in the gallbladder and bile ducts.

Hernia

A protrusion or displacement of an organ through a structure that normally holds it in place. Herniae of the digestive tract occur when the abdominal muscles are unable to hold the intestines in place because of a weakness. The weakness can be congenital (present at birth) or acquired from lifting heavy objects or straining on defecation.

A common hernia is the inguinal hernia, which is the displacement of intestine into the groin area (Figure 11-8).

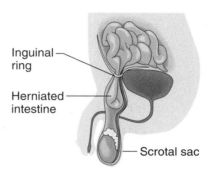

FIGURE 11-8   Inguinal hernia.

Crohn's Disease (CD) (KROHNZ)

A form of inflammatory bowel disease that can involve any part of the digestive tract. It is most often found in the ileum. The inflammation causes obstruction of intestinal contents.

In severe cases, the diseased bowel is removed and an artificial opening is created between the intestine and abdominal wall. (Figure 11-6). If the artificial opening is between the colon and abdominal wall, the operation is called a colostomy (koh-**LOSS**-toh-mee). If the artificial opening is between the ileum and abdominal wall, the operation is called an ileostomy (ill-ee-**OSS**-toh-mee).

Ulcers

Wearing away of the mucous membrane lining the digestive tract. This creates an open sore. The ulcer can literally eat a hole through the mucous membrane, causing bleeding to the digestive tract. Antibiotics are used to treat ulcers caused by the bacteria *Helicobacter pylori.*

11.11 REVIEW EXERCISES

| Exercise 11-1 | LOOK-ALIKE AND SOUND-ALIKE WORDS |

Below is a list of look-alike and sound-alike words. Study the definitions of each set of words, then read the sentences carefully and circle the word in parentheses that correctly completes the meaning.

acidic	pertaining to an acid
acetic	sour
ascitic	pertaining to ascites (accumulation of fluid in the abdomen)
aphagia	inability to swallow
aphasia	inability to speak or write
aplasia	lack of development
cirrhosis	a liver disease
scirrhous	pertaining to a hard cancer
dysphagia	difficulty swallowing
dysphasia	difficulty speaking
hepatoma	tumor of the liver
hematoma	bruise
ingestion	taking food or liquid into the body
injection	the placement of a substance into the body via a needle
ileum	the distal portion of the small intestine
ilium	the hip bone
labial	pertaining to the lip
labile	unstable
liver	large organ of the digestive system
livor	discoloration on different parts of the body after death
palate	roof of the mouth
pallet	a moveable platform for transporting objectives
pallette	a thin board with a thumb holes, used by artists to mix their paint
pellet	a small round ball of food

reflux	to flow backward
reflex	involuntary response to a stimulus

1. On examination of the gastrointestinal tract, there were no signs of (**dysphasia/dysphagia**), nausea, vomiting, or hematemesis. However, on neurological exam some (**aphasia/aphagia**) was noted due to the stroke.

2. She complained of tiredness and malaise as well as symptoms of (**reflux/reflex**) and heartburn.

3. Chronic hepatitis and (**cirrhosis/scirrhous**) are possible (**liver/livor**) diseases. Suggest (**liver/livor**) biopsy.

4. The physician's impression was that a (**cirrhosis/scirrhous**) mass was in the distal (**ileum/ilium**).

5. This patient has been admitted with dyspeptic symptoms due to multiple drug (**ingestions/injections**).

6. She has no abdominal distention, vomiting, (**acidic/acetic/ascitic**) regurgitation, or dyspepsia.

7. The disease is characterized by enlarged lips and (**labial/labile**) glands.

8. The patient was admitted with a large (**hepatoma/hematoma**) due to multiple wounds to the neck and back.

Exercise 11-2 MATCHING WORD PARTS WITH MEANING

Match the word part in Column A *with its meaning in* Column B.

Column A	Column B
_____ 1. -tripsy	A. gallbladder
_____ 2. cholecyst/o	B. common bile duct
_____ 3. stomat/o	C. gums
_____ 4. -flux	D. crushing
_____ 5. cholangi/o	E. lips
_____ 6. lapar/o	F. mouth
_____ 7. choledoch/o	G. liver
_____ 8. hepat/o	H. bile duct
_____ 9. gingiv/o	I. flow
_____ 10. labi/o	J. abdomen

| Exercise 11-3 | MATCHING–PATHOLOGY |

Match the disease in Column A *with its description in* Column B.

Column A	Column B
_____ 1. cholelithiasis	A. inflammatory bowel disease
_____ 2. hernia	B. wearing away of the mucous membrane lining of the digestive tract
_____ 3. melanemesis	
_____ 4. gingivitis	C. inflammation of the gums
_____ 5. Crohn's disease	D. stones in the gallbladder
_____ 6. ulcer	E. black vomit
	F. displacement of an organ through a structure that normally contains it

| Exercise 11-4 | LABELING–DIGESTIVE TRACT |

Write the name of each numbered structure on the corresponding line below the diagram (Figure 11-9). Use the body structures listed below.

appendix _____

esophagus _____

gallbladder _____

large intestine _____

liver _____

oral cavity _____

pancreas _____

pharynx _____

rectum _____

salivary gland _____

small intestine _____

stomach _____

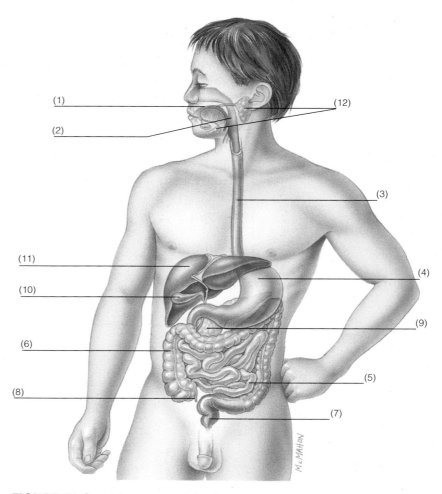

FIGURE 11-9   Major organs of the digestive system.

1. _____

2. _____

3. _____

4. _____

5. _____

6. _____

7. _____

8. _____

9. _____

10. _____

11. _____

12. _____

| **Exercise 11-5** | DEFINITIONS—ANATOMY |

Define the following terms. Use your medical dictionary if necessary.

1. oral cavity _____

2. pharynx _____

3. duodenum _____

4. cecum _____

5. gallbladder _____

6. bowel _____

7. jejunum _____

8. biliary tract _____

9. insulin _____

10. gingiva _____

| **Exercise 11-6** | DEFINITIONS—LEARNING THE TERMS |

Define the following terms.

1. glossitis _____

2. anorexia _____

3. colic _____

4. colostomy _____

5. malaise _____

6. dyspepsia _____

7. gastroesophageal reflux _____

8. hyperemesis _____

9. **sublingual** _____

10. **lithotripsy** _____

| Exercise 11-7 | BUILDING MEDICAL WORDS |

I. *Use lith/o to build medical words for the following definitions.*

   a. condition of stones in the gallbladder

      _____

   b. condition of stones in the common bile ducts

      _____

   c. crushing of gallstones _____

II. *Use -emesis to build medical words for the following definitions.*

   a. excessive vomiting _____

   b. vomiting of blood _____

   c. black vomit _____

III. *Use -phagia to build medical words for the following definitions.*

   a. no eating _____

   b. difficulty in eating _____

   c. excessive eating _____

IV. *Use -itis to build medical words for the following definitions*

   a. inflammation of the appendix _____

   b. inflammation of the gallbladder _____

   c. inflammation of the colon _____

   d. inflammation of the stomach and intestines

      _____

   e. inflammation of the gums _____

   f. inflammation of the tongue _____

   g. inflammation of the liver _____

   h. inflammation of the mouth _____

| Exercise 11-8 | **DEFINITIONS IN CONTEXT** |

Define the bolded terms in context. Use your medical dictionary if necessary.

1. The patient had an x-ray while in the emergency department that showed a normal pharynx, esophagus, stomach, and duodenum.

   a. x-ray _____

   b. pharynx _____

   c. duodenum _____

2. On his last admission, a colonoscopy showed worsening of his Crohn's disease. He also had a gastroscopy showing mild gastritis but no ulcer disease.

   d. colonoscopy _____

   e. Crohn's disease _____

   f. gastroscopy _____

   g. gastritis _____

   h. ulcer disease _____

3. The patient was admitted with epigastric pain, at which time she was diagnosed with cholecystolithiasis. We therefore decided to proceed with a cholecystectomy.

   i. epigastric pain _____

   j. cholecystolithiasis _____

   k. cholecystectomy _____

4. He has no visible emesis or gastroesophageal reflux.

   l. emesis _____

   m. gastroesophageal reflux _____

5. There was no dysphagia, nausea, malaise, or hematemesis.

   n. dysphagia _____

   o. nausea _____

   p. malaise _____

   q. hematemesis _____

| Exercise 11-9 | SPELLING |

Circle any words that are spelled incorrectly in the list below. Then correct the spelling in the space provided.

1. duodenum _____

2. malaise _____

3. Chron's disease _____

4. melanemesis _____

5. cholitis _____

6. appendix _____

7. jegunum _____

8. peritoneum _____

9. coledocholithiasis _____

10. disphagia _____

11.12 PRONUNCIATION AND SPELLING

Listen, read, and study, so you can speak and write.

1. Listen to each word on the audio CD.

2. Pronounce each word carefully.

3. Spell each word in the space provided.

Word	Pronunciation	Spelling
anorexia	an-oh-**RECK**-see-ah	
appendicitis	ah-**pen**-dih-**SIGH**-tis	
biliary	**BILL**-ee-air-ee	
cholecystectomy	koh-lee-sis-**TECK**-toh-mee	
choledochotomy	koh-led-oh-**KOT**-oh-mee	
colitis	koh-**LYE**-tis	
colostomy	koh-**LOSS**-toh-mee	
diarrhea	**dye**-ah-**REE**-ah	

Word	Pronunciation	Spelling
dyspepsia	dis-**PEP**-see-ah	
dysphagia	dis-**FAY**-jee-ah	
esophagus	eh-**SOF**-ah-gus	
gastroenteritis	**gas**-troh-**en**-ter-**EYE**-tis	
gingivitis	**jin**-jih-**VYE**-tis	
hematemesis	**hem**-ah-**TEM**-eh-sis	
hyperemesis	**high**-per-**EM**-eh-sis	
ileectomy	**ill**-ee-**ECK**-toh-mee	
ileum	**ILL**-ee-um	
insulin	**IN**-suh-lin	
jejunum	jeh-**JOO**-num	
labial	**LAY**-bee-al	
malaise	mah-**LAYZ**	
melanemesis	**mel**-ah-**NEM**-eh-sis	
oral	**OR**-al	
peritoneum	**per**-ih-toh-**NEE**-um	
stomatitis	**sto**-mah-**TYE**-tis	
sublingual	sub-**LING**-gwal	

CHAPTER 12

Cardiovascular System

LEARNING OBJECTIVES

After studying this chapter and completing the review exercises, you should be able to:

1. Name and locate the major organs of the cardiovascular system.
2. Name, locate, and describe the structures of the heart and associated blood vessels.
3. Describe the function of the heart and blood vessels.
4. Name the blood vessels.
5. Pronounce, spell, define, and write the medical terms related to the cardiovascular system.
6. Describe common diseases related to the cardiovascular system.
7. Listen, read, and study so you can speak and write.

INTRODUCTION

The human body is made up of 70 to 80 trillion cells. All of these cells need to be fed oxygen and nutrients. These are provided by the cardiovascular system (CVS), which is illustrated in Figure 12-1.

The body's cells must also get rid of waste materials. The CVS does this job too, at the same time it delivers oxygen and nutrients.

249

12.1 MAJOR ORGANS OF THE CARDIOVASCULAR SYSTEM

PRACTICE FOR LEARNING: MAJOR ORGANS OF THE CVS

Write the words below in the correct spaces on Figure 12-1. To help you, the number beside the word tells you where it goes on the figure. Be sure to pronounce each word as you write it. Repeat the pronunciation several times if you find the word hard to say.

1. heart (**HART**)

2. arteries (**AR-ter-eez**)

3. arterioles (**ar-TEER-ee-ohlz**)

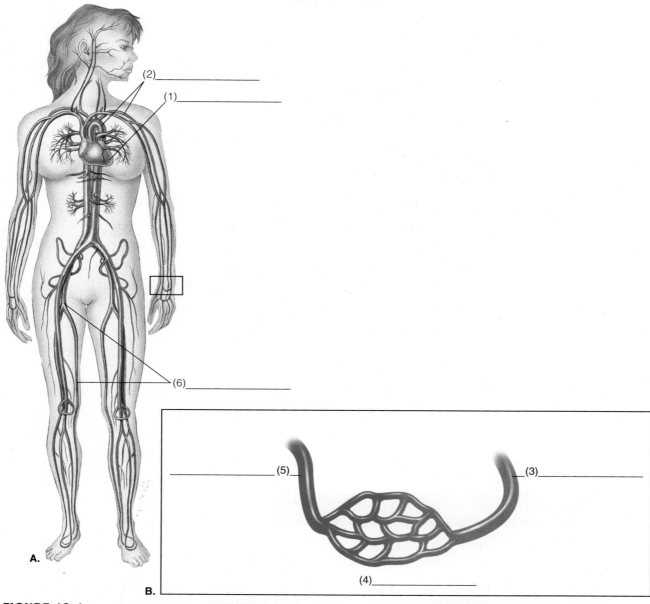

FIGURE 12-1 A, Structures of the cardiovascular system. B, Arteries, arterioles, capillaries, venules, and veins.

4. capillaries (kah-**PILL**-ah-reez)

5. venules (**VEN**-yoolz)

6. veins (**VAYNZ**)

The heart pumps blood. It beats 60 to 90 times every minute for your whole life. Each beat pumps blood throughout the body. The blood flows through blood vessels. Numbers 2 through 6 on Figure 12-1 are the different types of blood vessels.

12.2 STRUCTURES OF THE HEART

PRACTICE FOR LEARNING: THE HEART

Write the structures listed below on the correct spaces in Figure 12-2. To help you, the number beside the word tells you where it goes on the figure. Be sure to pronounce each word as you write it. Repeat the word several times if you find the word hard to say.

1. superior vena cava (**VEE**-nah **KAY**-vah)

2. pulmonary semilunar valve (**POOL**-mon-ayr-ee seh-me-**LOO**-nar **VALV**)

3. right atrium (**AY**-tree-um)

4. tricuspid valve (trigh-**KUS**-pid)

5. right ventricle (**VEN**-trih-kul)

6. inferior vena cava (**VEE**-nah **KAY**-vah)

7. septum (**SEP**-tum)

8. left ventricle (**VEN**-trih-kul)

9. bicuspid (bye-**KUS**-pid) or mitral (**MY**-tral) valve

10. aortic semilunar valve (ay-**OR**-tick seh-mee-**LOO**-nar **VALV**)

11. left atrium

12. aorta (ay-**OR**-tah)

Figure 12-2 shows you a big picture of the heart and the large blood vessels attached to it (aorta, superior vena cava, inferior vena cava, and pulmonary artery). Review it before you move on to the diagrams of parts of the heart, which come later.

Heart Chambers

Look at Figure 12-3. It shows that the heart contains four cavities. They are called chambers. The upper chambers are called atria

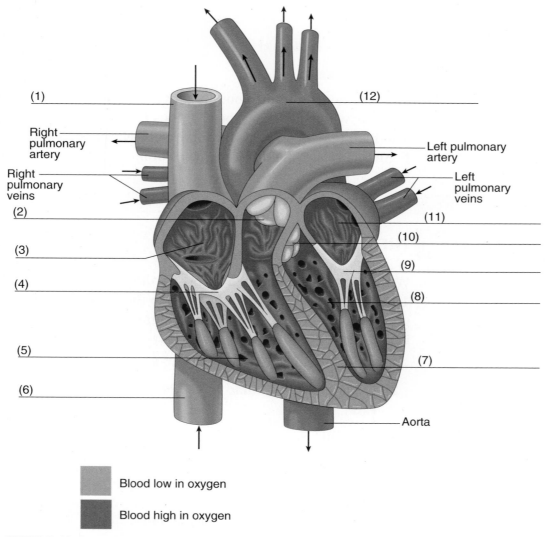

(1)

Right pulmonary artery

Right pulmonary veins

(2)

(3)

(4)

(5)

(6)

(12)

Left pulmonary artery

Left pulmonary veins

(11)

(10)

(9)

(8)

(7)

Aorta

Blood low in oxygen

Blood high in oxygen

FIGURE 12-2 Heart and major blood vessels.

(**AY-tree-ah**) (singular is atrium). The lower chambers are called ventricles (singular is ventricle).

Figure 12-3 also illustrates that the heart is separated into the right and left sections. The wall dividing them is called the septum.

IN BRIEF

Atria are the upper chambers.

Ventricles are the lower chambers

Septum separates the right and left sides of the heart

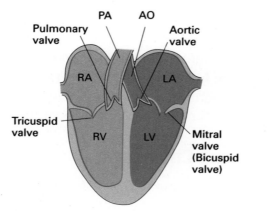

PA   AO

Pulmonary valve

Aortic valve

RA   LA

Tricuspid valve

RV   LV

Mitral valve (Bicuspid valve)

Legend:
AO = Aorta
PA = Pulmonary artery
RA = Right atrium
LA = Left atrium
RV = Right ventricle
LV = Left ventricle

FIGURE 12-3 Heart chambers.

PRACTICE FOR LEARNING: HEART CHAMBERS

Fill in the blanks with the correct answer.

1. Write the name for the upper chambers.

   _____

2. Write the name for the lower chambers.

   _____

3. Write the name for the partition that separates the right side of the heart from the left side._____

Answers: **1.** atria. **2.** ventricles. **3.** septum.

Heart Valves

There are four valves in the heart. They open to let blood in, and then they close tightly to ensure there is no backward flow of blood (Figure 12-4).

Two of the valves are called semilunar valves (Figure 12-4A). The semilunar valve at the entrance of the pulmonary artery is called the pulmonary valve. The one at the entrance of the aorta is called the aortic valve.

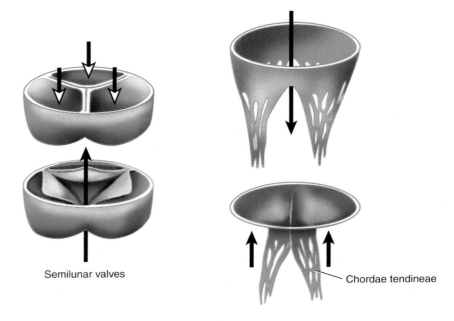

Semilunar valves

Chordae tendineae

Atrioventricular valves

FIGURE 12-4 Heart valves. A, Semilunar valves. B, Atrioventricular valves.

IN BRIEF

Semilunar valves
pulmonary valve
aortic valve

**Atrioventricular
(AV) valves**
bicuspid valve
tricuspid valve

The other two valves are called atrioventricular (**ay-tree-oh-ven-TRICK-yoo-lar**) valves, or AV valves (Figure 12-4B). The AV valve between the right atrium and ventricle is called the tricuspid valve because it has three cusps, or flaps. The AV valve between the left atrium and ventricle has two cusps and is referred to as the bicuspid, or mitral, valve.

Tough fibers called chordae tendineae (**KOR-dee TEN-din-ee**) attach the flaps of the AV valves to the heart wall. They ensure that the flaps close tightly.

PRACTICE FOR LEARNING: VALVES AND CHORDAE TENDINEAE

Write the correct answer in the space provided.

1. Name the valve that separate the atria from the ventricles.

   _____

2. How many flaps does the tricuspid valve have?

   _____

3. Write another name for the bicuspid valve.

   _____

4. Write the name of the fibrous cords that attach the atrioventricular flaps to the heart wall.

   _____

5. Write the name of the valve located at the entrance to the pulmonary artery. _____

6. Write the name of the valve located at the entrance to the aortic artery. _____

Answers: **1.** atrioventricular (AV) valve. **2.** three. **3.** mitral valve. **4.** chordae tendineae. **5.** pulmonary valve. **6.** aortic valve.

Walls of the Heart

The heart has three walls (Figure 12-5). The outer wall is the epicardium (**ep-ih-KAR-dee-um**). The middle wall is the myocardium (**my-oh-KAR-dee-um**). It is composed of the muscle that contracts the ventricles, pumping the blood out of the heart. The inner wall is the endocardium (**en-do-KAR-dee-um**).

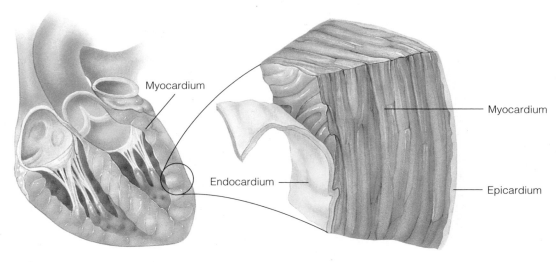

FIGURE 12-5 Walls of the heart.

Pericardium

The heart is surrounded by a sac called the pericardium (Figure 12-6). It has two layers. Pericardial fluid lies between the layers.

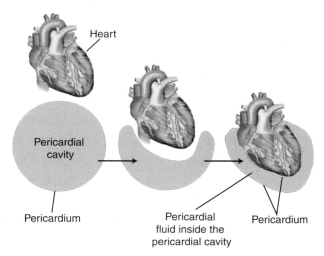

FIGURE 12-6 Pericardium.

PRACTICE FOR LEARNING: HEART WALLS

1. Name the three heart walls illustrated in Figure 12-5.

   _____ , _____ ,

   _____ .

2. Using the terminology you have learned, write the meaning of the following word parts.

   a. my/o _____

   b. cardi/o _____

   c. -um _____

   d. epi- _____

   e. endo- _____

3. Mark the following statements as True or False.

   a. The pericardium surrounds the heart. _____

   b. The endocardium is a sac filled with fluid. _____

   c. The pericardium is responsible for muscular contraction. _____

   d. The pericardium has two layers. _____

> *Answers:* **1.** epicardium, myocardium, endocardium. **2.** a. muscle, b. heart, c. structure, d. on; upon, e. within. **3.** a. True. b. False. c. False. d. True.

12.3 HOW THE HEART BEATS

IN BRIEF

Electrical impulses travel through the heart from the pacemaker to the Purkinje fibers, causing the ventricles to contract and the heart to beat. An **ECG** monitors the electrical impulses as they travel through the heart.

Electrical impulses stimulate the heart to beat. Unlike other nerve impulses, they do not come from the brain. They are created in special tissue in the atrium called the pacemaker. They then follow a trail through the heart to the Purkinje (per-**KIN**-jee) fibers, which extend throughout the ventricles. When the impulses reach the Purkinje fibers, the ventricles contract and push blood out of the heart into arteries.

The trail the impulses follow from the pacemaker to the ventricles is called the conduction pathway. It is illustrated in Figure 12-7. When the electrical impulses follow the conduction pathway properly, the heart will beat in a regular way, 60 to 90 beats per minute. This is called **normal sinus rhythm.**

The electrical activity of the heart can be recorded in a procedure called an electrocardiogram (ee-**leck**-troh-**KAR**-dee-oh-gram). It is usually referred to as an ECG or EKG. Figure 12-8 shows a normal ECG. The spikes or waves on the record represent the strength of contraction of the atria and ventricles.

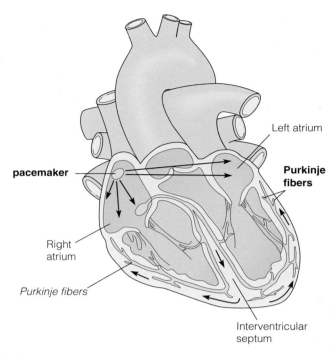

FIGURE 12-7 Arrows indicate electrical impulses as they travel from the pacemaker to the Purkinje fibers.

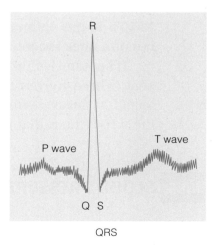

FIGURE 12-8 Normal electrocardiogram. P wave indicates strength of atrial contraction. QRS wave indicates strength of ventricular contraction. T wave indicates ventricular relaxation.

PRACTICE FOR LEARNING: HOW THE HEART BEATS AND ECGS

1. What is the purpose of an electrocardiogram?

   _____

2. When electrical impulses reach the Purkinje fibers, what contracts?

   _____

Answers: **1.** to record the electrical activity through the heart.
2. the ventricles.

12.4 BLOOD PRESSURE AND PULSE

When blood flows through an artery, it pushes on the artery wall. The pressure this creates is called blood pressure.

Blood pressure is measured with an instrument called a **sphygmomanometer** (**sfig-moh-man-OM-eh-ter**). Figure 12-9 shows you what that instrument looks like.

A normal blood pressure reading is written like this: 120/80 mm Hg. The first number shows the pressure against the arterial wall when the ventricles contract, pumping the blood out of the heart, and the second number shows the pressure against the arterial wall when the ventricles relax. High blood pressure is called **hypertension** (**high-per-TEN-shun**). Low blood pressure is called **hypotension** (**high-poh-TEN-shun**).

Hypertension is defined as 140/90 mm Hg or greater. Hypotension is lower than 120/80. Many experts now suggest that 115/75 is the optimum. Thus, a new category called **prehypertension** (**pree-high-per-TEN-shun**) is defined as 120/80 to 139/89.

The arteries dilate and constrict in unison with the heartbeat. These movements, known as a pulse, can be readily detected at several sites. Figure 12-10 illustrates the pulse site in the wrist (the radial pulse) and the neck (the carotid pulse).

IN BRIEF

Sphygmomanometer
A device used to measure blood pressure. Normal blood pressure reading is 120/80 mm Hg.

PRACTICE FOR LEARNING: BLOOD PRESSURE AND PULSE

1. Write the name of the device used to measure blood pressure. _____ .

2. The radial pulse is felt at the _____ .

3. The carotid pulse is felt at the _____ .

Answers: **1.** sphygmomanometer. **1.** wrist (over the radius). **3.** neck.

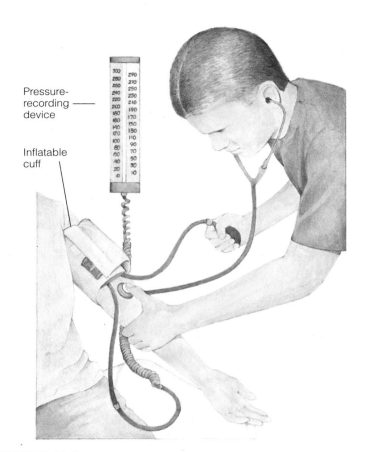

Pressure-recording device

Inflatable cuff

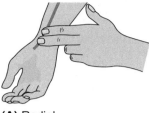

(A) Radial

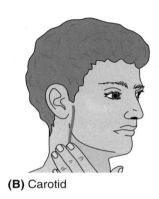

(B) Carotid

FIGURE 12-9 Blood pressure reading using a sphygmomanometer.

FIGURE 12-10 Pulse points.

12.5 BLOOD VESSELS AND CIRCULATION

Figure 12-11 outlines the circulatory system. Blood containing carbon dioxide and waste materials is pumped out of the right side of the heart to the lungs. There, the carbon dioxide and waste are absorbed by the lungs and breathed out. Oxygen is breathed in and absorbed by the blood. This oxygenated (**OCK-see-jeh-nay-ted**) blood then flows back to the left side of the heart, where it is pumped out into arteries. It flows from the arteries into smaller arteries called arterioles until it reaches an organ.

In each organ are the smallest blood vessels, called capillaries. The blood flows into the capillaries. Cells in the organ absorb the oxygen from the blood in the capillaries, as well as nutrients that the blood has picked up from the digestive system before it reaches the organ. At the same time, the organ cells release carbon dioxide and waste into the capillaries. This blood then leaves the capillaries and flows through tiny vessels called venules (small veins) into bigger vessels called veins. The veins lead into the inferior and superior venae cavae (**VEE-nee KAY-vee**), which are large veins. They carry the blood back to the heart. The blood is then pumped to the lungs where the cycle is repeated.

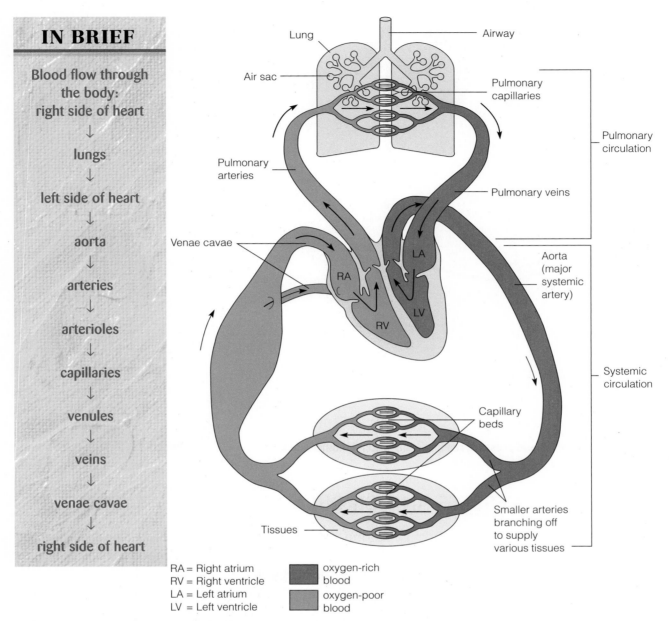

IN BRIEF	
Blood flow through the body: right side of heart	
↓	
lungs	
↓	
left side of heart	
↓	
aorta	
↓	
arteries	
↓	
arterioles	
↓	
capillaries	
↓	
venules	
↓	
veins	
↓	
venae cavae	
↓	
right side of heart	

RA = Right atrium
RV = Right ventricle
LA = Left atrium
LV = Left ventricle

oxygen-rich blood
oxygen-poor blood

FIGURE 12-11   Circulation of blood through the body.

PRACTICE FOR LEARNING: BLOOD VESSELS AND CIRCULATION

1. Name the three types of blood vessels. _____ , _____ , and _____ .

2. What are small arteries called? _____

3. What are small veins called? _____

Answers: **1.** arteries, veins, capillaries. **2.** arterioles. **3.** venules.

12.6 NEW ROOTS AND PREFIX

Use these additional roots and prefix when studying the terms in this chapter.

Root	Meaning
constrict/o	to draw together; constrict
dilat/o	to expand; widen
ech/o	sound

Prefix	Meaning
pan-	all

12.7 LEARNING THE TERMS

Following these steps will make it easier for you to learn medical terms:

1. Pronounce the term repeatedly until it is easy for you.

2. Write it down. Ensure the spelling is correct.

3. Also write the definition. If possible, relate the word to a word, thought, or picture that will help you remember it.

4. Analyze the term with the method taught in this text.

Root		Meaning	
angi/o		blood vessel	
Term	Term Analysis		Definition
angioplasty (**AN**-jee-oh-**plas**-tee)	-plasty = surgical repair; surgical reconstruction		surgical repair of a blood vessel

Root	Meaning
arteri/o	artery

Term	Term Analysis	Definition
arteriosclerosis (ar-**teer**-ee-oh-skleh-**ROH**-sis)	-sclerosis = hardening	hardening of the arteries due to the loss of elasticity in the arterial wall
arteriostenosis (ar-**teer**-ee-oh-steh-**NOH**-sis)	-stenosis = narrowing	narrowing of an artery

Root	Meaning
ather/o	fatty debris

Term	Term Analysis	Definition
atheroma (ath-er-**OH**-mah)	-oma = mass; tumor	fatty mass or debris on the wall of the artery
atherosclerosis (ath-er-oh-skleh-**ROH**-sis)	-sclerosis = hardening	accumulation of fatty debris on the arterial wall

Root	Meaning
cardi/o	heart

Term	Term Analysis	Definition
cardiologist (kar-dee-**OL**-oh-jist)	-logist = specialist in the study of	specialist in the study of the heart including its diseases and treatment
echocardiograph (eck-oh-**KAR**-dee-oh-graf)	-graph = instrument used to record ech/o = sound	an instrument used to record an image of the heart using ultrasound (Figure 12-12)

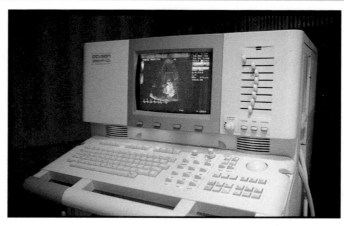

FIGURE 12-12 Echocardiograph. (Photograph by Marcia Butterfield. Courtesy of W. A. Foote Memorial Hospital, Jackson, MI.)

Term	Term Analysis	Definition
cardiomyopathy (**kar**-dee-oh-my-**OP**-ah-thee)	-pathy = disease my/o = muscle	disease of the heart muscle
pancarditis (**pan**-kar-**DYE**-tis)	-itis = inflammation pan- = all	inflammation of all the walls of the heart, including the epicardium, myocardium, and endocardium

Root	Meaning
coron/o	crown

Term	Term Analysis	Definition
coronary arteries (**KOR**-uh-**nehr**-ee)	-ary = pertaining to	the arteries that supply the heart with blood

Root	Meaning
embol/o	plug

Term	Term Analysis	Definition
embolus (**EM**-boh-lus)	-us = condition; thing	a blood clot or clump of foreign material moving through a blood vessel obstructing blood flow. Can be fatal.

Root	Meaning
isch/o	hold back

Term	Term Analysis	Definition
myocardial ischemia (my-oh-**KAR**-dee-al iss-**KEE**-me-ah)	-emia = blood condition -al = pertaining to my/o = muscle cardi/o = heart	deficiency of blood in the heart muscle

Root	Meaning
phleb/o (see also ven/o)	vein

Term	Term Analysis	Definition
thrombophlebitis (**throm-boh-fleh-BYE**-tis)	-itis = inflammation thromb/o = clot	inflammation of a vein with clot formation

Root	Meaning
rhythm/o	rhythm

Term	Term Analysis	Definition
arrhythmia (ah-**RITH**-mee-ah)	-ia = state of; condition; process an- = no; not	deviation from the normal heart rhythm

NOTE: The "n" changes to "r" when the root starts with an "r."

Root	Meaning
thromb/o	clot

Term	Term Analysis	Definition
thrombus (**THROM**-bus)	-us = condition; thing	a blood clot that obstructs a blood vessel

Root	Meaning	
vas/o	vessel	
Term	**Term Analysis**	**Definition**
vasoconstriction (**vas**-oh-kon-**STRICK**-shun)	-ion = process constrict/o = to draw together; constrict	constriction or narrowing of the walls of a vessel
vasodilation (**vas**-oh-dye-**LAY**-shun)	-ion = process dilat/o =expand; widen	widening of the walls of a vessel

Root	Meaning	
ven/o	vein	
Term	**Term Analysis**	**Definition**
venous (**VEE**-nus)	-ous = pertaining to	pertaining to a vein

Prefix	Meaning	
brady-	slow	
Term	**Term Analysis**	**Definition**
bradycardia (**brad**-ee-**KAR**-dee-uh)	-ia = condition; state of cardi/o = heart	slow heartbeat

Prefix	Meaning	
tachy-	fast	
Term	**Term Analysis**	**Definition**
tachycardia (**tack**-ee-**KAR**-dee-ah)	-ia = condition; state of cardi/o = heart	fast heartbeat

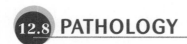

12.8 PATHOLOGY

Aneurysm (AN-yoo-rizm)

An abnormal bulge in the wall of an artery (Figure 12-13). It occurs most often in the aorta or in the brain.

A ruptured aneurysm occurs when the wall of the artery bursts. This causes internal hemorrhaging, which may result in death.

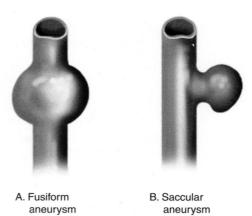

A. Fusiform
aneurysm

B. Saccular
aneurysm

FIGURE 12-13   Aneurysms. A, Fusiform—bulging on both sides of the artery. B, Saccular—bulging on one side of the artery.

Coronary Artery Disease (CAD)

Complete or partial blockage of the coronary arteries resulting in decreased blood flow to the heart muscle (Figure 12-14). A common cause of CAD is atherosclerosis.

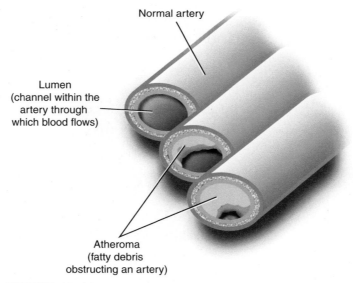

Normal artery

Lumen
(channel within the
artery through
which blood flows)

Atheroma
(fatty debris
obstructing an artery)

FIGURE 12-14   Coronary artery disease caused by atherosclerosis.

Cerebrovascular Accident (CVA); Stroke

Lack of blood to the brain, depriving it of oxygen and nutrients (Figure 12-15). May be caused by a burst aneurysm or atherosclerosis.

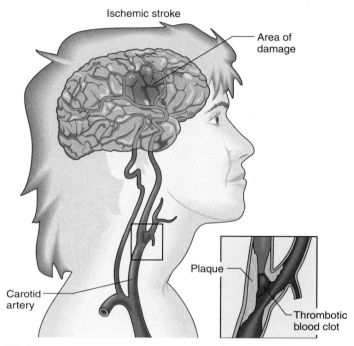

FIGURE 12-15 An ischemic stroke is caused by the lack of blood to the brain. The obstruction is due to plaque (atheroma) or thrombus.

Cardiac Arrest

The heart suddenly stops pumping blood.

Myocardial Infarction (MI); Heart Attack

Myocardial infarction means death of the heart muscle. Look at Figure 12-16. When one or more of the coronary arteries are blocked because of coronary heart disease, blood flow to the heart muscle stops and the tissue dies. The heart is unable to function properly, and not enough blood is pumped to the body's tissues.

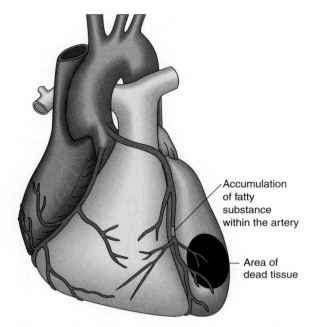

FIGURE 12-16 Myocardial infarction (heart attack).

The primary symptom is **angina pectoris,** which means "pain over the chest area."

Varicose Veins

Dilated and twisted veins, usually the saphenous veins of the lower leg (Figure 12-17). The cause is damaged valves in the veins. They do not close, allowing the blood to flow backwards. The blood forms pools, which dilate the veins.

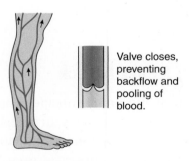

Valve closes, preventing backflow and pooling of blood.

A. Normal veins

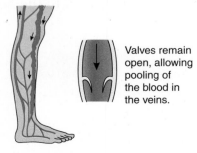

Valves remain open, allowing pooling of the blood in the veins.

B. Varicose veins

C.

FIGURE 12-17 Varicose veins.

12.9 REVIEW EXERCISES

Exercise 12-1 | LOOK-ALIKE AND SOUND-ALIKE WORDS

Below is a list of look-alike and sound-alike words. Study the definitions of each set of words, then read the sentences carefully and circle the word in parentheses that correctly completes the meaning.

arrhythmia	abnormal heart rhythm
erythremia	increase in the number of red blood cells
infarction	death of tissue
infection	to contaminate with a disease
venous	pertaining to a vein
venus	one of the planets around the earth
palpation	to feel
palpitation	fast heartbeat
pericardium	structure around the heart
precordium	area in front of the heart
vain	unsuccessful, conceited
vane	a device used to show the way the wind blows; weathervane
vein	a type of blood vessel

1. This 53-year-old-man is admitted with an upper respiratory (**infection/infarction**) and pneumonia of two days' duration.

2. A diagnosis of renal (**infection/infarction**) due to narrowing of the renal arteries was made.

3. There are abnormal jugular (**venus/venous**) pulses; the carotid arterial pulses are normal.

4. On (**palpation/palpitation**) there was a mass noted over the breastbone.

5. The patient was admitted with shortness of breath and (**palpations/palpitations**).

6. In open-heart surgery, a segment of the saphenous (**vain/vane/vein**) is removed and used as a graft.

7. In a (**vain/vane/vein**) attempt at hemostasis, the artery was clamped and ligated.

8. Previous pancarditis has resulted in inflammation of the (**precordium/pericardium**), the structure surrounding the heart.

| Exercise 12-2 | MATCHING WORD PARTS WITH MEANING |

Match word part in Column A *with meaning in* Column B.

	Column A	Column B
_____	1. dilat/o	A. fatty debris
_____	2. -sclerosis	B. vessel
_____	3. -stenosis	C. crown
_____	4. pan-	D. narrowing
_____	5. endo-	E. hold back
_____	6. isch/o	F. widen
_____	7. vas/o	G. vein
_____	8. coron/o	H. hardening
_____	9. phleb/o	I. all
_____	10. ather/o	J. within

Exercise 12-3 LABELING

Using the body structures listed below, write the name of each numbered structure in Figure 12-18 on the corresponding line on page 272.

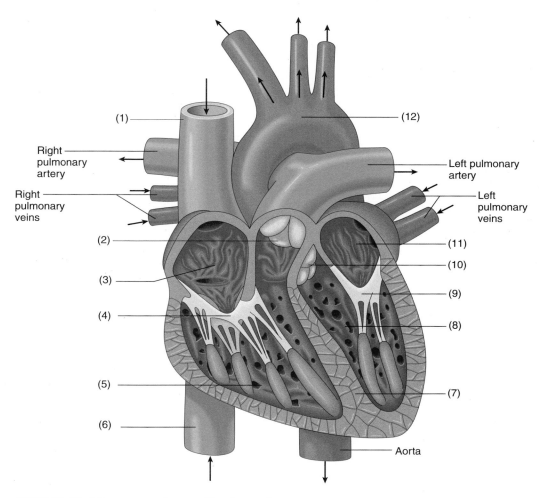

FIGURE 12-18 Heart and major blood vessels.

aorta
_____

aortic semilunar valve
_____

inferior vena cava
_____

interventricular septum
_____

left atrium
_____

left ventricle
_____

mitral valve
_____

pulmonary semilunar valve
_____

right atrium
_____

right ventricle
_____

superior vena cava _____

tricuspid valve _____

    1. _____

    2. _____

    3. _____

    4. _____

    5. _____

    6. _____

    7. _____

    8. _____

    9. _____

   10. _____

   11. _____

   12. _____

| Exercise 12-4 | **DEFINITIONS—LEARNING THE TERMS** |

Define the following terms.

    1. **arteriosclerosis** _____

    2. **atheroma** _____

    3. **arteriostenosis** _____

    4. **embolus** _____

    5. **thrombus** _____

    6. **ischemia** _____

    7. **vasoconstriction** _____

    8. **bradycardia** _____

    9. **angioplasty** _____

   10. **coronary arteries** _____

| Exercise 12-5 | MATCHING—ANATOMY |

Match the terms below with their descriptions that follow.

atria	bicuspid
chordae tendineae	electrocardiograph
epicardium	pericardium
pulmonary valve	sphygmomanometer
tricuspid	ventricles

1. outermost wall of the heart _____

2. lower chamber of the heart _____

3. left atrioventricular valve _____

4. right atrioventricular valve _____

5. sac surrounding the heart _____

6. anchors atrioventricular valves to the heart wall

   _____

7. instrument that measures blood pressure

   _____

8. upper chambers of the heart _____

9. instrument that records electrical impulses

   _____

10. semilunar valve _____

| Exercise 12-6 | DEFINITIONS—PATHOLOGY |

Match the following conditions with their descriptions below and on page 274.

aneurysm	angina pectoris
cardiac arrest	cerebrovascular accident
hypertension	myocardial infarction
myocardial ischemia	varicose veins

1. chest pains _____

2. dilated, twisted veins of the leg _____

3. abnormal bulge in the wall of the artery

   _____

4. interruption of blood to the brain _____

5. condition where the heart muscle dies because of a lack of oxygen _____

6. hold back of blood to heart muscle _____

7. sudden stoppage of the heart _____

8. high blood pressure _____

Exercise 12-7   DEFINITIONS IN CONTEXT

Define the bolded terms in context. Use your medical dictionary if necessary.

Report #1 ECHOCARDIOGRAPHY REPORT

No **arrhythmia**. The right **atrium** is at the upper limits of normal. The **ventricle** is also normal. The **aortic valve** and **tricuspid** function normally. There was no evidence of a **thrombus** within the **coronary arteries**.

    a. echocardiography _____

    b. arrhythmia _____

    c. atrium _____

    d. ventricle _____

    e. aortic valve _____

    f. tricuspid _____

    g. thrombus _____

    h. coronary arteries _____

Report #2 HISTORY AND PHYSICAL EXAMINATION

This patient says she had a severe attack of **angina pectoris** about two years ago and was hospitalized for **myocardial ischemia.**

About one day ago, she started having difficulty breathing plus **nausea** and vomiting. Because her breathing was very difficult, she went to the emergency department of the hospital and was found to have a **myocardial infarction.**

On physical examination, the patient does appear older than her stated age of 56. Her **blood pressure** is **182/80.** Her **pulse** is 130, and she has **tachycardia.**

Neck veins are **distended.** Abdomen is soft, not distended. No masses can be felt. There is **edema** in the lower extremities.

DIAGNOSES

1. MYOCARDIAL INFARCTION

2. ATHEROSCLEROSIS

3. CARDIOVASCULAR DISEASE DUE TO HYPERTENSION

   a. angina pectoris_____

   b. myocardial ischemia _____

   c. nausea _____

   d. myocardial infarction _____

   e. blood pressure _____

   f. 182/80 _____

   g. pulse _____

   h. tachycardia _____

   i. distended _____

   j. edema _____

   k. atherosclerosis _____

   l. cardiovascular disease _____

  m. hypertension _____

Exercise 12-8

SPELLING

Circle any words that are spelled incorrectly in the list below. Then correct the spelling in the space provided.

1. anurysm _____

2. arhythmia _____

3. atherosclerosis _____

4. ischemia _____

5. thromboflebitis _____

6. vesoconstriction _____

7. chordae tendineae _____

8. coronery _____

9. sphygmomanometer _____

10. embolous _____

12.10 PRONUNCIATION AND SPELLING

Listen, read, and study, so you can speak and write.

1. Listen to each word on the audio CD.

2. Pronounce each word carefully.

3. Spell each word in the space provided.

Word	Pronunciation	Spelling
aneurysm	**AN**-yoo-rizm	
angioplasty	**AN**-jee-oh-**plas**-tee	
aorta	ay-**OR**-tah	
arrhythmia	ah-**RITH**-mee-ah	
arteries	**AR**-ter-eez	
arterioles	ar-**TEER**-ee-ohlz	
arteriosclerosis	ar-**teer**-ee-oh-skleh-**ROH**-sis	
atheroma	**ath**-er-**OH**-mah	
atherosclerosis	**ath**-er-oh-skleh-**ROH**-sis	
atrioventricular	ay-tree-oh-ven-**TRICK**-yoo-lar	
bicuspid	bye-**KUS**-pid	
bradycardia	brad-ee-**KAR**-dee-uh	
capillaries	ka-**PILL**-ah-reez	
cardiologist	kar-dee-**OL**-oh-jist	
cardiomyopathy	kar-dee-oh-my-**OP**-ah-thee	
chordae tendineae	**KOR**-dee **TEN**-din-ee	
coronary	**KOR**-uh-**nehr**-ee	
embolus	**EM**-boh-lus	
endocardium	en-doh-**KAR**-dee-um	
epicardium	ep-ih-**KAR**-dee-um	
infarction	in-**FARK**-shun	
ischemia	iss-**KEE**-me-ah	

Word	Pronunciation	Spelling
myocardium	my-oh-**KAR**-dee-um	
sphygmomanometer	**sfig**-moh-man-**OM**-eh-ter	
tachycardia	**tack**-ee-**KAR**-dee-ah	
thrombophlebitis	**throm**-boh-fleh-**BYE**-tis	
thrombus	**THROM**-bus	
tricuspid	trigh-**KUS**-pid	
vasoconstriction	**vas**-oh-kon-**STRICK**-shun	
vasodilation	**vas**-oh-dye-**LAY**-shun	
veins	**VAYNZ**	
vena cava	**VE**-nah **KAY**-vah	
ventricle	**VEN**-trih-kul	
venules	**VEN**-yoolz	

CHAPTER 13

Blood

LEARNING OBJECTIVES

After studying this chapter and completing the review exercises, you should be able to:

1. Name and describe the components of blood.
2. Pronounce, spell, define, and write the medical terms related to the blood.
3. Describe common diseases of the blood.
4. Listen, read, and study so you can speak and write.

INTRODUCTION

In the chapter on the skeletal system, you learned that blood cells are formed in the red bone marrow. In studying the cardiovascular system, you learned that blood carries oxygen and nutrients to the cells and carries away waste products. In this chapter, you will learn about the makeup of blood and the role it plays in fighting disease.

13.1 MAJOR COMPONENTS OF BLOOD

PRACTICE FOR LEARNING: **MAJOR COMPONENTS OF BLOOD**

Write the words below in the correct spaces on Figure 13-1. To help you, the number beside the word tells you where it goes on the figure. Be sure to pronounce each word as you write it. Repeat the pronunciation several times if you find the word hard to say.

1. plasma (**PLAZ**-mah)

2. formed elements

3. erythrocyte (eh-**RITH**-roh-sight)

4. thrombocyte (**THROM**-boh-sight)

5. basophil (**BAY**-soh-fill)

6. neutrophil (**NEW**-troh-fill)

7. eosinophil (ee-oh-**SIN**-oh-fill)

8. lymphocyte (**LIM**-foh-sight)

9. monocyte (**MON**-oh-sight)

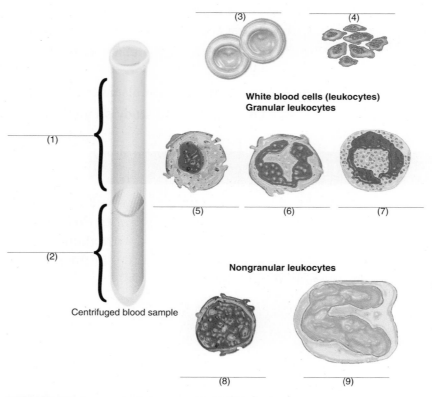

FIGURE 13-1   Formed elements of the blood.

13.2 BLOOD COMPOSITION

IN BRIEF

Blood consists of
formed elements
and plasma

Whole blood is about 45% solid and 55% liquid, as illustrated in Figure 13-1. The solid portion is referred to as formed elements. Formed elements are produced in the bone marrow and consist of three types of blood cells: red blood cells (RBCs), white blood cells (WBCs), and platelets. RBCs are also called erythrocytes, WBCs are called leukocytes, and platelets are called thrombocytes.

The liquid portion of blood is called plasma. Because plasma is more than 90% water, it is thin and almost colorless when it is separated from the blood cells.

Formed Elements

IN BRIEF

Formed elements
erythrocytes
leukocytes
thrombocytes

Granular leukocytes
basophils
neutrophils
and eosinophils

Nongranular leukocytes
lymphocytes
monocytes

Erythrocytes transport
oxygen and carbon
dioxide

Leukocytes fight
infection

Thrombocytes are
important in blood
clotting

Erythrocytes contain a protein called hemoglobin (**HEE-moh-gloh-bin**) (Hgb). It has the ability to bind with oxygen and carbon dioxide. As erythrocytes circulate in the body, the hemoglobin in them transports oxygen to the organ cells and carries carbon dioxide away from the organ cells.

Leukocytes fight infections. They have the ability to move from the bloodstream into the site of infection in the tissues. New white blood cells replace old white cells that are destroyed in the fight. As illustrated in Figure 13-1, leukocytes are classified as either granular or nongranular. The granular leukocytes are further classified as either eosinophils, basophils, or neutrophils. The agranular leukocytes are classified as either monocytes or lymphocytes.

Thrombocytes (platelets) initiate blood clotting when bleeding occurs. Platelets gather at the cut and combine with clotting factors in the plasma. This action causes a platelet plug to be formed where the vessel wall has been cut, thus forming a seal to stop bleeding.

Plasma

IN BRIEF

Plasma is the liquid
portion of the blood.

Serum is plasma
without the clotting
elements

Plasma carries many important solids. It transports proteins, fats, gases, salts, and hormones to their various places throughout the body and picks up waste materials from organ cells.

Proteins in the plasma function to maintain water balance in the blood. If too much water escapes from the blood and accumulates in the body tissues, it will cause pooling of water in body tissues. This is called edema (**eh-DEE-mah**).

Other proteins in plasma prevent excessive bleeding by making the blood clot. These proteins are called clotting factors. When clotting factors are removed from the plasma, the liquid that is left is called serum (**SEER-um**). In other words, serum is the clear fluid of plasma minus the clotting elements. Many blood tests are performed on serum.

PRACTICE FOR LEARNING: **BLOOD COMPOSITION**

Underline the correct answer in each sentence.

1. Red blood cells are also known as (leukocytes/platelets/erythrocytes).

2. The liquid portion of the blood is called (plasma/serum).

3. Plasma minus the clotting factors is called (formed elements/serum/blood).

4. Accumulation of water in body tissue is called (anemia/edema/congestion).

5. Platelets are also called (leukocytes/thrombocytes/ erythrocytes).

6. The oxygen-carrying component of red blood cells is (plasma/serum/hemoglobin).

7. The function of white blood cells is (blood clotting/fighting infections).

8. The function of thrombocytes is (blood clotting/fighting infections).

Answers: **1.** erythrocytes. **2.** plasma. **3.** serum. **4.** edema.
5. thrombocytes. **6.** hemoglobin. **7.** fighting infections. **8.** blood clotting.

13.3 BLOOD TYPES

IN BRIEF

type A blood has only
A antigens

type B blood has only B
antigens

type AB blood has
both antigens

type O has neither
antigen

Most people are
Rh positive—they
have Rh antigen

The body's immune system produces antibodies (**AN-tee-bah-deez**) to protect it against invaders such as viruses and bacteria. Any substance that stimulates the body's immune response to produce antibodies is referred to as an antigen (**AN-tih-jen**). (Antigen is an abbreviation for the term "antibody generator.")

There are two antigens that may or may not be on the surface of red blood cells. They are referred to as type A and type B antigens. Blood is classified according to the presence or absence of these antigens. Type A blood has only type A antigens. Type B blood has only type B antigens. Type AB blood has both antigens. Type O blood has neither.

Persons who require a blood transfusion must receive the correct type of blood. If they receive blood that has an antigen that their blood does not recognize, antibodies will be formed because the antigen is seen as a foreign body. This reaction is called an antigen-antibody reaction.

The antigen-antibody reaction causes clumping of red blood cells and can be fatal. Blood must therefore be cross-matched before it is transfused into a patient.

There are several other blood antigens. The most important is the Rh antigen, which was first discovered by examining the blood of Rhesus monkeys. Most people are Rh positive (Rh+), meaning they have the Rh antigen. Those who lack it are Rh negative (Rh−).

PRACTICE FOR LEARNING: BLOOD TYPES

Answer the following questions on the space provided.

1. Define antigen._____
   _____
   _____

2. Name four blood types. _____
   _____

3. What happens when a person is transfused with the wrong type of blood? _____
   _____

Answers: **1.** any substance that stimulates the body's immune response to produce antibodies. **2.** A, B, AB, O. **3.** antigen-antibody reaction occurs, causing the red blood cells to clump.

13.4 NEW SUFFIXES

Use these additional suffixes when studying the terms in this chapter.

Suffix	Meaning
-lysis	destruction; breakdown
-poietin	hormone regulating the production of blood cells

13.5 LEARNING THE TERMS

Root	Meaning
erythr/o	red

Term	Term Analysis	Definition
erythropoietin (eh-**rith**-roh-**POI**-eh-tin)	-poietin = hormone regulating the production of blood cells	hormone in the kidney that stimulates the production of red blood cells in the bone marrow

Root	Meaning
hemat/o; hem/o	blood

Term	Term Analysis	Definition
hemolysis (hee-**MOL**-ih-sis)	-lysis = breakdown; separation; destruction	breakdown of blood
hematology (hee-mah-**TOL**-oh-jee)	-logy = study of	study of blood, blood disorders, and their treatment

Root	Meaning
leuk/o	white

Term	Term Analysis	Definition
leukocyte (**LOO**-koh-sight)	-cyte = cell	white blood cell

Root	Meaning
myel/o	bone marrow (also spinal cord)

Term	Term Analysis	Definition
myelogenous (my-eh-**LOJ**-en-us)	-genous = produced by	produced in the bone marrow

Root	Meaning
thromb/o	clot

Term	Term Analysis	Definition
thrombosis (throm-**BOH**-sis)	-osis = abnormal condition	abnormal condition of blood clots
thrombolysis (throm-**BOL**-ih-sis)	-lysis = destruction; breakdown; separation	breakdown of clots

Suffix	Meaning
-blast	immature; growing thing

Term	Term Analysis	Definition
hemocytoblast (**hee**-moh-**SIGHT**-oh-blast)	hem/o = blood cyt/o = cell	an immature blood cell that can develop into any type of mature blood cell. Also known as stem cells.

Suffix	Meaning
-cytosis	abnormal condition of cells; abnormal increase in the number of cells

Term	Term Analysis	Definition
leukocytosis (**loo**-koh-sigh-**TOH**-sis)	leuk/o = white	abnormal increase in the number of white blood cells
NOTE: Usually a sign of an inflammation occurring inside the body		

Suffix		Meaning	
-emia		blood condition	
Term	**Term Analysis**		**Definition**
anemia (ah-**NEE**-mee-ah)	an- = lack of; no; not		lack of red blood cells or hemoglobin content in the blood
erythremia (er-ih-**THREE**-mee-ah)	erythr/o = red		abnormal increase in the number of red blood cells

Suffix		Meaning	
-penia		deficient; decrease	
Term	**Term Analysis**		**Definition**
erythrocytopenia; erythropenia (eh-**rith**-roh-**sigh**-toh-**PEE**-nee-ah); (eh-**rith**-roh-**PEE**-nee-ah)	erythr/o = red cyt/o = cell		decrease in the number of red blood cells
pancytopenia (**pan**-sigh-toh-**PEE**-nee-ah)	pan- = all cyt/o = cell		decrease in the number of all blood cells

Suffix		Meaning	
-poiesis		production; manufacture; formation	
Term	**Term Analysis**		**Definition**
erythropoiesis (eh-**rith**-roh-poi-**EE**-sis)	erythr/o = red		production of red blood cells

Suffix		Meaning	
-stasis		stopping; controlling	
Term	**Term Analysis**		**Definition**
hemostasis (**hee**-moh-**STAY**-sis)	hem/o = blood		stopping of bleeding

13.6 PATHOLOGY

Anemia

Insufficient red blood cells and hemoglobin in the blood. The lack of hemoglobin makes the blood unable to carry enough oxygen to tissues. As a result, the patient becomes tired and pale. There are many different types of anemia. Some can be fatal, and others are benign.

Hemophilia (hee-moh-FEE-lee-ah)

Spontaneous or traumatic bleeding into skin, joints, or mouth.

A genetic condition characterized by a lack of clotting factors VIII and IX, which are necessary for blood to clot. The blood does not clot quickly and bleeding is prolonged. The patient can lose a large amount of blood, which can be fatal.

Leukemia (loo-KEE-mee-ah)

A form of bone marrow cancer that results in a malignant increase in the number of white blood cells.

The white blood cells eventually replace red blood cells, platelets, and normal functioning white blood cells. Oxygen delivery to tissues, blood clotting, and immunity are impaired as a result. Leukemic cells may spread to other organs such as the spleen, lymph nodes, and central nervous system.

Multiple Myeloma (my-eh-LOH-mah)

Malignant neoplasm of the bone marrow. This results in bone destruction, as the tumor replaces bone.

13.7 REVIEW EXERCISES

Exercise 13-1 | LOOK-ALIKE AND SOUND-ALIKE

Below is a list of look-alike and sound-alike words. Study the definitions of each set of words, then read the sentences carefully and circle the word in parentheses that correctly completes the meaning.

hemostasis	stoppage of blood
homeostasis	balanced yet varied state
leukopenia	deficiency of white blood cells
leukemia	malignant increase in the number of white blood cells

hyperchromic	excessively pigmented red blood cells
hypochromic	underpigmented red blood cells
myogenous	produced in muscle tissue
myelogenous	produced by bone marrow
erythremia	abnormal increase in the number of red blood cells
erythema	redness of the skin

1. At the end of the operation, the arteries were tied and (**homeostasis/hemostasis**) was obtained. The patient left the operating room in good condition.

2. In a certain type of anemia, there is underdevelopment of the bone marrow with associated (**leukemia/leukopenia**).

3. In iron deficiency anemia, the erythrocytes are less than their normal color, they are (**hyperchromic/hypochromic**).

4. This 61-year-old man was admitted with a diagnosis of acute (**myelogenous/myogenous**) leukemia.

5. The patient was admitted with (**erythremia/erythema**) to the entire body because of a rash due to a drug allergy.

Exercise 13-2   MATCHING WORD PARTS WITH MEANING

Match the word part in Column A *with its meaning in* Column B.

	Column A		Column B
_____	1. hem/o	A.	destruction
_____	2. -lysis	B.	abnormal condition of cells
_____	3. -stasis		
_____	4. -poiesis	C.	clot
_____	5. pan-	D.	blood
_____	6. -penia	E.	deficient
_____	7. thromb/o	F.	blood condition
_____	8. -emia	G.	stopping
_____	9. -cytosis	H.	all
_____	10. -blast	I.	production
		J.	immature

Exercise 13-3 | DEFINITIONS—ANATOMY AND PATHOLOGY

Define the following terms.

1. formed elements _____

2. plasma _____

3. hemophilia _____

4. edema _____

5. anemia _____

6. multiple myeloma _____

7. type A blood _____

8. hemoglobin _____

9. antibodies _____

10. antigens _____

11. leukemia _____

Exercise 13-4 | DEFINITIONS—LEARNING THE TERMS

Define the following terms.

1. hematology _____

2. myelogenous _____

3. thrombosis _____

4. thrombocyte _____

5. thrombus _____

6. hemocytoblast _____

7. leukocytosis _____

8. erythremia _____

9. pancytopenia _____

10. hemostasis _____

| **Exercise 13-5** | SPELLING |

Circle any words that are spelled incorrectly in the list below.
Then correct the spelling in the space provided.

1. cerum _____

2. hemolysis _____

3. plattelets _____

4. myelogenous _____

5. arithrocytes _____

6. leukopoiesis _____

7. hemostasis _____

8. hemopillia _____

9. adema _____

10. myeloma _____

13.8 PRONUNCIATION AND SPELLING

1. Listen to each word on the audio CD.

2. Pronounce each word carefully.

3. Spell each word in the space provided.

Word	Pronunciation	Spelling
anemia	ah-**NEE**-mee-ah	
antibodies	**AN**-tee-**bah**-deez	
edema	eh-**DEE**-mah	
erythremia	er-ih-**THREE**-mee-ah	
erythrocytopenia	eh-**rith**-roh-**sigh**-toh-**PEE**-nee-ah	
erythropoiesis	eh-**rith**-roh-poi-**EE**-sis	
hematology	hee-mah-**TOL**-oh-jee	
hemoglobin	**HEE**-moh-**gloh**-bin	

Word	Pronunciation	Spelling
hemolysis	hee-**MOL**-ih-sis	
hemophilia	**hee**-moh-**FEE**-lee-ah	
hemostasis	**hee**-moh-**STAY**-sis	
leukemia	loo-**KEE**-mee-ah	
leukocytes	**LOO**-koh-sights	
leukocytosis	**loo**-koh-sigh-**TOH**-sis	
myelogenous	**my**-eh-**LOJ**-en-us	
pancytopenia	**pan**-sigh-toh-**PEE**-nee-ah	
plasma	**PLAZ**-mah	
serum	**SEER**-um	
thrombocyte	**THROM**-boh-sight	
thrombolysis	throm-**BOL**-ih-sis	
thrombosis	throm-**BOH**-sis	

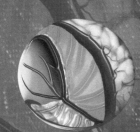

CHAPTER 14

Lymphatic and Immune Systems

CHAPTER OUTLINE

LEARNING OBJECTIVES

After studying this chapter and completing the review exercises, you should be able to:

1. Locate and describe the organs of the lymphatic system.
2. Define terms relating to the immune system.
3. Pronounce, spell, define, and write the medical terms related to the lymphatic and immune systems.
4. Describe common diseases of the lymphatic and immune systems.
5. Listen, read, and study so you can speak and write.

INTRODUCTION

The **lymphatic** (lim-**FAH**-tick) system is the body's other circulatory system. It works with the blood system to fight infection and disease, transport nutrients, and drain excess fluid from tissues.

14.1 MAJOR ORGANS OF THE LYMPHATIC SYSTEM

PRACTICE FOR LEARNING: MAJOR ORGANS OF THE LYMPHATIC SYSTEM

Write the words below in the correct spaces on Figure 14-1. To help you, the number beside the word tells you where it goes on the figure. Be sure to pronounce each word as you write it. Repeat the pronunciation several times if you find the word hard to say.

1. tonsils (**TON**-silz)

2. lymph vessels (**LIMF VESS**-elz)

3. thymus (**THIGH**-mus)

4. spleen (**SPLEEN**)

5. lymph nodes

14.2 LYMPHATIC SYSTEM

As you saw in Figure 14-1, the lymphatic system consists of a vascular system, the lymph nodes, the thymus gland, the spleen, and the tonsils. The fluid traveling through the vascular system is called lymph.

The lymphatic system serves a number of important functions in the body. Of primary importance is the task of draining excess fluids away from body tissues and delivering them to the bloodstream. This system also transports nutrients to body tissues. Because of the presence of lymphocytes and monocytes, the lymphatic system also plays an important role in the body's defense against infection.

IN BRIEF

Parts of the lymphatic system

vascular system
lymph
lymph nodes
thymus gland
spleen

Functions of the lymphatic system

immunity
drains excess fluid
carries nutrients

Lymphatic Vessels

Look at Figure 14-2. You will see that the vascular system consists of three types of vessels: lymphatic capillaries, lymphatic vessels (lymphatics), and the right and left lymphatic ducts.

The lymphatic capillaries are the smallest of these vessels. They are present in body tissues. Excess fluid and bacteria from body tissues seep into the lymphatic capillaries. Once inside the capillaries, the fluid is called lymph.

As illustrated in Figure 14-2, the lymph flows from the lymphatic capillaries, into larger vessels called lymphatics. The lymphatics ultimately drain into the largest vessels of the lymphatic system, called lymphatic ducts.

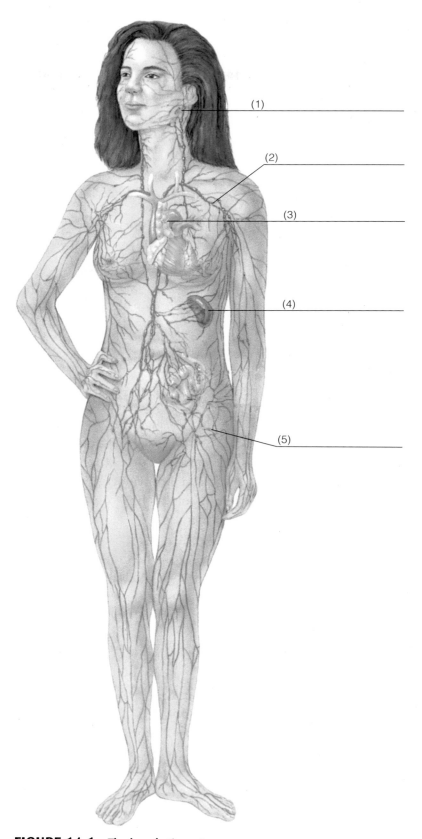

(1) _____

(2) _____

(3) _____

(4) _____

(5) _____

FIGURE 14-1   The lymphatic system.

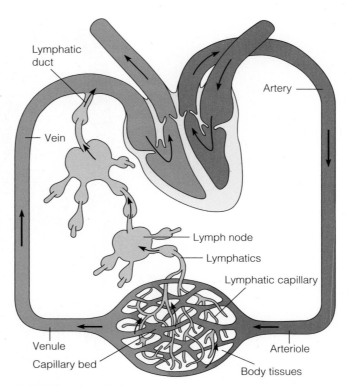

FIGURE 14-2 Lymph vessels.

IN BRIEF

Lymph flows from the
lymphatic capillaries
↓
lymphatics
↓
right and left
lymphatic ducts
↓
bloodstream

Lymph node clusters

cervical
submandibular
axillary
inguinal
mediastinal

Lymph nodes digest
unwanted material

The two lymphatic ducts are shown in Figure 14-3. Lymph from the right side of the head, neck, and chest and from the right arm drains into the right lymphatic duct. Lymph from the rest of the body drains into the left lymphatic duct. Both of the lymphatic ducts drain into the bloodstream.

Lymph is cleaned by lymph nodes before it drains into the bloodstream. These nodes are located in clusters at various sites in the body. Look at Figure 14-3. You will see the principal clusters of nodes. They are called the cervical, submandibular, axillary, mediastinal, and inguinal nodes.

The lymph nodes act as filtration devices for lymph and contain a great number of white blood cells called **phagocytes** (**FAG-oh-sights**). Phagocytes (phag/o = to eat; -cyte = cell) eat bacteria.

You can see the thymus gland in Figure 14-1. It is located near the heart in the thoracic cavity. It is important because it protects the body from disease. It also plays a role in the development of lymphocytes. Remember from Chapter 13 that lymphocytes are white blood cells that fight against foreign substances such as viruses and bacteria.

The spleen is also shown in Figure 14-1. It is located in the left side of the abdominal cavity. It produces and stores red blood cells and gets rid of old red blood cells. It also eliminates bacteria from the blood.

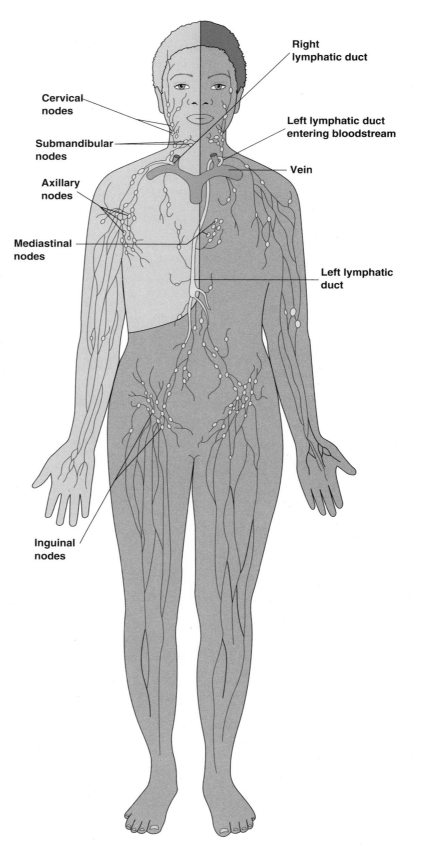

FIGURE 14-3 Lymphatic ducts and lymph nodes. Notice the body areas served by the two lymphatic ducts.

Tonsils are made of lymphatic tissue. Three pairs are located in the throat. The palatine (**PAL**-ah-tine) tonsils are normally referred to simply as tonsils. The pharyngeal (far-**IN**-jee-al) tonsils are commonly called the adenoids (**AD**-eh-noids). The lingual (**LING**-gwal) tonsils are at the base of the tongue. Because of their location, they filter bacteria from food and air.

PRACTICE FOR LEARNING: **LYMPHATIC SYSTEM**

Write the answers to the following statements in the space provided.

1. Write the name of the fluid circulating through the lymphatic vessels. _____

2. Write three functions of the lymphatic system.

   _____

   _____

   _____

3. Lymph node clusters under the lower jaw are called

   _____

4. The pharyngeal tonsils are commonly known as _____

5. List three functions of the spleen.

   _____

   _____

   _____

6. Where is the thymus located? _____

Answers: **1.** lymph. **2.** immunity, drains excess fluid, carries nutrients. **3.** submandibular. **4.** adenoids. **5.** stores red blood cells; produces red blood cells; rids the body of old red blood cells and bacteria. **6.** thoracic cavity.

14.3 IMMUNE SYSTEM

<table>
<tr><td>

IN BRIEF

Lymphocytes are important in the immune response

Types of lymphocytes

T lymphocytes (T-cells)

B lymphocytes (B-cells)

T cells kill virus-infected cells and cancerous cells

B cells produce antibodies

</td><td>

The immune system is our protection against disease. This system includes the lymphoid organs (lymph nodes, spleen, and thymus). It also includes lymphocytes and antibodies. When an infectious agent invades the body, the immune response is turned on by two types of lymphocytes: T lymphocytes (T-cells) and B lymphocytes (B-cells).

T-cells recognize and kill cells that have been infected with a virus. They also recognize and kill cancerous cells.

B-cells produce antibodies. These antibodies travel through the blood. They have the ability to attach to foreign cells, labeling them for destruction by phagocytes.

</td></tr>
</table>

PRACTICE FOR LEARNING: IMMUNE SYSTEM

Underline the correct answer in each sentence.

1. (T-cells/B-cells) produce antibodies.

2. (T-cells/B-cells) recognize cells infected with a virus.

3. Lymphocytes are (red blood cells/white blood cells/platelets).

Answers: **1.** B-cells. **2.** T-cells. **3.** white blood cells.

14.4 NEW SUFFIXES

Use these additional suffixes when studying the terms in this chapter.

Suffix	Meaning
-edema	accumulation of fluid in body tissues
-stitial	to place

14.5 LEARNING THE TERMS

Following these steps will make it easier for you to learn medical terms:

1. Pronounce the term repeatedly until it is easy for you.

2. Write it down. Ensure the spelling is correct.

3. Also write the definition. If possible, relate the word to a word, thought, or picture that will help you remember it.

4. Analyze the term with the method taught in this text.

Root	Meaning	
immun/o	immunity; safe	
Term	**Term Analysis**	**Definition**
immuno-deficiency (im-yoo-no-dee-**FISH**-en-see)	deficiency = lacking	inadequate immune response
immunology (im-yoo-**NOL**-oh-jee)	-logy = study of	study of the immune system

Root	Meaning	
lymphaden/o	lymph node	
Term	**Term Analysis**	**Definition**
lymphadenitis (lim-**fad**-eh-**NIGH**-tis)	-itis = inflammation	inflammation of the lymph nodes
lymphadenopathy (lim-**fad**-eh-**NOP**-ah-**thee**)	-pathy = disease	disease of the lymph nodes, especially enlargement of the lymph nodes

Root	Meaning	
lymphangi/o	lymph vessels	
Term	**Term Analysis**	**Definition**
lymphangitis (**lim**-fan-**JIGH**-tis)	-itis = inflammation	inflammation of the lymph vessels

Root	Meaning
lymph/o	lymph

Term	Term Analysis	Definition
lymphedema (lim-feh-**DEE**-mah)	-edema = accumulation of fluid in body tissues	accumulation of fluid in body tissues due to obstruction of lymphatic structures
lymphoid tissue (**LIM**-foyd)	-oid = resembling; pertaining to	pertaining to lymph tissue

NOTE: Includes tissue of the bone marrow, thymus, lymph nodes, spleen, and tonsils.

Root	Meaning
splen/o	spleen

Term	Term Analysis	Definition
splenomegaly (**splee**-noh-**MEG**-ah-lee)	-megaly = enlargement	enlargement of the spleen
splenorrhagia (**splee**-noh-**RAY**-jee-ah)	-rrhagia = bursting forth	hemorrhage from the spleen
splenorrhaphy (splee-**NOR**-ah-fee)	-rrhaphy = suture	suture of the spleen

Root	Meaning
thym/o	thymus gland

Term	Term Analysis	Definition
thymectomy (thigh-**MECK**-toh-mee)	-ectomy = excision; surgical removal	excision of the thymus

Root	Meaning
tonsill/o	tonsils

Term	Term Analysis	Definition
tonsillectomy (ton-sih-**LECK**-toh-mee)	-ectomy = excision; surgical removal	excision of the tonsils

Suffix	Meaning
-immune	immunity; safe

Term	Term Analysis	Definition
autoimmune disease (aw-toh-ih-**MYOON**)	auto- = self	an immune response to one's own body tissue; destruction of one's cells by the immune system

Suffix	Meaning
-stitial	to place

Term	Term Analysis	Definition
interstitial fluid (in-ter-**STISH**-al)	inter- = between	fluid placed between the tissue spaces

14.6 PATHOLOGY

HIV; AIDS

Infection with the human immunodeficiency virus (HIV). This virus obstructs the body's ability to fight off microorganisms that cause disease such as bacteria, viruses, parasites, and fungi.

With the appropriate treatment, a person can live with HIV for many years, functioning normally without major problems. As the disease progresses, however, the immune system becomes weakened and incapacitated. A diagnosis of AIDS (**AYDZ**) is given at this time. HIV infection and AIDS are the same disease. The label HIV is used when the disease is in its early stages. The label AIDS is used in the late stages of the disease.

Hypersensitivity/Allergic Reactions

Abnormal inflammatory response or hypersensitivity to an allergen (any substance causing an allergic reaction such as pollen, dander, and bee stings).

Allergic reactions occur when the body is exposed to a substance that causes an immune response that is harmful to the body. The body's response can be mild or severe. It can include asthma, hay fever, hives (urticaria), allergic dermatitis, and allergic rhinitis. The most severe reaction is anaphylactic (**an-ih-fih-**

LACK-tick) shock. This is an extreme reaction to the allergen. It can be fatal.

Lymphoma

Lymphomas are tumors of lymphoid tissue. The major categories of malignant lymphoma are Hodgkin's (**HOJ-kinz**) disease and non-Hodgkin's lymphoma. Although possessing similar names, these conditions have different characteristics. Non-Hodgkin's lymphoma is the more common condition.

14.7 REVIEW EXERCISES

Exercise 14-1   MATCHING WORD PARTS WITH MEANING

Match the word part in Column A *with its meaning in* Column B.

Column A		Column B
_____ 1. -edema		A. lymph vessel
_____ 2. -rrhaphy		B. bursting forth
_____ 3. -immune		C. self
_____ 4. lymphangi/o		D. between
_____ 5. lymphaden/o		E. accumulation of fluid in body tissues
_____ 6. -rrhagia		F. to place
_____ 7. auto-		G. lymph gland
_____ 8. inter-		H. enlargement
_____ 9. -stitial		I. suture
_____ 10. -megaly		J. safe

Exercise 14-2   ANATOMY AND PATHOLOGY

Fill in the blanks with the most appropriate term listed below.
Not all terms are used.

allergen
_____

allergy
_____

autoimmune disease
_____

B-cells
_____

edema
_____

HIV _____

Hodgkin's disease _____

lymph nodes _____

phagocytes _____

spleen _____

T-cells _____

thymus _____

tonsils _____

1. Organ that filters lymph of unwanted material

   _____

2. Leukocytes that eat unwanted material

   _____

3. Lymphoid organ that stores red blood cells

   _____

4. Structure in the throat that filters bacteria

   _____

5. White blood cells that kill cancerous cells

   _____

6. Cells that produce antibodies _____

7. Accumulation of fluid in body tissues _____

8. Any substance causing an allergic reaction

   _____

9. Abnormal hypersensitivity to an allergen

   _____

10. Type of lymphoma _____

11. Microorganism causing AIDS _____

| **Exercise 14-3** | **FILL IN THE BLANK—LYMPH NODES** |

Write the location of the following lymph nodes.

    a. **submandibular** _____

    b. **axillary** _____

    c. **inguinal** _____

    d. **cervical** _____

| Exercise 14-4 | DEFINITIONS—LEARNING THE TERMS |

Define the following terms.

1. immunodeficiency _____

2. lymphadenopathy _____

3. splenomegaly _____

4. lymphedema _____

5. interstitial fluid _____

| Exercise 14-5 | BUILDING MEDICAL TERMS |

Build the medical words.

1. study of the immune system _____

2. inflammation of the lymph glands _____

3. hemorrhage from the spleen _____

4. suture of the spleen _____

5. excision of the thymus _____

| Exercise 14-6 | SPELLING |

Circle any words that are spelled incorrectly in the list below. Then correct the spelling in the space provided.

1. interstial fluid _____

2. lymphadenitis _____

3. imunology _____

4. lymphangiitis _____

5. thymectomy _____

6. spleenorrhagia _____

5. **Listen, read, and study so you can speak and write.**

INTRODUCTION

When you studied the cardiovascular system, you learned that blood travels to the lungs to pick up oxygen and give off wastes and carbon dioxide. It then carries the oxygen to the body's cells and picks up more wastes and carbon dioxide. This chapter is about the respiratory system. It is responsible for the ongoing process of respiration (**res-pih-RAY-shun**). Respiration means taking in oxygen and giving off carbon dioxide.

The lungs get oxygen by breathing it in from the air. This is called inhalation. It is also called inspiration. The lungs get rid

PRONUNCIATION AND SPELLING

1. Listen to each word on the audio CD.

2. Pronounce each word carefully.

3. Spell each word in the space provided.

Word	Pronunciation	Spelling
adenoids	**AD-eh-noids**	

of the carbon dioxide by breathing out. This is called exhalation. It is also called expiration.

Various structures work together to make the passage of air into and out of the lungs possible. Together they are called the respiratory tract. As you will learn below, these structures are divided into two further categories: the upper respiratory tract (URT) and the lower respiratory tract (LRT).

15.1 MAJOR ORGANS OF THE RESPIRATORY SYSTEM

PRACTICE FOR LEARNING: MAJOR ORGANS OF THE RESPIRATORY SYSTEM

Write the words below in the correct spaces on Figure 15-1. To help you, the number beside the word tells you where it goes on the figure. Be sure to pronounce each word as you write it. Repeat the pronunciation several times if you find the word hard to say.

1. nasal cavity (**NAY-zal**)

2. nares (**NAH-reez**) (nostrils)

3. pharynx (**FAR-inks**)

4. larynx (**LAR-inks**)

5. trachea (**TRAY-kee-ah**)

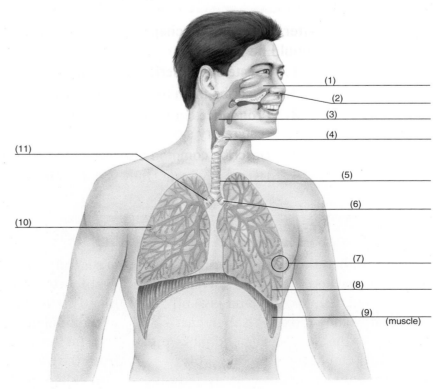

FIGURE 15-1   Major organs of the respiratory system.

6. left bronchus (**BRONG**-kus)

7. alveoli (al-**VEE**-oh-lye)

8. bronchiole (**BRONG**-kee-ohl)

9. diaphragm (**DYE**-ah-fram)

10. right lung

11. right bronchus

15.2 UPPER RESPIRATORY TRACT (URT)

PRACTICE FOR LEARNING: UPPER RESPIRATORY TRACT

Write the words below in the correct spaces on Figure 15-2. To help you, the number beside the word tells you where it goes on the figure. Be sure to pronounce each word as you write it. Repeat the pronunciation several times if you find the word hard to say.

1. nasal cavity (**NAY**-zal)

2. epiglottis (**ep**-ih-**GLOT**-is)

3. vocal cords (**VOH**-kal **KORDZ**)

4. trachea (**TRAY**-kee-ah)

5. pharynx (**FAR**-inks)

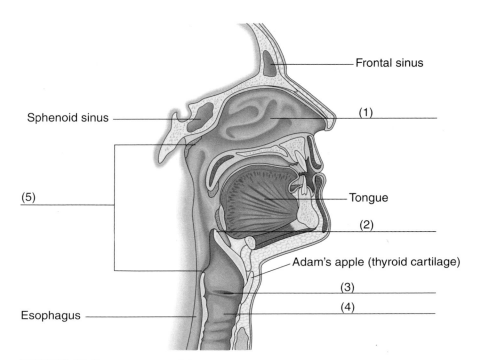

FIGURE 15-2   Structures of the upper respiratory tract.

The URT is illustrated in Figure 15-2. It includes the respiratory structures located outside the thoracic cavity. These are the nasal cavity, pharynx, larynx, and upper trachea. Mucous membrane lines the URT.

Nasal Cavity

Air enters the nasal cavity through the nares (nostrils). The hairs inside the nares filter out dust particles from the air as it is inhaled. These hairs are called **cilia** (**SIL-ee-ah**). The nasal septum divides the cavity into right and left. The nasal cavity warms and moistens air. It is lined with nerve cells called **olfactory** (**ol-FACK-toh-ree**) **neurons** that provide us with our sense of smell. From the nares, the cavity extends to the pharynx.

Pharynx

As you can see in Figure 15-2, the pharynx is the throat. It contains the tonsils and adenoids, which function as part of the immune system as they fight off microorganisms that may be harmful to the body.

Larynx

The larynx is the voice box. It consists of the vocal cords, the epiglottis, and the Adam's apple (thyroid cartilage).

The vocal cords are folds of mucous membrane. As air moves out of the lungs, it goes past the vocal cords. They vibrate and produce sound.

The epiglottis swings up and down like a lid. It covers the opening of the larynx during swallowing so that food from the pharynx does not go down the respiratory tract.

The Adam's apple is a large shield of cartilage that protects the inner structures. It is a bump that you can feel on the front of the neck.

IN BRIEF

External nares are the nostrils

Pharynx is the throat

Larynx is the voicebox

PRACTICE FOR LEARNING: UPPER RESPIRATORY TRACT

Fill in the blanks with the most appropriate answer.

1. Name the structure in the larynx that prevents food from entering the respiratory tract. _____

2. Write the function of the tonsils.

   _____

3. Write another name for nares. _____

4. Write one function of cilia. _____

Answers: **1.** epiglottis. **2.** immunity. **3.** nostrils. **4.** filters out dust particles.

15.3 LOWER RESPIRATORY TRACT

PRACTICE FOR LEARNING: LOWER RESPIRATORY TRACT

Write the words below in the correct spaces on Figure 15-3. To help you, the number beside the word tells you where it goes on the figure. Be sure to pronounce each word as you write it. Repeat the pronunciation several times if you find the word hard to say.

1. trachea (**TRAY**-kee-ah)

2. primary bronchi (**BRONG**-keye)

3. bronchiole (**BRONG**-kee-ohl)

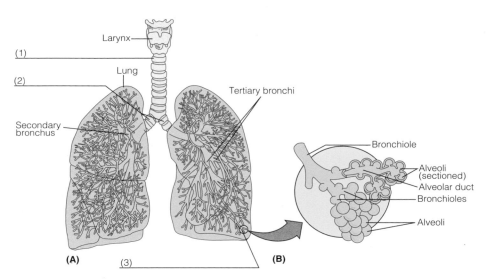

FIGURE 15-3 Lower respiratory tract. A, Trachea, bronchi, and bronchioles. B, Bronchioles, alveolar duct, and alveoli.

Trachea, Bronchi, Bronchioles

The lower respiratory tract is illustrated in Figure 15-3. It includes the lower trachea, bronchi, and bronchioles. The trachea is the windpipe. It extends from the larynx to the bronchi. It is lined with mucous membrane and cilia, which filter the air.

The trachea branches into two tubes called the primary bronchi. Like the trachea, the primary bronchi (singular = bronchus) (**BRONG**-kus) are lined with mucous membrane and cilia. Each extends into a lung, and then branches into smaller and smaller bronchi. These small bronchi extend to tiny structures called bronchioles. The trachea and bronchi together form the tracheobronchial system. As you can see in Figure 15-3, the

IN BRIEF

Trachea is the windpipe

Trachea branches into the primary bronchi, which eventually connect to bronchioles

whole structure looks like an upside-down tree. As a result, it is often referred to as the tracheobronchial tree.

The tracheobronchial tree normally secretes mucus. This functions as a lubricant and protects against infection. When mucus and other matter are expelled from the trachea and the bronchus and through the mouth, it is called sputum (**SPYOO**-tum). Laboratory examination of the sputum is helpful in diagnosing respiratory problems.

Lungs and Alveoli

PRACTICE FOR LEARNING: LUNGS

Write the words below in the correct spaces on Figure 15-4. To help you, the number beside the word tells you where it goes on the figure. Be sure to pronounce each word as you write it. Repeat the pronunciation several times if you find the word hard to say.

1. right superior lobe

2. right inferior lobe

3. right middle lobe

4. left inferior lobe

5. left superior lobe

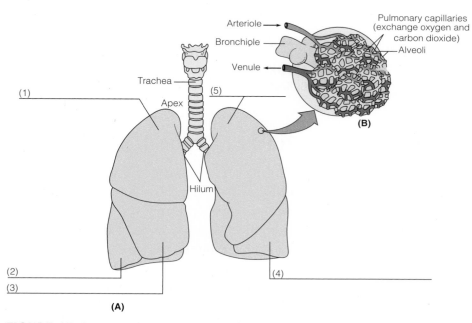

FIGURE 15-4   The lungs and alveoli. A, Structures of the lung. B, Pulmonary capillaries surrounding the alveoli.

IN BRIEF

Right lung has three lobes

Left lung has two lobes

Alveoli are responsible for gas exchange with the pulmonary capillaries

The lungs lie in the thoracic cavity. The top of each lung is called the apex, and the bottom is the base. The right lung is divided into three lobes called the superior, middle, and inferior lobes. The left lung has no middle lobe (Figure 15-4A).

Inside each lung are approximately 300 million **alveoli** (al-**VEE**-oh-lye). They are like tiny balloons. When you inhale, the air goes down through the bronchioles and into the alveoli. They expand and fill up with air. The oxygen in the air is absorbed by the **pulmonary** (**PUL**-moh-ner-ee) **capillaries** that surround the alveoli (Figure 15-4B). The oxygenated blood continues on to the heart, to be pumped to the cells of the body. While the alveoli are giving off oxygen to the capillaries, they are also absorbing carbon dioxide from them. The carbon dioxide is expelled from the lungs during exhalation.

PRACTICE FOR LEARNING: RESPIRATORY TRACT

Answer the following question.

Name in sequence the structures through which air passes to the lungs. Start with the nasal cavity.

_____

_____

_____

_____

Answer: nasal cavity, pharynx, larynx, trachea, bronchi, lungs.

15.4 PARANASAL SINUSES

Paranasal (**par-ah-NAY-zal**) **sinuses** (Figure 15-5) are hollow spaces in the skull bones. They are named after the bones in which they lie. There are four paranasal sinuses: frontal, ethmoid, sphenoid, and maxillary. They are lined with mucous membrane, which helps moisten and warm the air that is breathed in. The paranasal sinuses also help in producing voice sounds.

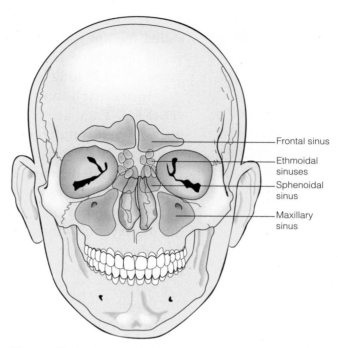

Figure 15-5 Paranasal sinuses.

15.5 PLEURAL AND MEDIASTINAL CAVITIES

IN BRIEF

Pleural cavity surrounds the lungs

Mediastinal cavity is between the lungs

The thoracic cavity contains two smaller cavities called the **pleural** (**PLOOR-al**) and **mediastinal** (**me-dee-as-TYE-nal**) cavities (Figure 15-6). The pleural cavity surrounds the lungs. It has two layers. Between these two layers is the pleural cavity, filled with pleural fluid. The fluid prevents friction between the two layers. The mediastinal cavity lies between the lungs and contains the heart, aorta, trachea, and esophagus.

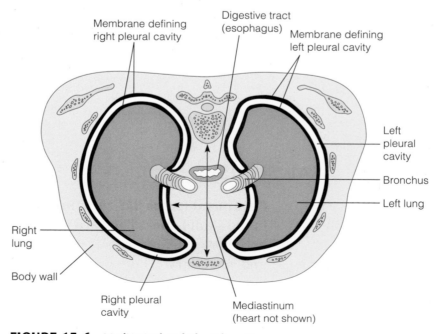

FIGURE 15-6 Mediastinal and pleural cavities.

PRACTICE FOR LEARNING: PARANASAL SINUSES, PLEURAL AND MEDIASTINAL CAVITIES

Fill in the blanks with the most appropriate answer.

1. Write the functions of the paranasal sinuses.

   _____

2. Where is the pleural cavity?

   _____

3. Where is the mediastinal cavity?

   _____

4. What does the pleural cavity contain?

   _____

5. What organs are in the mediastinal cavity?

   _____

Answers: **1.** warms and moistens air and aids in producing voice sounds. **2.** around the lungs. **3.** between the lungs. **4.** fluid. **5.** heart, aorta, trachea, and esophagus.

15.6 NEW PREFIX

Use this additional prefix when studying the medical terms in this chapter.

Prefix	Meaning
oligo-	scanty; few

15.7 LEARNING THE TERMS

Following these steps will make it easier for you to learn medical terms:

1. Pronounce the term repeatedly until it is easy for you.

2. Write it down. Ensure the spelling is correct.

3. Also write the definition. If possible, relate the word to a word, thought, or picture that will help you remember it.

4. Analyze the term with the method taught in this text.

Root	Meaning
adenoid/o	adenoids

Term	Term Analysis	Definition
adenoidectomy (**ad**-eh-noid-**ECK**-toh-mee)	-ectomy = excision	excision of the adenoids

NOTE: If the adenoids become enlarged, airflow is obstructed, necessitating adenoidectomy.

Root	Meaning
bronchi/o; bronch/o	bronchus

Term	Term Analysis	Definition
chronic bronchitis (**KRAH**-nick brong-**KYE**-tis)	-itis = inflammation chronic = disease lasting over a long period of time	inflammation of the bronchus lasting over a long period of time
bronchodilator (**brong**-koh-**DYE**-lay-tor)	-or = person or thing that does something dilat/o = dilatation; widening	drugs used to dilate the bronchus to relieve bronchospasm
bronchospasm (**BRONG**-koh-spazm)	-spasm = sudden, involuntary contraction	sudden, involuntary contraction of the bronchus

Root	Meaning
laryng/o	larynx

Term	Term Analysis	Definition
laryngotrache-obronchitis (lah-**ring**-goh-**tray**-kee-oh-brong-**KYE**-tis)	-itis = inflammation trache/o = trachea	inflammation of the larynx and trachea. Also known as croup (**KROOP**).

NOTE: Croup is a disease of infants and young children.

Root	Meaning
muc/o	**mucus** (a sticky, thick secretion of mucous membrane)

Term	Term Analysis	Definition
mucolytic (**myoo**-koh-**LIH**-tick)	-lytic = breakdown; destruction; separate	drugs used to break down thick mucus so it can be coughed up

Root	Meaning
nas/o (see also rhin/o)	nose

Term	Term Analysis	Definition
nasopharyngeal (**nay**-zoh-far-**INN**-jee-al)	-eal = pertaining to pharyng/o = pharynx; throat	pertaining to the nasopharynx (the portion of the pharynx located behind the nose)

Root	Meaning
ox/o	oxygen

Term	Term Analysis	Definition
hypoxia (high-**POCK**-see-ah)	-ia = state of; condition hypo- = deficient; abnormal decrease	deficiency of oxygen to tissues

Root	Meaning
pector/o (see also **thorac/o**)	chest

Term	Term Analysis	Definition
pectoral (**PECK**-toh-rahl)	-al = pertaining to	pertaining to the chest

Root	Meaning
pharyng/o	throat; pharyng/o

Term	Term Analysis	Definition
oropharyngeal (**or**-oh-far-**IN**-jee-al)	-eal = pertaining to or/o = mouth	throat; pharynx

Root	Meaning
phren/o	diaphragm

Term	Term Analysis	Definition
phrenic (**FREN**-ick)	-ic = pertaining to	pertaining to the diaphragm

Root	Meaning
pleur/o	pleura; pleural cavity

Term	Term Analysis	Definition
pleuritis (ploor-**EYE**-tis)	-itis = inflammation	inflammation of the pleura. Also known as pleurisy.

Root	Meaning
pneumon/o; pulmon/o	lungs

Term	Term Analysis	Definition
pneumonia (noo-**MOH**-nee-ah)	-ia = condition	inflammation of the lung. Also known as pneumonitis.
pulmonary edema (**PUL**-moh-ner-ee eh-**DEE**-mah)	-ary = pertaining to edema = accumulation of fluid in body tissues	accumulation of fluid in the lung tissue

Root	Meaning
rhin/o	nose

Term	Term Analysis	Definition
otorhinolar-yngology (**oh**-toh-**rye**-no-**lar**-in-**GOL**-oh-jee)	-logy = study of ot/o = ear laryng/o = voice box; larynx	the study of the ears, nose, and throat. Abbreviated ENT.
rhinorrhea (rih-noh-**REE**-ah)	-rrhea = discharge	discharge from the nose
rhinoplasty (**RYE**-noh-**plas**-tee)	-plasty = surgical reconstruction; surgical repair	surgical repair of the nose; plastic surgery on the nose for cosmetic or reconstructive purposes; a nose job

Root	Meaning
steth/o	chest

Term	Term Analysis	Definition
stethoscope (**STETH**-oh-skope)	-scope = instrument used to examine	instrument used to listen to chest sounds

Root	Meaning
thorac/o	chest

Term	Term Analysis	Definition
thoracocentesis (**thoh**-rah-koh-sen-**TEE**-sis)	-centesis = surgical puncture	surgical puncture to remove fluid from the pleural cavity (Figure 15-7).

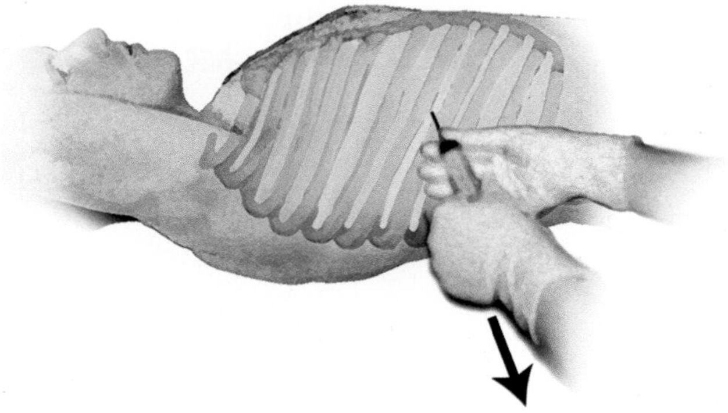

FIGURE 15-7 Thoracocentesis.

Term	Term Analysis	Definition
thoracotomy (**thor**-ah-**KOT**-oh-mee)	-tomy = process of cutting	process of cutting into the chest

Root	Meaning
tonsill/o	tonsils

Term	Term Analysis	Definition
tonsillectomy (**ton**-sih-**LECK**-toh-mee)	-ectomy = surgical excision; removal	excision of the tonsils
tonsillitis (**ton**-sih-**LYE**-tis)	-itis = inflammation	inflammation of the tonsils

Root	Meaning
trache/o	trachea; windpipe

Term	Term Analysis	Definition
endotracheal (**en**-doh-**TRAY**-kee-al)	-eal = pertaining to endo- = within	pertaining to within the trachea
tracheostomy (**tray**-kee-**OS**-toh-mee)	-stomy = new opening	new opening into the trachea is created through the neck and a tube is inserted to assist breathing. The tracheostomy tube may be temporary or permanent (Figure 15-8)

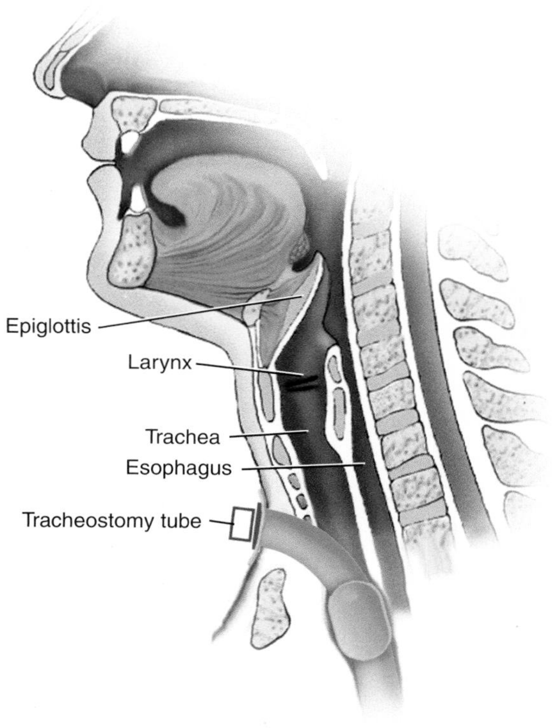

Epiglottis
Larynx
Trachea
Esophagus
Tracheostomy tube

FIGURE 15-8 Tracheostomy.

tracheotomy (**tray**-kee-**OT**-oh-mee)	-tomy = process of cutting	process of cutting into the trachea (Figure 15-9)

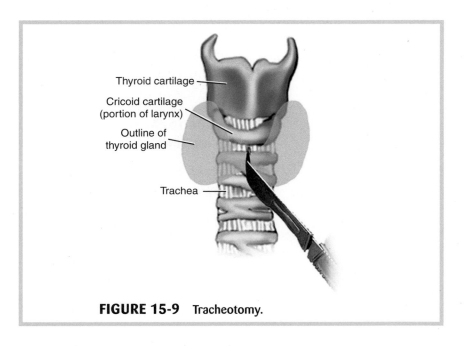

FIGURE 15-9 Tracheotomy.

Suffix	Meaning
-ectasis	dilatation; stretching; widening

Term	Term Analysis	Definition
atelectasis (at-eh-LECK-tah-sis)	atel/o = imperfect	incomplete expansion of the lung; collapsed lung (Figure 15-10)

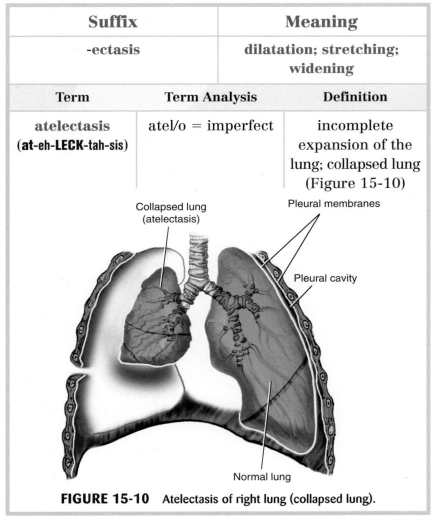

FIGURE 15-10 Atelectasis of right lung (collapsed lung).

(continued)

bronchiectasis (**brong-kee-ECK-**tah-sis)	bronchi/o = bronchus	dilation of the bronchus (Figure 15-11)

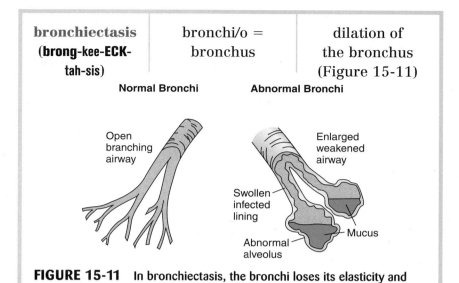

FIGURE 15-11 In bronchiectasis, the bronchi loses its elasticity and widens. Mucus accumulates in the alveoli, making breathing difficult.

Suffix	Meaning
-phonia	voice

Term	Term Analysis	Definition
aphonia (ah-**FOH**-nee-ah)	a- = no; not; lack of	loss of voice
dysphonia (dis-**FOH**-nee-ah)	dys- = difficult; bad; painful	difficulty in speaking

Suffix	Meaning
-pnea	breathing

Term	Term Analysis	Definition
eupnea (yoop-**NEE**-ah)	eu- = normal	normal breathing (Figure 15-12A)
tachypnea (**tack-ip-NEE**-ah)	tachy- = fast	fast breathing (Figure 15-12B)
bradypnea (**brad-ip-NEE**-ah)	brady- = slow	slow breathing (Figure 15-12C)
apnea (**AP**-nee-ah)	a- = no; not; lack of	no breathing (Figure 15-12D)
dyspnea (**DISP**-nee-ah)	dys- = painful; difficult; bad	painful breathing

(continued)

hyperpnea (**high**-perp-**NEE**-ah)	hyper- = abnormal increase; excessive	abnormal increase in depth and rate of breathing (Figure 15-12E)
oligopnea (**ol**-ih-gop-**NEE**-ah)	oligo- = scanty; few	infrequent breathing (resulting in a reduction of air entering the lungs)
orthopnea (**or**-thop-**NEE**-ah)	ortho- = straight	difficulty breathing except in the upright position

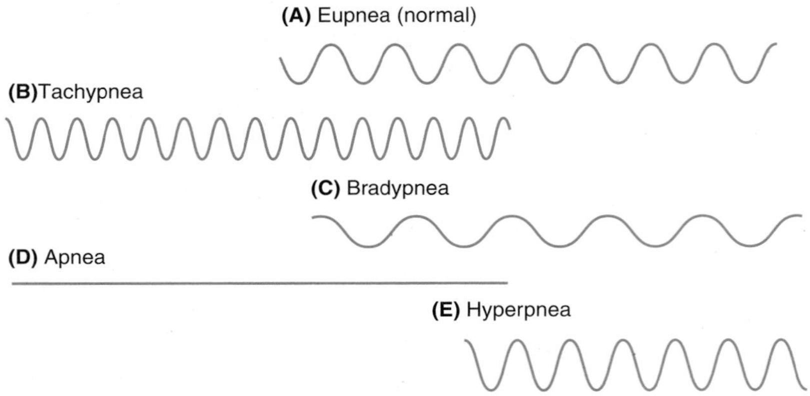

FIGURE 15-12 Breathing patterns.

Suffix	Meaning
-ptysis	spitting

Term	Term Analysis	Definition
hemoptysis (hee-**MOP**-tih-sis)	hem/o = blood	spitting up of blood

Suffix	Meaning
-sphyxia	pulse

Term	Term Analysis	Definition
asphyxia (as-**FICK**-see-ah)	a- = no; not; lack of	lack of oxygen to body tissues; can interfere with respiration and eventually lead to a loss of pulse

Suffix		Meaning	
-thorax		chest	
Term	**Term Analysis**	**Definition**	
hemothorax (**hee**-moh-**THOR**-acks)	hem/o = blood	blood in the pleural cavity	
hydrothorax (**high**-droh-**THOR**-acks)	hydr/o = water	fluid in the pleural cavity	
pneumothorax (**noo**-moh-**THOR**-acks)	pneum/o = air	collection of air in the pleural cavity (Figure 15-13)	
pyothorax (**pye**-oh-**THOR**-acks)	py/o = pus	pus in the pleural cavity (Figure 15-13). Also known as empyema (**em-pye-EE-mah**)	

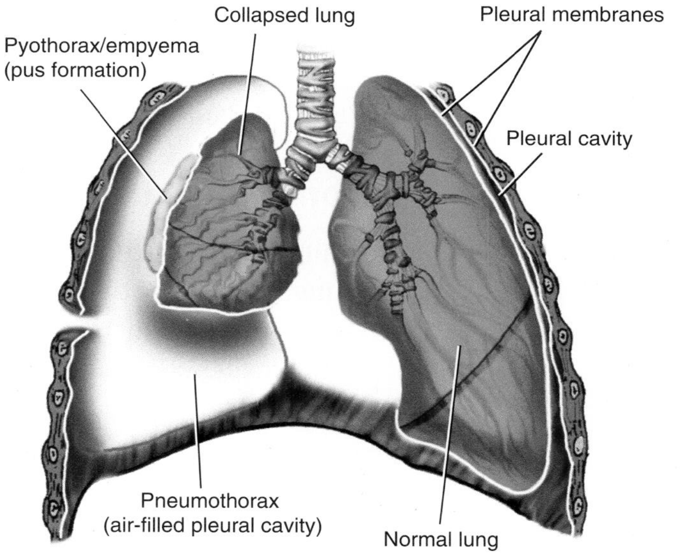

FIGURE 15-13 Pneumothorax and pyothorax. External pressure from air or pus causes the lung to collapse.

15.8 PATHOLOGY

Asthma (AZ-mah)

A bronchospasm that results in airway obstruction (Figure 15-14). Although the bronchospasm can be reversed with the proper treatment, prolonged spasm of the bronchus can be fatal.

Inhaled allergens such as chemicals, pollen, dust, or mold can irritate the airways. This can cause bronchospasm, which obstructs the airways and makes breathing difficult.

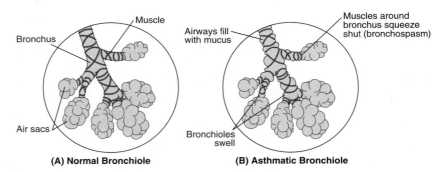

FIGURE 15-14   Asthma. A, Normal bronchiole: muscles are relaxed and the airways are open. B, Asthmatic bronchiole: muscles tighten and airways fill with mucus.

Bronchogenic Carcinoma

Malignant neoplasm of the lung arising from the bronchus or bronchioles.

Cigarette smoking is the cause of most lung cancers. Other factors may be radiation exposure and inhalation of carcinogenic agents such as asbestos.

Treatment includes surgery to remove the tumor. Radiotherapy and chemotherapy are also used to kill cancer cells.

Chronic Obstructive Pulmonary Disease (COPD)

Chronic disease of the respiratory tract that obstructs air flow to the lungs and body tissues. Chronic bronchitis, asthma, and emphysema (described below) are diseases associated with COPD. Over time, they weaken the lung, making breathing difficult.

Emphysema (em-fih-SEE-mah)

Overexpansion (dilation) of the alveoli. Once this happens, they do not return to their normal size and the air becomes trapped in them. This obstructs the passage of oxygen from the lungs into body tissues. This leads to eventual destruction of the alveoli and loss of pulmonary function. Cigarette smoking is a major risk factor.

Pneumonia; Pneumonitis

Inflammation and infection of the lung. As the condition progresses, the effects of the inflammatory process deteriorates the lung. This hinders the exchange of oxygen and carbon dioxide between blood vessels.

15.9 REVIEW EXERCISES

Exercise 15-1 LOOK-ALIKE AND SOUND-ALIKE WORDS

Below is a list of look-alike and sound-alike words. Study the definitions of each set of words, then read the sentences carefully and circle the word in parentheses that correctly completes the meaning

breath	air taken into the lungs (noun). Pronounced BREHTH
breathe	to take air into the lungs (verb). Pronounced BREETH
expiration	to breathe out from the lung
inspiration	to draw air into the lungs
perfusion	to pour through (to perfuse blood through blood vessels)
profusion	abundance; excess
hoarse	harsh and rough in sound
horse	a four-legged, hoofed animal
course	sequence of events
coarse	rough; abrasive
intracostal	within the ribs
intercostal	between the ribs
infracostal	below the ribs
rales	abnormal crackling sound heard on respiration
rails	a bar extending from one support to another to form a railing or guardrail

1. Decreased (**breath/breathe**) sounds in the lower third of the right lung.

2. He has recurring pain when he tries to (**breath/breathe**).

3. (**Inspiratory/Expiratory**) wheezing was noted when the patient took a deep (**breath/breathe**).

4. The head injury caused a (**perfusion/profusion**) of blood.

5. The lung scan showed normal (**profusion/perfusion**) of blood through the lungs.

6. The child was seen two days ago, and at that time had a barky cough and sounded (**hoarse/horse**).

7. The disease took its normal (**course/coarse**), and the patient was discharged seven days following admission.

8. Chest x-ray showed the lung tissue to be (**course/coarse**) and granular.

9. Lungs were noted to have (**rails/rales**) at the left base with decreased (**breath/breathe**) sounds.

10. Place the (**rales/rails**) in the upright position.

Exercise 15-2 | MATCHING WORD PARTS WITH MEANING

Match the word part in Column A *with its meaning in* Column B.

Column A	Column B
_____ 1. ox/o	A. pertaining to
_____ 2. -ectasis	B. diaphragm
_____ 3. pector/o	C. voice
_____ 4. phren/o	D. straight
_____ 5. oligo-	E. normal
_____ 6. pulmon/o	F. nose
_____ 7. rhin/o	G. oxygen
_____ 8. -ar	H. dilation
_____ 9. eu-	I. chest
_____ 10. ortho-	J. few; scanty
_____ 11. -phonia	K. lung
_____ 12. -pnea	L. pulse
_____ 13. -sphyxia	M. breathing

Exercise 15-3 | MATCHING—ANATOMY

Match the structure in Column A *with its description in* Column B.

Column A	Column B
_____ 1. cilia	A. exchanges oxygen and carbon dioxide
_____ 2. olfactory neurons	B. prevents food from entering the respiratory tract

	Column A		Column B
_____	3. pharynx	C.	nostrils
_____	4. paranasal sinuses	D.	mucus and other matter ejected from the mouth
_____	5. larynx		
_____	6. alveoli	E.	throat
_____	7. trachea	F.	filters out dust particles
_____	8. sputum		
_____	9. epiglottis	G.	voice box
_____	10. nares	H.	windpipe
		I.	warms and moistens air
		J.	sense of smell

Exercise 15-4   PATHOLOGY

Select the disease from the list below that best fits its description that follows.

pneumonia _____

asthma _____

atelectasis _____

bronchiectasis _____

croup _____

emphysema _____

pleurisy _____

1. Bronchospasm resulting in airway obstruction

   _____

2. Overexpansion of the alveoli _____

3. Inflammation of the pleura _____

4. Widening of the bronchi traps mucus in the bronchial tubes, causing obstructed airflow _____

5. Inflammation of the lung _____

6. Inflammation of the larynx, trachea, and bronchus in young children _____

7. Incomplete expansion of the alveoli _____

| Exercise 15-5 | LABELING—RESPIRATORY TRACT |

Using the body structures listed below, write the name of each numbered structure in Figure 15-15 on the corresponding line on page 331.

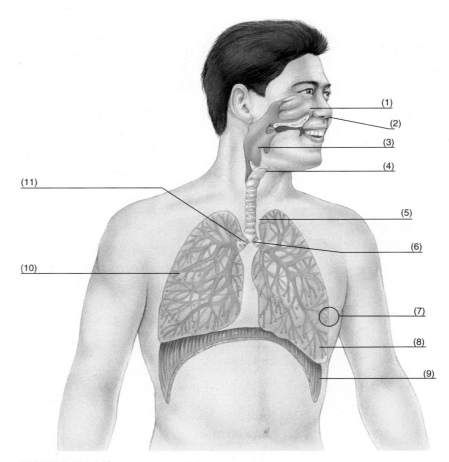

FIGURE 15-15   Structures of the respiratory system.

alveoli _____

bronchiole _____

diaphragm _____

naris _____

larynx _____

left bronchus _____

nasal cavity _____

pharynx _____

right bronchus _____

right lung _____

trachea _____

1. _____

2. _____

3. _____

4. _____

5. _____

6. _____

7. _____

8. _____

9. _____

10. _____

11. _____

| Exercise 15-6 | **DEFINITIONS—ANATOMY** |

Define the following terms in the space provided.

1. upper respiratory tract _____

2. paranasal sinuses. Name these sinuses. _____

    _____

    _____

3. sputum _____

4. mediastinum _____

5. nasal septum _____

6. nares _____

7. pulmonary capillaries _____

    _____

    _____

8. alveoli _____

| **Exercise 15-7** | DEFINITIONS—LEARNING THE TERMS |

Define the following terms.

1. **bronchodilator** _____

2. **mucolytic** _____

3. **phrenic** _____

4. **pulmonary edema** _____

5. **otorhinolaryngology** _____

6. **rhinorrhea** _____

7. **stethoscope** _____

8. **thoracotomy** _____

9. **aphonia** _____

10. **dysphonia** _____

11. **orthopnea** _____

12. **bradypnea** _____

13. **hemoptysis** _____

14. **asphyxia** _____

15. **nasopharyngeal** _____

16. **eupnea** _____

17. **oligopnea** _____

18. **tonsillitis** _____

| **Exercise 15-8** | BUILDING MEDICAL WORDS |

I. *Use the suffix -pnea to build medical words for the following definitions.*

   a. fast breathing _____

   b. breathing only in the upright position

      _____

    c. no breathing _____

    d. slow breathing _____

    e. infrequent breathing _____

    f. abnormal increase in depth and rate of breathing
_____

    g. difficult breathing _____

    h. normal breathing _____

II. *Use rhin/o to build medical words for the following definitions.*

    a. discharge from the nose _____

    b. surgical reconstruction of the nose
_____

III. *Use trache/o to build medical words for the following definitions.*

    a. new opening into the trachea _____

    b. process of cutting into the trachea _____

    c. pertaining to within the trachea _____

IV. *Use -thorax to build medical words for the following definitions.*

    a. blood in the pleural cavity _____

    b. pus in the pleural cavity _____

    c. water in the pleural cavity _____

    d. air in the pleural cavity _____

Exercise 15-9 | DEFINITIONS IN CONTEXT

Define the bolded terms in context. Use your medical dictionary if necessary.

This 64-year-old female with advanced **COPD** was admitted to the hospital with a five-day history of increased **dyspnea** to the point that she was **SOB** at rest.

There was evidence of right **inferior lobe pneumonia** on x-ray. Laboratory tests including **hemoglobin** and white blood cell count were normal. **Sputum** taken from the **oropharynx** was examined for growth of **microorganisms.**

    a. COPD _____

    b. dyspnea _____

    c. SOB _____

    d. inferior lobe pneumonia _____

    e. hemoglobin _____

    f. sputum _____

    g. oropharynx _____

    h. microorganisms _____

Exercise 15-10 SPELLING

Circle any words that are spelled incorrectly in the list below. Then correct the spelling in the space provided.

1. diaphram _____

2. epiglottis _____

3. dispnea _____

4. plurisy _____

5. mediastinum _____

6. stethoscope _____

7. tackypnea _____

8. emphysema _____

9. tonsilectomy _____

10. asphixia _____

15.10 PRONUNCIATION AND SPELLING

1. Listen to each word on the audio CD.

2. Pronounce each word carefully.

3. Spell each word in the space provided.

Word	Pronunciation	Spelling
adenoidectomy	**ad-eh-noid-ECK-toh-mee**	
asthma	**AZ-mah**	

Word	Pronunciation	Spelling
atelectasis	at-eh-**LECK**-tah-sis	
bradypnea	**brad**-ip-**NEE**-ah	
bronchiectasis	**brong**-kee-**ECK**-tah-sis	
bronchiole	**BRONG**-kee-ohl	
bronchus	**BRONG**-kus	
cilia	**SIL**-ee-ah	
croup	**KROOP**	
diaphragm	**DYE**-ah-fram	
dysphonia	dis-**FOH**-nee-ah	
emphysema	**em**-fih-**SEE**-mah	
empyema	**em**-pye-**EE**-mah	
endotracheal	**en**-doh-**TRAY**-kee-al	
epiglottis	**ep**-ih-**GLOT**-is	
eupnea	yoop-**NEE**-ah	
hemothorax	**hee**-moh-**THOR**-acks	
hydrothorax	**high**-droh-**THOR**-acks	
hyperpnea	**high**-perp-**NEE**-ah	
hypoxia	high-**POCK**-see-ah	
laryngotracheobronchitis	lah-**ring**-goh-**tray**-kee-oh-brong-**KYE**-tis	
larynx	**LAR**-inks	
mucolytic	**myoo**-koh-**LIH**-tick	
nares	**NAH**-reez	
olfactory	ol-**FACK**-toh-ree	
oligopnea	**ol**-ih-**GOP**-nee-ah	
orthopnea	**or**-thop-**NEE**-ah	
otorhinolaryngology	**oh**-toh-**rye**-no-**lar**-in-**GOL**-oh-jee	
pharynx	**FAR**-inks	

Word	Pronunciation	Spelling
pleurisy	**PLOOR**-ih-see	
pneumonia	noo-**MOH**-nee-ah	
stethoscope	**STETH**-oh-skope	
tonsillectomy	ton-sih-**LECK**-toh-mee	
trachea	**TRAY**-kee-ah	
tracheostomy	tray-kee-**OS**-toh-mee	

CHAPTER 16

The Urinary System

LEARNING OBJECTIVES

After studying this chapter and completing the review exercises, you should be able to:

1. Locate the organs of the urinary system.
2. Describe the structure and functions of the kidney, ureters, bladder, and urethra.
3. Describe how the kidneys produce urine.
4. Pronounce, spell, define, and write the medical terms related to the urinary system.
5. Describe common diseases of the urinary system.
6. Listen, read, and study so you can speak and write.

INTRODUCTION

In previous chapters you learned that when the blood delivers oxygen to the cells, it also picks up carbon dioxide and other waste products. Through the process of respiration, the carbon dioxide goes from the blood into the alveoli. It is then exhaled from the body. The other waste products remain in the blood. The urinary system filters these waste products from the blood and excretes them from the body.

16.1 MAJOR ORGANS OF THE URINARY SYSTEM

PRACTICE FOR LEARNING: **MAJOR ORGANS OF THE URINARY SYSTEM**

Write the words below in the correct spaces on Figure 16-1. To help you, the number beside the word tells you where it goes on the figure. Be sure to pronounce each word as you write it. Repeat the pronunciation several times if you find the word hard to say.

1. kidney (**KID**-nee)

2. ureter (yoo-**REE**-ter)

3. urinary bladder (**YOO**-rih-**nar**-ee **BLAH**-der)

4. urethra (yoo-**REE**-thrah)

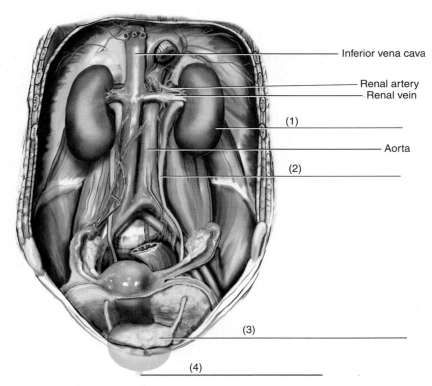

FIGURE 16-1   Major organs of the urinary system.

The urinary system is illustrated in Figure 16-1. It consists of two kidneys, two tubes called ureters, a sac called the urinary bladder, and another tube called the urethra.

16.2 STRUCTURE AND FUNCTION OF THE URINARY SYSTEM

Kidneys

The kidneys are shaped like a bean. They are about the size of your fist. They are located at the back of the abdomen, one on each side of the lumbar vertebrae. The kidneys filter the blood to remove waste products. These waste products combine with water to form urine (**YOO-rin**). Urine flows out of the kidneys into the renal pelvis (**REE-nal PEL-vis**), which is the dilated portion of the ureter.

Ureters, Bladder, and Urethra

As you can see in Figure 16-1, the ureters are long, narrow tubes that connect the kidneys to a sac called the urinary bladder. Urine constantly flows through the ureters to the urinary bladder. The bladder stores urine. When the bladder is full, the urine is squeezed out into the urethra.

The urethra (Figure 16-1) carries urine out of the body. This is called urination or voiding. In females, the urethra is about 1.6 inches (4.1 cm) long. In males, it runs along the length of the penis and also serves as part of the reproductive system for the transport of sperm. The external opening of the urethra is called the urinary meatus (**MEE-ah-tus**).

IN BRIEF

Urine moves from the kidneys

↓

ureters

↓

urinary bladder

↓

urethra

↓

out of the body

PRACTICE FOR LEARNING: **KIDNEYS, URETERS, BLADDER, AND URETHRA**

Complete the sentence by underlining the correct answer.

1. The (bladder/ureter/urethra) is a long, narrow tube extending from the kidney for the passage of urine.

2. Urine is stored in the (ureter/urethra/bladder/kidney).

3. The (kidneys/ureters/bladder/urethra) filter waste products from the blood.

4. All blood goes to the (kidneys/ureters/bladder/urethra).

5. The (kidneys/ureters/bladder/urethra) (are) is also part of the male reproductive system.

Answers: **1.** ureter. **2.** bladder. **3.** kidneys. **4.** kidneys. **5.** urethra.

16.3 URINE PRODUCTION IN THE KIDNEY

Inside each kidney, there are approximately one million nephrons (**NEF-ronz**) (Figure 16-2). These microscopic structures are responsible for producing urine. As the blood flows through the kidneys, part of the nephron called the **glomerulus** (gloh-**MER**-yoo-lus) filters the blood of waste products and unnecessary nutrients. The clean blood continues through the blood vessels returning to the heart. The unwanted material combines with water to form urine. The urine travels the length of the nephron and is excreted through the urinary structures to the outside of the body.

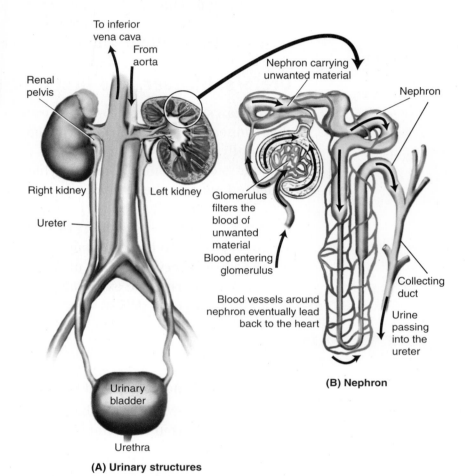

(A) Urinary structures

FIGURE 16-2   The nephron.

16.4 NEW ROOTS

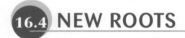

Use these additional roots when studying the medical terms in this chapter.

Root	Meaning
noct/o	night
urin/o	urine

16.5 LEARNING THE TERMS

Following these steps will make it easier for you to learn medical terms:

1. Pronounce the term repeatedly until it is easy for you.

2. Write it down. Ensure the spelling is correct.

3. Also write the definition. If possible, relate the word to a word, thought, or picture that will help you remember it.

4. Analyze the term with the method taught in this text.

Root	Meaning
cyst/o (see also **vesic/o**)	**bladder**

Term	Term Analysis	Definition
cystitis (sis-**TYE**-tis)	-itis = inflammation	inflammation of the bladder
cystoscopy (sis-**TOS**-koh-pee)	-scopy = process of visually examining	process of visually examining the bladder (Figure 16-3).

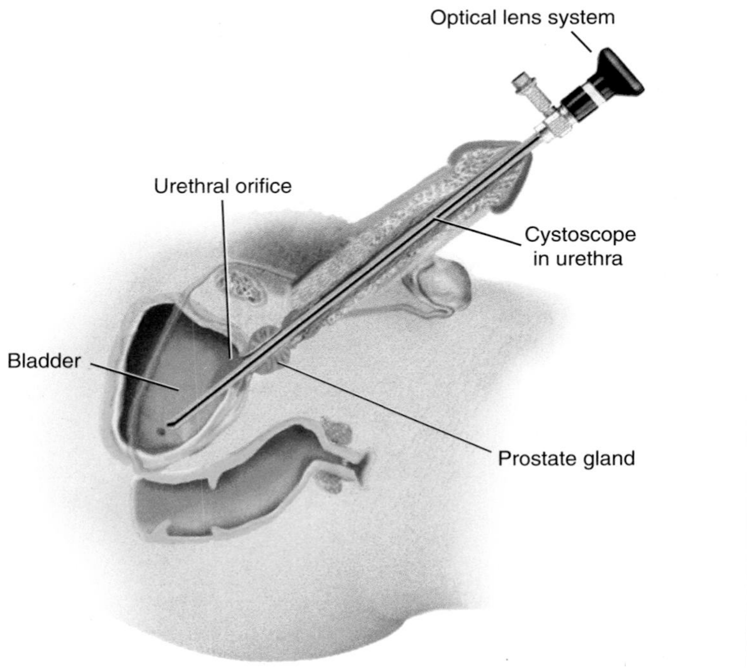

FIGURE 16-3 Cystoscopy.

(continued)

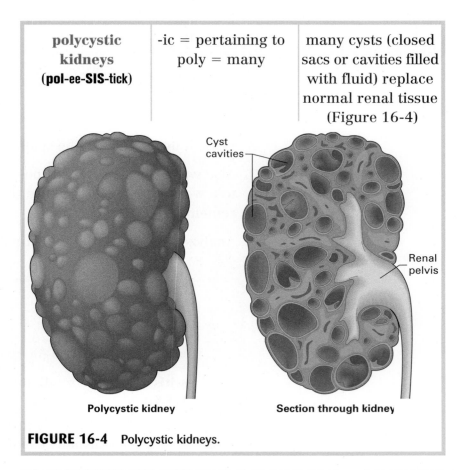

polycystic kidneys (**pol**-ee-**SIS**-tick)	-ic = pertaining to poly = many	many cysts (closed sacs or cavities filled with fluid) replace normal renal tissue (Figure 16-4)

Cyst cavities

Renal pelvis

Polycystic kidney

Section through kidney

FIGURE 16-4   Polycystic kidneys.

Root	Meaning
glomerul/o	**glomerulus** (portion of the nephron that filters blood)

Term	Term Analysis	Definition
glomerulo-nephritis (gloh-**mer**-yoo-loh-neh-**FRY**-tis)	-itis = inflammation nephr/o = kidney	inflammation of the glomerulus and kidney; Bright's disease

Root	Meaning
meat/o	**meatus** (opening at the tip of the urethra)

Term	Term Analysis	Definition
meatotomy (**mee**-ah-**TOT**-oh-me)	-tomy = process of cutting	process of cutting into the urinary meatus (to widen the meatus)

Root	Meaning
nephr/o (see also **ren/o**)	**kidney**

Term	Term Analysis	Definition
hydronephrosis (**high-droh-neh-FROH**-sis)	-osis = abnormal condition hydr/o = water	accumulation of urine in the renal pelvis (due to narrowing of the ureter) (Figure 16-5)

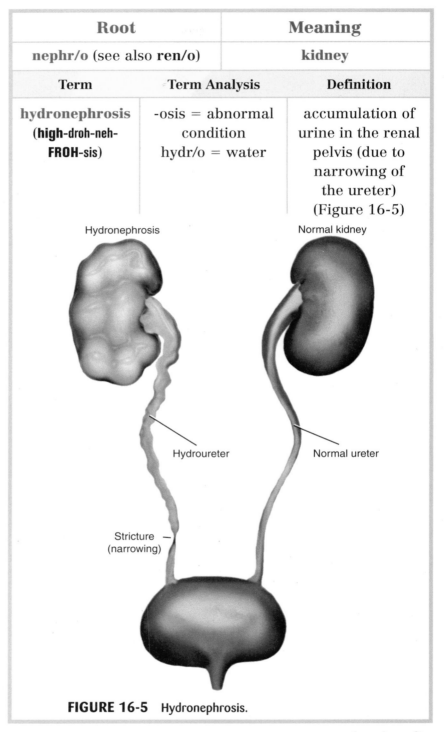

Hydronephrosis

Normal kidney

Hydroureter

Normal ureter

Stricture (narrowing)

FIGURE 16-5 Hydronephrosis.

(continued)

nephrolithiasis (**nef**-roh-lih-**THIGH**-ah-sis)	-iasis = abnormal condition lith/o = stones	kidney stones (Figure 16-6)

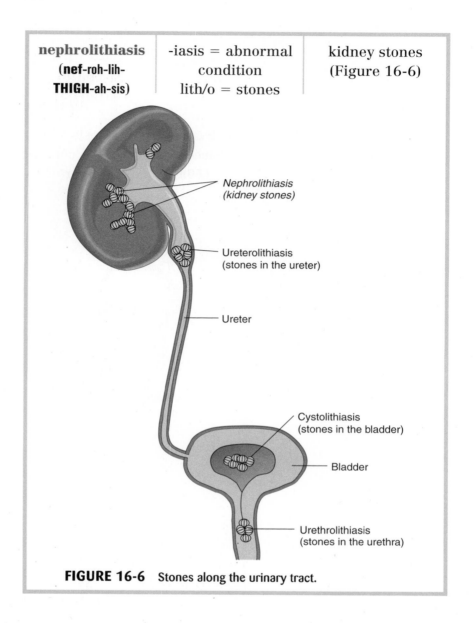

FIGURE 16-6   Stones along the urinary tract.

Root	Meaning	
pyel/o	renal pelvis; kidney pelvis	
Term	**Term Analysis**	**Definition**
pyelonephritis (**pye**-eh-loh-neh-**FRY**-tis)	-itis = inflammation nephr/o = kidney	inflammation of the kidney pelvis and kidney

Root	Meaning
ren/o	kidney

Term	Term Analysis	Definition
renal hypoplasia (**REE**-nal **high**-poh-**PLAY**-zee-ah)	-al = pertaining to -plasia = formation; development hypo- = under; below normal; deficient	underdeveloped kidney

Root	Meaning
ureter/o	ureter

Term	Term Analysis	Definition
ureteral (yoo-**REE**-ter-al)	-al = pertaining to	pertaining to the ureter

Root	Meaning
urethr/o	urethra

Term	Term Analysis	Definition
transurethral (**tranz**-yoo-**REE**-thral)	-al = pertaining to trans- = through; across	pertaining to something moving through the urethra

Root	Meaning
ur/o	urinary tract; urine; urination

Term	Term Analysis	Definition
uremia (yoo-**REE**-mee-ah)	-emia = blood condition	accumulation of waste products in the blood; also known as azotemia

(continued)

urologist (yoo-**ROL**-oh-jist)	-logist = specialist	specialist in the study of the urinary system in females and the urinary and reproductive systems in males
urogram (**YOO**-roh-gram)	-gram = record	record of the urinary tract (Figure 16-7)

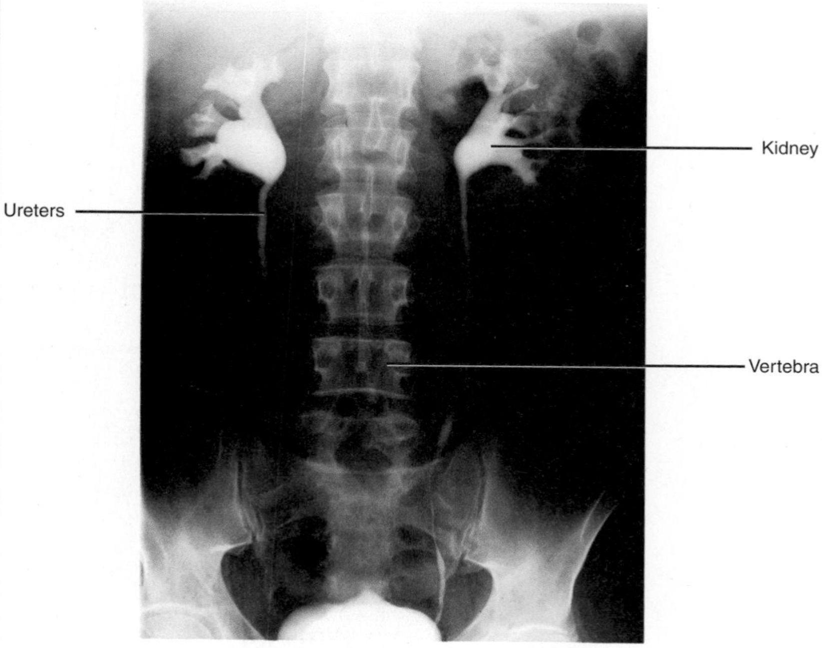

FIGURE 16-7   An excretory urogram showing the kidneys and ureters.

HELPING YOU REMEMBER

Although they are pronounced the same, do not confuse vesical with vesicle. Vesical means "pertaining to the bladder." Vesicle means a "small sac containing liquid; a blister."

Root	Meaning	
vesic/o	bladder	
Term	**Term Analysis**	**Definition**
vesical (**VES**-ih-kal)	-al = pertaining to	pertaining to the bladder

Suffix	Meaning
-lysis	separate; break down

Term	Term Analysis	Definition
dialysis (dye-AL-ih-sis)	dia- = through; complete	mechanical replacement of kidney function when the kidney is not working (Figure 16-8)

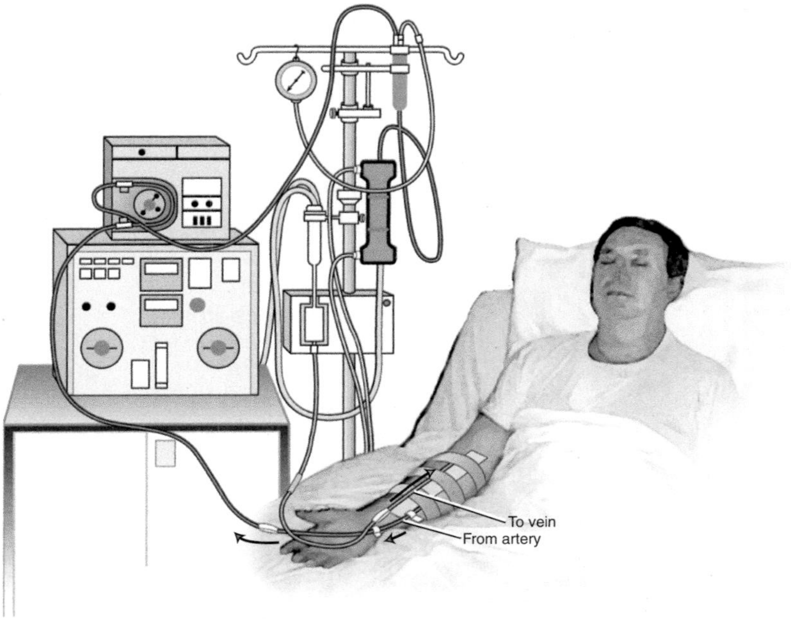

FIGURE 16-8 Hemodialysis.

Term	Term Analysis	Definition
urinalysis (yoo-rih-NAL-ih-sis)	urin/o = urine ana- = apart	laboratory analysis of urine

Suffix	Meaning
-uria	urine; urination

Term	Term Analysis	Definition
anuria (ah-**NOO**-ree-ah)	an- = no; not; lack of	no urine formation; also known as suppression
dysuria (dis-**YOO**-ree-ah)	dys- = painful; difficult; bad	painful urination
hematuria (**hem**-ah-**TOO**-ree-ah)	hemat/o = blood	blood in the urine
nocturia (nock-**TOO**-ree-ah)	noct/o = night	frequent urination at night
oliguria (**ol**-ih-**GOO**-ree-ah)	oligo- = scanty; deficient; few	decreased urination
pyuria (pye-**YOO**-ree-ah)	py/o = pus	pus in the urine
polyuria (**pol**-ee-**YOO**-ree-ah)	poly- = many	excretion of large amounts of urine

16.6 PATHOLOGY

Renal Failure

Loss of kidney function. Acute renal failure comes on suddenly and is of short duration. Chronic renal failure comes on gradually and is of long duration. End-stage renal disease (ESRD) is the final stage of renal failure. Without adequate filtration, the waste products build up in the blood and death occurs because of uremia.

Voiding Disorders

Urinary Incontinence *(in-**KON**-tih-nens)*

Involuntary outflow of urine. Stress incontinence occurs when there is pressure on the bladder from coughing or laughing. Urge incontinence is the inability to stop the flow of urine once the urge has been felt.

Urinary Retention

Inability of the bladder to empty completely during urination. If urine needs to be removed from the bladder before an effective treatment has been established, catheterization (**kath**-eh-ter-eye-

ZAY-shun) may be done. This involves the insertion of a flexible tube (catheter) into the bladder to withdraw urine. The catheter is placed through the urethra and into the bladder (Figure 16-9A, and 9B).

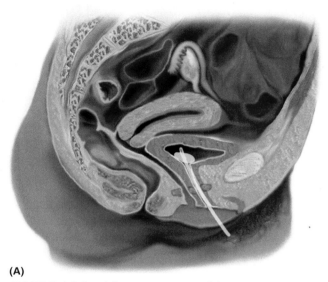

(A)

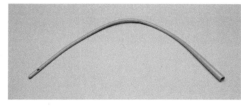

(B)

FIGURE 16-9   (A) Catheterization, (B) Catheter is placed in the bladder to drain urine.

16.7 REVIEW EXERCISES

Exercise 16-1   LOOK-ALIKE AND SOUND-ALIKE WORDS

Below is a list of look-alike and sound-alike words. Study the definitions of each set of words, then read the sentences carefully and circle the word in parentheses that correctly completes the meaning.

anuresis	retention of urine in the bladder
enuresis	bedwetting at night
creatine	an amino acid found in tissues, especially muscles
creatinine	waste product excreted in the urine; elevated in kidney disease
ureteral	pertaining to the ureter
urethral	pertaining to the urethra
vesical (adj)	pertaining to the bladder
vesicle (noun)	blister

1. The patient complains of severe (**anuresis/enuresis**) to the point that he was wearing pads at night.

2. Mr. Chavez was admitted with glomerulonephritis. His laboratory tests showed abnormal levels of urine (**creatine/creatinine**).

3. This woman has had three previous attacks of right (**urethral/ureteral**) pain.

4. Repeat cystoscopies resulted in multiple (**vesicals/vesicles**) in the bladder.

5. After elevation of the (**vesical/vesicle**) neck, incontinence stopped.

Exercise 16-2 — MATCHING WORD PARTS WITH MEANING

Match the word part in Column A *with its meaning in* Column B.

Column A	Column B
_____ 1. dia-	A. opening at the tip of the urethra
_____ 2. -plasia	
_____ 3. py/o	B. kidney
_____ 4. pyel/o	C. pus
_____ 5. vesic/o	D. stone
_____ 6. meat/o	E. night
_____ 7. noct/o	F. through; complete
_____ 8. lith/o	G. bladder
_____ 9. oligo-	H. scanty
_____ 10. nephr/o	I. formation; development
	J. renal pelvis

Exercise 16-3 — LABELING—URINARY TRACT

Write the name of each numbered structure on the corresponding line below the diagram (Figure 16-10). Use the body structures listed below.

kidney
_____

urinary bladder

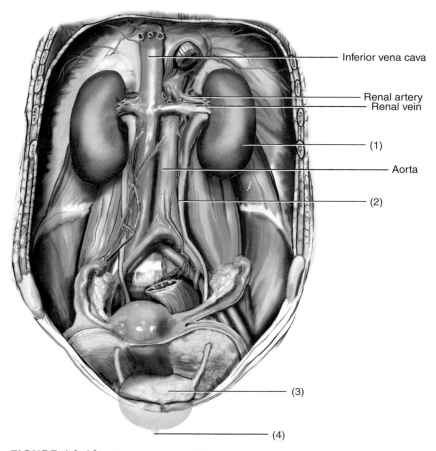

Inferior vena cava

Renal artery
Renal vein

(1)

Aorta

(2)

(3)

(4)

FIGURE 16-10 Major organs of the urinary system.

ureter _____

urethra _____

1. _____

2. _____

3. _____

4. _____

Exercise 16-4 DEFINITIONS—LEARNING THE TERMS

Define the following terms.

1. **cystoscope** _____

2. **meatotomy** _____

3. **nephrolithiasis** _____

4. **renal hypoplasia** _____

5. dialysis _____

6. urethral _____

7. azotemia _____

8. anuria _____

9. dysuria _____

10. suppression _____

11. polyuria _____

12. pyuria _____

13. urologist _____

Exercise 16-5 BUILDING MEDICAL WORDS

I. *Use the suffix -uria to build medical words for the following definitions.*

a. no urine formation _____

b. painful urination _____

c. blood in the urine _____

d. frequent urination at night _____

e. decreased urination _____

f. pus in the urine _____

g. excretion of large amounts of urine

_____

II. *Use the combining form cyst/o to build medical words for the following definitions.*

a. inflammation of the bladder _____

b. instrument used to visually examine the inside of the bladder _____

Exercise 16-6 DEFINITIONS—PATHOLOGY

Define the following diseases.

1. polycystic kidneys

_____

_____

2. incontinence

_____

_____

3. nephrolithiasis

_____

_____

4. renal failure

_____

_____

5. pyelonephritis

_____

_____

6. urinary retention

_____

_____

| Exercise 16-7 | DEFINITIONS IN CONTEXT |

Define the bolded terms in the spaces provided. Use your medical dictionary if necessary.

ADMISSION DIAGNOSIS: RIGHT HYDROURETER AND
HYDRONEPHROSIS

HISTORY OF PRESENT ILLNESS

A 65-year-old man was admitted with abdominal pain. He had been having this pain off and on for the past two years. On admission, he was found to have **renal calculi**. An **urography** was performed that showed poor function on the right with a **hypoplastic** scarred kidney. The patient therefore underwent a **cystoscopy** and **MRI,** revealing a poorly positioned right kidney with a **stricture** involving the **distal** one-third of the ureter. The patient was admitted at this time for consideration of **nephrectomy.**

a. **hydronephrosis** _____

b. **renal calculi** _____

c. **urography** _____

d. **hypoplastic** _____

e. **cystoscopy** _____

    f. **MRI** _____

    g. **stricture** _____

    h. **distal** _____

    i. **nephrectomy** _____

Exercise 16-8   SPELLING

Circle any words that are spelled incorrectly in the list below.
Then correct the spelling in the space provided.

1. glomairulus _____

2. cistitis _____

3. retention _____

4. urineation _____

5. nephrolithiasis _____

6. dialisis _____

7. vesical _____

8. incontinance _____

9. cathaterization _____

10. excretion _____

16.8 PRONUNCIATION AND SPELLING

1. Listen to each word on the audio CD.

2. Pronounce each word carefully.

3. Spell each word in the space provided.

Word	Pronunciation	Spelling
anuria	ah-**NOO**-ree-ah	
cystitis	sis-**TYE**-tis	
cystoscope	**SIS**-toh-skope	
dialysis	dye-**AL**-ih-sis	
dysuria	dis-**YOO**-ree-ah	

Word	Pronunciation	Spelling
glomerulonephritis	glow-**mer**-yoo-loh-neh-**FRY**-tis	
glomerulus	gloh-**MER**-yoo-lus	
hematuria	**hem**-ah-**TOO**-ree-ah	
hydronephrosis	**high**-droh-neh-**FROH**-sis	
kidney	**KID**-nee	
meatotomy	**me**-ah-**TOT**-oh-me	
nephrolithiasis	**nef**-roh-lith-**THIGH**-ah-sis	
nocturia	nock-**TOO**-ree-ah	
oliguria	**ol**-ih-**GOO**-ree-ah	
polyuria	**pol**-ee-**YOO**-ree-ah	
pyuria	pye-**YOO**-ree-ah	
renal hypoplasia	**REE**-nal **high**-poh-**PLAY**-zee-ah	
uremia	yoo-**REE**-mee-ah	
ureter	yoo-**REE**-ter	
ureteral	yoo-**REE**-ter-al	
urethra	yoo-**REE**-thrah	
urinalysis	**yoo**-rih-**NAL**-ih-sis	
urologist	yoo-**ROL**-oh-jist	

CHAPTER 17

Male Reproductive System

LEARNING OBJECTIVES

After studying this chapter and completing the review exercises, you should be able to:

1. Locate the organs of the male reproductive system.
2. Describe the structure and function of the male reproductive system.
3. Pronounce, spell, define, and write the medical terms related to the male reproductive system.
4. Describe common diseases of the male reproductive system.
5. Listen, read, and study so you can speak and write.

INTRODUCTION

The male reproductive system performs three basic tasks. The first is to manufacture sperm that carries the genetic code of the male. The second is to produce the hormone testosterone (tes-**TOS**-ter-ohn). The third is to deliver the sperm and semen out of the male's body.

17.1 MAJOR ORGANS OF THE MALE REPRODUCTIVE SYSTEM

PRACTICE FOR LEARNING: MAJOR ORGANS OF THE MALE REPRODUCTIVE SYSTEM

Write the words below in the correct spaces on Figure 17-1. To help you, the number beside the word tells you where it goes on the figure. Be sure to pronounce each word as you write it. Repeat the pronunciation several times if you find the word hard to say.

1. vas deferens (**VASS DEF**-er-enz)

2. penis (**PEE**-nis)

3. glans penis (**GLANZ**)

4. testis (**TEST**-tis)

5. scrotum (**SKROH**-tum)

6. epididymis (**ep**-ih-**DID**-ih-mis)

7. bulbourethral gland (**bul**-boh-yoo-**REE**-thral **GLAND**)

8. prostate (**PROS**-tayt)

9. ejaculatory duct (ee-**JACK**-yoo-lah-tor-ee **DUCT**)

10. seminal vesicle (**SEM**-ih-nal **VESS**-ih-kal)

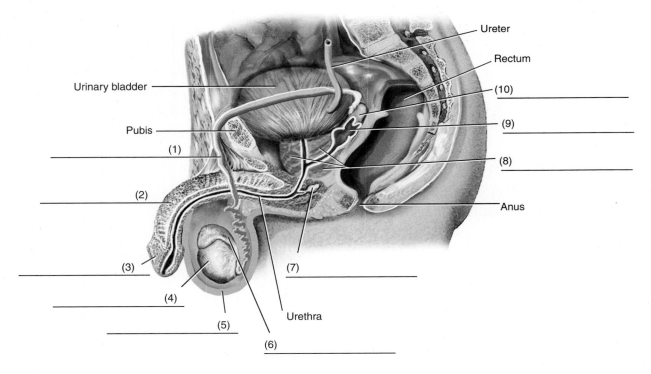

A.

FIGURE 17-1 (A) Major organs of the male reproductive system.

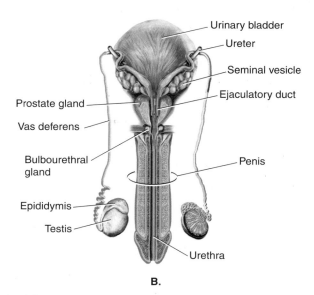

Urinary bladder

Ureter

Seminal vesicle

Ejaculatory duct

Prostate gland

Vas deferens

Bulbourethral gland

Penis

Epididymis

Testis

Urethra

B.

FIGURE 17-1 (B) The testicles and vas deferens are bilateral.

STRUCTURE AND FUNCTION OF THE MALE REPRODUCTIVE SYSTEM
17.2

Sperm is produced in the testes (**TEST-tees**) (singular = testis). The testes are also called the testicles (**TEST-ick-els**). The sperm is mixed with semen (**SEE-men**), a fluid produced by the male reproductive organs and then delivered out of the body through the reproductive tract. The other components of the male reproductive system are the accessory reproductive organs and external genitalia (**jen-ih-TAIL-ee-yah**). The entire male reproductive system is illustrated in Figure 17-1.

Testes

The testes are located in an external skin sac called the scrotum (**SKROH-tum**). The production of sperm is called spermatogenesis (**sper-mah-toh-jen-EE-sis**). The testes also produce the hormone testosterone. It is essential for spermatogenesis and for the development of secondary male gender characteristics such as facial hair, muscularity, and voice change at puberty.

Epididymis, Vas Deferens, Seminal Vesicle, and Ejaculatory Duct

You can trace the entire reproductive tract on Figure 17-1. It begins with the epididymis (**ep-ih-DID-ih-mis**), which is a coiled tube on the superior surface of each testicle. Sperm are stored there. The epididymis leads into a duct called the ductus deferens or vas deferens. This duct encircles the urinary bladder and joins another duct from the seminal vesicle to form the ejaculatory duct. This duct joins the urethra, which passes through a hole in the prostate gland.

Accessory Organs

The accessory organs can also be seen in Figure 17-1. They are the seminal vesicles, the prostate gland, and bulbourethral glands, which are also called **Cowper's glands**. The accessory organs secrete substances that combine to form semen, which nourishes and protects sperm.

External Genitalia

The scrotum and the penis are the external genitalia. The tip of the penis is called the glans penis. It contains the opening for urination and ejaculation, called the **urethral orifice (yoo-REE-thral OR-ih-fis)**. The urethral orifice is also called the urinary **meatus (ME-ah-tus)**. The glans is covered with loose skin called the foreskin or **prepuce (PRE-pyoos)**. This skin may be removed by a surgical process called **circumcision (ser-kum-SIZH-un)**.

IN BRIEF

Male reproductive organs

testes, epididymis, vas deferens, ejaculatory duct, and urethra

Functions

produces sperm and testosterone

Accessory organs

seminal vesicles, prostate, and bulbourethral glands

External genitalia

penis and scrotum

PRACTICE FOR LEARNING: MALE REPRODUCTIVE STRUCTURE AND FUNCTION

1. Write the function for the following structures:

   a. testicles _____

   b. epididymis _____

   c. vas deferens _____

   d. seminal vesicles, prostate gland, and bulbourethral glands _____

2. From the list of words below, complete sentences a, b, c, and d. Not all terms are used.

   Cowper's

   epididymis

   glans penis

   prepuce

   scrotum

   testicals

urethral orifice

ductus deferens

a. The tip of the penis is called the _____ .

b. The urinary meatus is also known as the

_____ .

c. The glans penis is covered with loose skin called

_____ .

d. A sac containing the testicles is _____ .

e. An another name for bulbourethral gland is

_____ .

Answers: **1. a.** produce sperm and testosterone. **b.** stores sperm. **c.** transports sperm. **d.** all of these structures secrete substances that together form semen, which nourishes and protects the sperm. **2. a.** glans penis. **b.** urethral orifice. **c.** prepuce. **d.** scrotum. **e.** Cowper's.

17.3 NEW ROOTS AND SUFFIXES

Root	Meaning
crypt/o	hidden
varic/o	varicose vein

Suffix	Meaning
-cidal	to kill
-genesis	production; formation

17.4 LEARNING THE TERMS

Following these steps will make it easier for you to learn medical terms:

1. Pronounce the term repeatedly until it is easy for you.

2. Write it down. Ensure the spelling is correct.

3. Also write the definition. If possible, relate the word to a word, thought or picture that will help you remember it.

4. Analyze the term with the method taught in this text.

Root	Meaning
andr/o	male

Term	Term Analysis	Definition
androgenic (**an**-droh-**JEN**-ick)	-genic = producing	producing masculinizing effects

Root	Meaning
balan/o	glans penis

Term	Term Analysis	Definition
balanorrhea (**bal**-an-oh-**REE**-ah)	-rrhea = flow; discharge	discharge from the glans penis

Root	Meaning
mast/o	breast

Term	Term Analysis	Definition
gynecomastia (**guy**-neh-koh-**MAS**-tee-ah)	-ia = condition gynec/o = woman	abnormal enlargement of the male breast

Root	Meaning
orchid/o; orchi/o (see also **testicul/o**)	testicle; testis

Term	Term Analysis	Definition
cryptorchidism (krip-**TOR**-kih-**diz**-um)	-ism = process crypt/o = hidden	undescended testicles (Figure 17-2).

NOTE: During fetal development, one or both testicles fail to descend into the scrotum, remaining instead in the abdominal cavity. If not treated, this condition results in sterility.

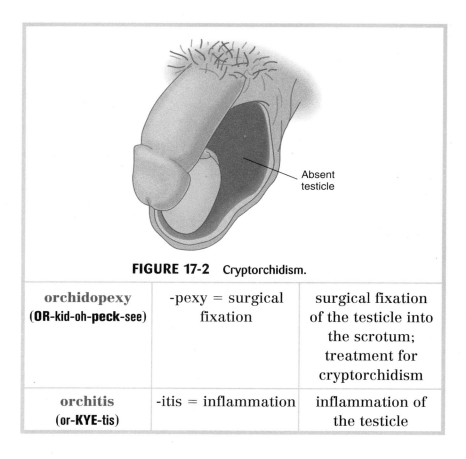

FIGURE 17-2   Cryptorchidism.

orchidopexy (**OR**-kid-oh-**peck**-see)	-pexy = surgical fixation	surgical fixation of the testicle into the scrotum; treatment for cryptorchidism
orchitis (or-**KYE**-tis)	-itis = inflammation	inflammation of the testicle

Root		Meaning	
prostat/o		prostate	
Term	**Term Analysis**	**Definition**	
prostatitis (**pros**-tah-**TYE**-tis)	-itis = inflammation	inflammation of the prostate	
transurethral prostatectomy (TUP) (**tranz**-yoo-**REE**-thral **pros**-teh-**TECK**- teh-mee)	-al = pertaining to trans- = through; across -ectomy = excision; surgical removal	partial removal of the prostate using a cystoscope passed through the urethra; also known as transurethral resection of the prostate (TURP) (Figure 17-3)	

(continued)

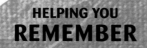

HELPING YOU
REMEMBER

Do not confuse
prostate, a male
reproductive gland,
with prostrate,
meaning "stretched
out on the ground."

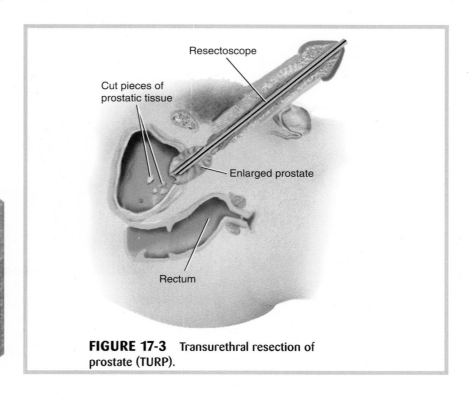

FIGURE 17-3 Transurethral resection of prostate (TURP).

Root	Meaning	
sperm/o; spermat/o	spermatozoa; sperm	
Term	**Term Analysis**	**Definition**
aspermatogenesis (ay-**sper**-mah-toh-**JEN**-eh-sis)	-genesis = production; formation a- = no; not; lack of	no production of spermatozoa
NOTE: The singular of spermatozoa is spermatozoon.		
oligospermia (**ol**-ih-goh-**SPER**-mee-ah)	-ia = condition oligo- = deficient; scanty; few	deficient number of spermatozoa
spermatocidal (**sper**-mah-toh-**SYE**-dal)	-cidal = to kill	to kill or destroy spermatozoa; spermicidal

Root	Meaning
testicul/o	testicle; testis

Term	Term Analysis	Definition
testicular (tes-**TICK**-yoo-lar)	-ar = pertaining to	pertaining to the testicle

Root	Meaning
vas/o	vessel; vas deferens

Term	Term Analysis	Definition
vasectomy (vah-**SECK**-toh-mee)	-ectomy = excision; surgical removal	excision of the vas deferens or a portion of it (Figure 17-4)

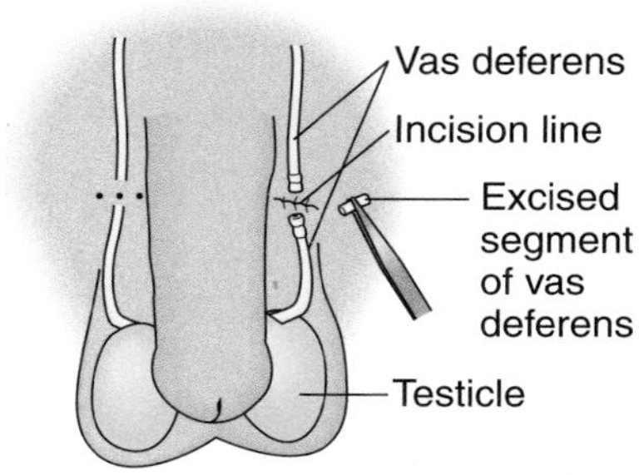

FIGURE 17-4 Vasectomy.

Suffix	Meaning
-cele	hernia; protrusion

Term	Term Analysis	Definition
hematocele (**HEE**-mah-toh-seel)	hemat/o = blood	accumulation of blood around the testicles
hydrocele (**HIGH**-droh-seel)	hydr/o = water	accumulation of fluid around the testicles (Figure 17-5)

(continued)

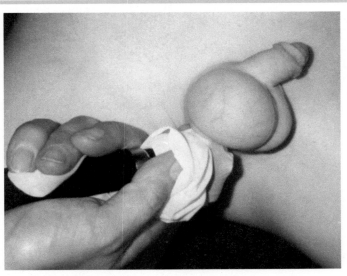

FIGURE 17-5 Hydrocele. A flashlight is shown behind the scrotum. If a hydrocele is present, a red glow will show up in the scrotum because the light will pass through it. If a tumor is present, no glow will show up.

varicocele (**VAR**-ih-koh-**seel**)	varic/o = varicose veins; dilated, twisted veins	dilation of the testicular veins inside the scrotum (Figure 17-6)

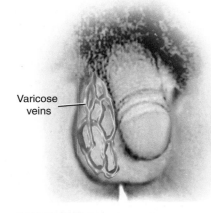

Varicose veins

FIGURE 17-6 Varicocele.

Suffix		Meaning
-potence		power
Term	**Term Analysis**	**Definition**
impotence (**IM**-poh-tens)	in- = no; not	inability to achieve or maintain an erection

Suffix	Meaning
-spadias	opening; split

Term	Term Analysis	Definition
hypospadias (**high**-poh-**SPAY**-dee-as)	hypo- = under	the urinary meatus is located on the underside of the penis; a congenital condition (Figure 17-7)

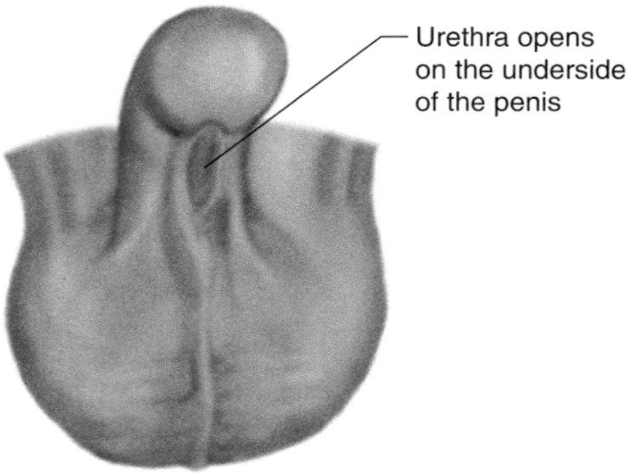

Urethra opens on the underside of the penis

FIGURE 17-7   Hypospadias.

Prefix	Meaning
circum-	around

Term	Term Analysis	Definition
circumcision (**ser**-kum-**SIZH**-un)	-ion = process cis/o = to cut	removal of the prepuce or foreskin (Figure 17-8)

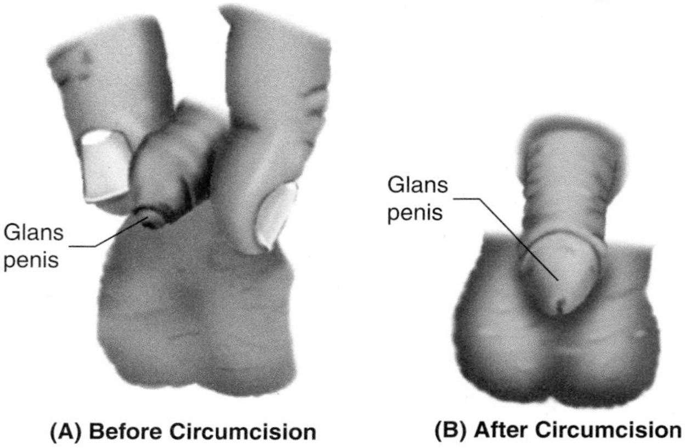

Glans penis

Glans penis

(A) Before Circumcision   (B) After Circumcision

FIGURE 17-8   Circumcision.

Benign Prostatic Hypertrophy (BPH)

Noncancerous enlargement of the prostate. The urethra goes through an opening in the prostate. If the prostate enlarges, it squeezes the urethra and obstructs the flow of urine (Figure 17-9). This causes urinary retention.

This condition commonly occurs in men over 50 years of age. Transurethral resection of the prostate (TURP) may be performed.

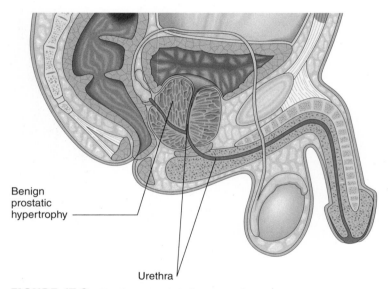

Benign prostatic hypertrophy

Urethra

FIGURE 17-9 Benign prostatic hypertrophy.

Carcinoma of the Prostate

Malignant tumor of the prostate, primarily affecting men over 50.

Phimosis (fih-**MOH**-sis)

Tightened foreskin that cannot be pulled back. Secretions can accumulate between the foreskin and the penis, causing inflammation. May lead to penile cancer. Circumcision is the method of treatment.

Sexually Transmitted Diseases (STDs)

Sexually transmitted diseases occur in both men and women. A list of the most common STDs is found in the pathology section on the female reproductive system. AIDS is also an STD. It is described in Chapter 14, Lymphatic and Immune Systems.

Testicular Cancer

Malignant tumor of the testicles. It is most common in men between the ages of 15 and 40. When treated early, the cancer is curable.

17.6 REVIEW EXERCISES

Exercise 17-1

LOOK-ALIKE AND SOUND-ALIKE WORDS

prostate	male reproductive gland
prostrate	stretched out on the ground
glans	refers to glans penis (tip of the penis)
glands	a group of cells whose function is the production and secretion of a particular substance
hyperplastic	pertaining to an abnormal increase in the number of cells in tissues
hypoplastic	pertaining to an underdevelopment of an organ or tissue

1. Physical examination at the time of admission revealed the (**prostrate/prostate**) to be smooth, benign, and enlarged.

2. The patient was found (**prostrate/prostate**) outside his apartment having suffered an apparent heart attack.

3. The (**glans/glands**) were swollen and there was evidence of lymphadenopathy.

4. Examination of the patient's thyroid revealed the gland to be approximately twice its normal size. The (**hyperplastic/hypoplastic**) thyroid was noted three months ago, shortly after she became pregnant.

Exercise 17-2

MATCHING WORD PARTS WITH MEANING

Match the word part in Column A *with the meaning in* Column B.

Column A		Column B	
_____	1. orchid/o	A.	male
_____	3. hemat/o	B.	glans penis
_____	3. varic/o	C.	power
_____	4. -potence	D.	opening

(Exercise continues on page 370)

Column A	Column B
_____ 5. crypt/o	E. protrusion; hernia
_____ 6. andr/o	F. around
_____ 7. -spadias	G. blood
_____ 8. circum-	H. dilated, twisted veins
_____ 9. -cele	I. hidden
_____ 10. balan/o	J. testicul/o

Exercise 17-3   DEFINITIONS—ANATOMY, PHYSIOLOGY, AND PATHOLOGY

In the space provided, write the medical term that is described below.

1. structure producing sperm and testosterone _____

2. structure that stores sperm _____

3. three structures that secrete substances to nourish sperm

   _____ , _____ ,

   _____

4. the medical term meaning sperm production

   _____

5. structure that encases the testicles _____

6. noncancerous enlargement of the prostate _____

7. tightened foreskin that cannot be pulled back

   _____

8. another term for foreskin _____

Exercise 17-4   LEARNING THE TERMS

Define the following medical words.

1. **androgenic** _____

2. **balanorrhea** _____

3. cryptorchidism _____

4. aspermatogenesis _____

5. vasectomy _____

6. transurethral _____

7. impotence _____

8. hypospadias _____

9. circumcision _____

10. congenital _____

Exercise 17-5 | **BUILDING MEDICAL WORDS**

Write the medical word for the following definitions.

    a. accumulation of fluid around the testicle

    _____

    b. surgical fixation of the testicle _____

    c. deficient number of spermatozoa _____

    d. pertaining to the testicle _____

    e. accumulation of blood around the testicles

    _____

    f. dilation of testicular veins inside the scrotum

    _____

    g. opening of the urinary meatus on the underside of the penis _____

    h. inflammation of the testicle _____

    i. to kill or destroy spermatozoa _____

    j. producing masculinizing effects _____

Exercise 17-6 | **LABELING—MALE REPRODUCTIVE SYSTEM**

Write the name of each numbered structure on the corresponding line below the diagram (Figure 17-10). Use the body structures listed on page 372.

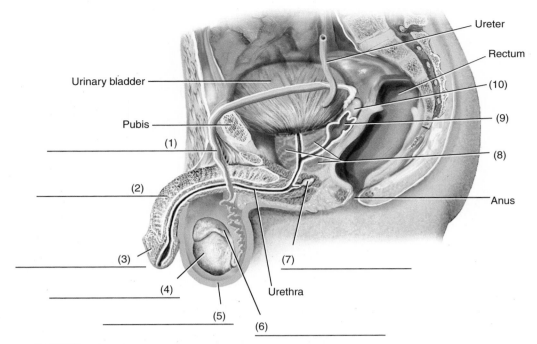

Ureter

Rectum

Urinary bladder

(10)

Pubis

(9)

(1)

(8)

(2)

Anus

(3)

(7)

(4)

Urethra

(5)

(6)

FIGURE 17-10 Major organs of the male reproductive system.

bulbourethral gland

ejaculatory duct

epididymis

glans penis

penis

prostate

scrotum

seminal vesicle

testis

vas deferens

1. _____

2. _____

3. _____

4. _____

5. _____

6. _____

7. _____

8. _____

9. _____

10. _____

Exercise 17-7   SPELLING

Circle any words that are spelled incorrectly in the list below. Then correct the spelling in the space provided.

1. prostratic _____

2. ressection _____

3. transillumination _____

4. epididmus _____

5. seminal vesicle _____

6. balanorhea _____

7. cryptorchidism _____

8. impotance _____

9. genitalia _____

10. orifce _____

17.7 PRONUNCIATION AND SPELLING

1. Listen to each word on the audio CD.

2. Pronounce each word carefully.

3. Spell each word in the space provided.

Word	Pronunciation	Spelling
androgenic	an-droh-**JEN**-ick	
aspermatogenesis	ay-**sper**-mah-toh-**JEN**-eh-sis	
balanorrhea	**bal**-an-oh-**REE**-ah	
benign prostatic hypertrophy	be-**NINE** proh-**STAT**-ick **HIGH**-per-troh-fee	

Word	Pronunciation	Spelling
circumcision	ser-kum-**SIZH**-un	
cryptorchidism	krip-**TOR**-kih-**diz**-um	
epididymis	ep-ih-**DID**-ih-mis	
glans penis	**GLANZ PEE**-nis	
hematocele	**HEE**-mah-toh-seel	
hypospadias	high-poh-**SPAY**-dee-as	
impotence	**IM**-poh-tens	
oligospermia	ol-ih-goh-**SPER**-mee-ah	
orchidopexy	**OR**-kid-oh-**peck**-see	
orchitis	or-**KYE**-tis	
prostatitis	pros-tah-**TYE**-tis	
scrotum	**SKROH**-tum	
spermatogenesis	sper-mah-toh-jen-**EE**-sis	
testicles	**TEST**-ick-els	
testicular	tes-**TICK**-yoo-lar	
varicocele	**VAR**-ih-koh-**seel**	
vas deferens	**VASS DEF**-er-enz	
vasectomy	vah-**SECK**-toh-mee	

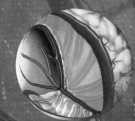

CHAPTER 18

Female Reproductive System

CHAPTER OUTLINE

18.1 Major Organs of the Female Reproductive System
18.2 Structure and Function of the Female Reproductive System
18.3 New Roots and Suffixes
18.4 Learning the Terms
18.5 Pathology
18.6 Review Exercises
18.7 Pronunciation and Spelling

LEARNING OBJECTIVES

After studying this chapter and completing the review exercises, you should be able to:

1. Locate the organs of the female reproductive system.
2. Describe the structures and functions of the female reproductive system.
3. Pronounce, spell, define, and write the medical terms related to the female reproductive system.
4. Describe common diseases of the female reproductive system.
5. Listen, read, and study so you can speak and write.

INTRODUCTION

The female reproductive system consists of the ovaries (**OH**-vah-rees), the uterus (**YOO**-ter-us), the uterine or fallopian (fah-**LOH**-pee-an) tubes, the vagina (vah-**JIGH**-nah), the external genitalia (**jen**-ih-**TAIL**-yah), and the mammary glands (**MAM**-ah-ree). Figure 18-1 illustrates these structures (except for the mammary glands).

18.1 MAJOR ORGANS OF THE FEMALE REPRODUCTIVE SYSTEM

PRACTICE FOR LEARNING: **MAJOR ORGANS OF THE FEMALE REPRODUCTIVE SYSTEM**

Write the words below in the correct spaces on Figure 18-1. (Some urinary structures are also included.) To help you, the number beside the word tells you where it goes on the figure. Be sure to pronounce each word as you write it. Repeat the pronunciation several times if you find the word hard to say.

1. ovary (**OH**-vah-ree)

2. rectouterine pouch (**reck**-toh-**YOO**-ter-in **POWCH**)

3. cervix uteri (**SER**-vicks **YOO**-ter-eye)

4. vagina (vah-**JIGH**-nah)

5. urethra (yoo-**REE**-thra)

6. urinary bladder (**YOO**-rih-**nar**-ee **BLAH**-der)

7. uterus (**YOO**-ter-us)

8. fallopian tubes (fal-**LOH**-pee-an **TOOBZ**)

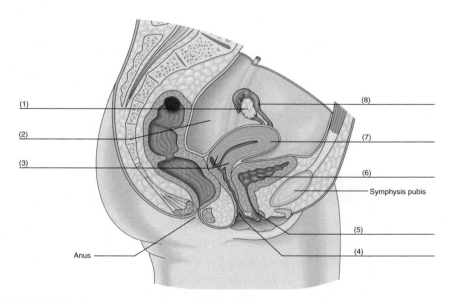

FIGURE 18-1 Major structures of the female reproductive system.

18.2 STRUCTURE AND FUNCTION OF THE FEMALE REPRODUCTIVE SYSTEM

Ovaries

The ovaries are almond-shaped glands. They are located in the pelvic cavity. There is one on each side of the uterus. As shown in Figure 18-2, they are held in place by ligaments. The ovaries discharge the egg or ovum (**OH-vum**) (plural = ova) and produce various hormones.

The ovaries of a newborn female contain a lifetime supply of immature eggs. Egg release begins at puberty, which is the age at which sexual reproduction is possible. One egg is released approximately every 28 days. This alternates from ovary to ovary each time. The process is called ovulation (**ahv-yoo-LAY-shun**).

The ovaries release the hormones estrogen (**ES-troh-jen**) and progesterone (**pro-JES-ter-on**). Estrogen helps develop the secondary female characteristics such as the breasts and pubic hair. Progesterone stimulates the growth of blood vessels in the uterus. Estrogen also stimulates the thickening of the uterine lining to prepare for the implantation of a fertilized egg. If no fertilization takes place, this buildup of tissue is sloughed off (discharged) in a process called menstruation (**men-stroo-AY-shun**) or menses (**MEN-seez**). Sometime between the ages of 45 and 55, all of the eggs either have been discharged or have degenerated. The reproductive cycle then ceases, and the woman is in menopause (**MEN-oh-pawz**).

Fallopian Tubes

The fallopian tubes are shown in Figure 18-2. They link the ovaries and the uterus. The distal end of each tube is equipped with tiny fingerlike projections called fimbriae (**FIM-bree-ee**). They sweep back and forth, creating waves in the fluid surrounding the ovary. The waves pull an ovum into the tube, and it is then transported to the uterus.

Fertilization is the union of the ovum and sperm. Sperm enters the female reproductive tract following ejaculation by the male. Fertilization usually takes place inside the fallopian tube. If the ovum is fertilized, it begins to grow into a fetus (**FEE-tus**), the name given to the unborn baby. If it is not fertilized, the ovum breaks down within 24 hours after ovulation.

IN BRIEF

Ovaries
discharge ova
and produce estrogen
and progesterone

Estrogen
important in
the development of
female secondary sex
characteristics.
It also thickens the
uterine lining

Progesterone
stimulates the growth
of blood vessels in the
endometrium

Fallopian tubes
transport the egg from
the ovary to the uterus.

Uterus
houses and protects
the developing fetus.

Vagina
birth canal and accepts
the penis during coitus.

Uterus

The uterus is a muscular, thick-walled organ. It is shaped like an inverted pear and is held in place in the pelvic cavity by ligaments (Figure 18-2). The superior, rounded portion of the uterus is called the fundus (**FUN-dus**). The middle portion is the body. The inferior portion is the cervix uteri (**SER-vicks YOO-ter-eye**), which projects into the vagina.

Inside the uterus is a hollow space in which the fetus develops. This space is enclosed by three walls: the endometrium (**en-doh-MEE-tree-um**), myometrium (**my-oh-MEE-tree-um**), and perimetrium (**per-ih-MEE-tree-um**). The endometrium is sloughed off during menstruation. The myometrium is the muscular wall. The perimetrium is the outermost wall.

In Figure 18-1, you can see the lowest point of the abdominal cavity. It is called the rectouterine (**reck-toh-YOO-ter-in**) pouch. It is also called the cul-de-sac of Douglas. It lies between the uterus and the rectum.

The uterine tubes, ovaries, and the ligaments holding the uterus in place are collectively called the adnexa (**ad-NECK-sah**).

Vagina

The vagina can be seen in Figure 18-2. It is a muscular tube leading from the cervix to the exterior. It is approximately 6 inches (15 cm) long and is lined with mucous membrane.

The vagina accepts the penis of the male during intercourse. It is also called the birth canal.

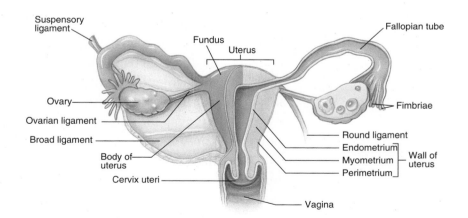

FIGURE 18-2   Uterus, fallopian tubes, ovaries, and related structures.

External Genitalia

The external genitalia, or vulva (**VUL**-vah), are illustrated in Figure 18-3.

The area from the vulva to the anus is called the perineum (**per**-ih-**NEE**-um).

The other parts of the external genitalia are the clitoris (**KLIT**-eh-ris), labia majora (**LAY**-bee-a mah-**JOR**-ah), labia minora (mih-**NOR**-ah), and mons pubis (**MONZ PYOO**-bis). Also included are Bartholin's (**BAR**-toh-linz) glands. They secrete lubricants for intercourse.

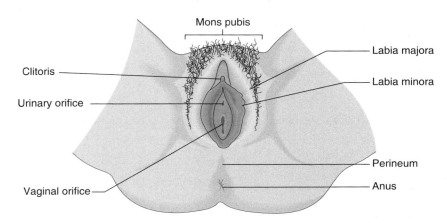

FIGURE 18-3   External genitalia.

Breasts

PRACTICE FOR LEARNING: **THE BREASTS**

Write the words below in the correct spaces on Figure 18-4. To help you, the number beside the word tells you where it goes on the figure. Be sure to pronounce each word as you write it. Repeat the pronunciation several times if you find the word hard to say.

1. lactiferous ducts (lack-**TIF**-er-us **DUKTS**)

2. lactiferous sinus (lack-**TIF**-er-us **SIGH**-nus)

3. nipple (**NIH**-pul)

4. areola (ah-**REE**-oh-lah)

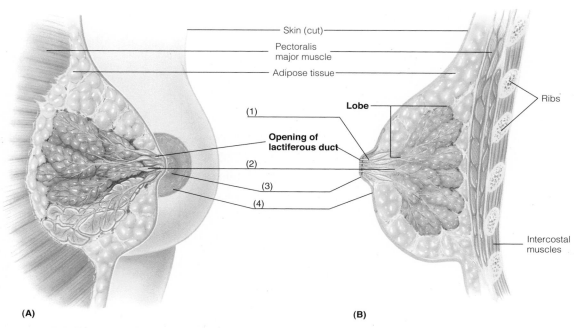

Skin (cut)
Pectoralis major muscle
Adipose tissue
Ribs
Lobe
(1)
Opening of lactiferous duct
(2)
(3)
(4)
Intercostal muscles

(A)   (B)

FIGURE 18-4   The breast. (A) Anterior view. (B) Sagittal view.

IN BRIEF

Breasts
include the nipple, areola, lactiferous sinuses, and lactiferous ducts.

Figure 18-4 illustrates the structures of the breast or mammary gland. The nipple is surrounded by a darker ring of skin called the **areola** (**ah-REE-oh-lah**).

The mammary glands produce milk after childbirth. Each gland consists of a number of **lobes** (**LOHBZ**), which contain many little sacs (lobules) that secrete milk. The milk is stored in **lactiferous** (**lack-TIF-er-us**) **sinuses**. It travels through the lacterifous (milk) ducts to tiny openings in the nipple. Oils produced by glands in the areola help minimize drying out of the skin around the nipple due to breastfeeding.

PRACTICE FOR LEARNING: FEMALE REPRODUCTIVE ORGANS

Write the structure responsible for the functions listed below.

1. holds the fetus during pregnancy _____

2. lubricates the vagina for intercourse _____

3. acts as the birth canal _____

4. transports the egg to the uterus _____

5. secretes estrogen and progesterone _____

6. ovulation _____

Answers: **1.** uterus. **2.** Bartholin's gland. **3.** vagina. **4.** fallopian tubes. **5.** ovaries. **6.** ovaries.

PRACTICE FOR LEARNING: **FEMALE REPRODUCTIVE ORGANS**

Write the location of the structures in the numbered list. Choose your answers from the list below.

abdominal cavity

breast

external genitalia

fallopian tubes

pelvic cavity

uterus

1. cul-de-sac of Douglas _____

2. perineum _____

3. areola _____

4. ovary _____

5. fundus _____

6. fimbriae _____

7. cervix _____

Answers: **1.** abdominal cavity. **2.** external genitalia. **3.** breast. **4.** pelvic cavity. **5.** uterus. **6.** fallopian tubes. **7.** uterus.

18.3 NEW ROOTS AND SUFFIXES

Use these additional roots and suffixes when studying the medical words in this chapter.

Root	Meaning
flex/o	bend
men/o	month
tub/o	tube
versi/o	tilting; turning; tipping

Suffix	Meaning
-an	pertaining to
-ine	pertaining to

18.4 LEARNING THE TERMS

Following these steps will make it easier for you to learn medical terms:

1. Pronounce the term repeatedly until it is easy for you.

2. Write it down. Ensure the spelling is correct.

3. Also write the definition. If possible, relate the word to a word, thought, or picture that will help you remember it.

4. Analyze the term with the method taught in this text.

Roots

Root	Meaning
cervic/o	cervix; cervix uteri; neck of the uterus

Term	Term Analysis	Definition
cervicitis (ser-vih-**SIGH**-tis)	-itis = inflammation	inflammation of the cervix
cervical polyp (**SER**-vih-kal **POL**-up)	-al = pertaining to polyp = protruding growth from the mucous membrane	abnormal growth extending from the mucous membrane of the cervix uteri (Figure 18-5)

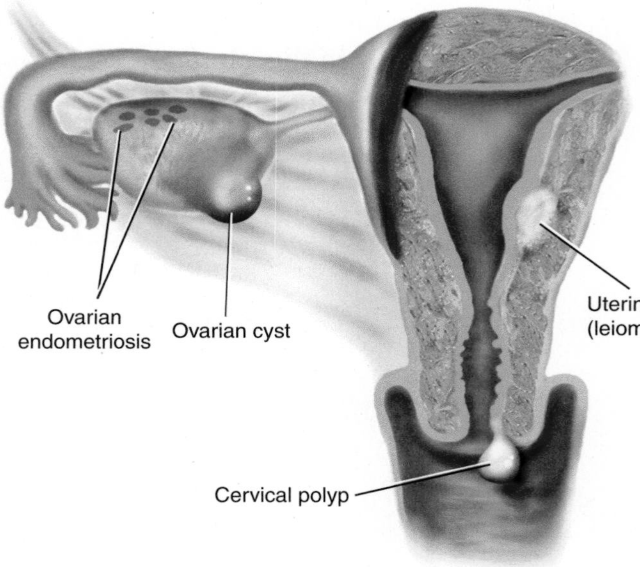

Ovarian endometriosis

Ovarian cyst

Uterine fibroid (leiomyoma)

Cervical polyp

FIGURE 18-5 Cervical polyp, endometriosis, ovarian cyst, uterine fibroid.

Root	Meaning
colp/o (see also **vagin/o**)	vagina

Term	Term Analysis	Definition
colporrhaphy (kohl-**POR**-ah-fee)	-rrhaphy = suture	suturing of the vagina

Root	Meaning
episi/o	vulva; external genitalia; pudendum

Term	Term Analysis	Definition
episiotomy (eh-**piz**-ee-**OT**-oh-mee)	-tomy = process of cutting	process of cutting the vulva

NOTE: An episiotomy is used to assist delivery of the fetus. It lengthens the vulvar area for delivery of the fetus.

Term	Term Analysis	Definition
episiorrhaphy (eh-**piz**-ee-**OR**-ah-fee)	-rrhaphy = suture	suturing of the vulva and perineum

Root	Meaning
fibr/o	fibers; fibrous tissue

Term	Term Analysis	Definition
fibroadenoma (**fye**-broh-**ad**-eh-**NOH**-mah)	-oma = mass, tumor aden/o = gland	abnormal masses in the breast that are round, firm, and rubbery.

NOTE: The condition involves fibrous (connective) tissue in a gland. Thus, the word parts aden/o and fibr/o are used.

(continued)

Root	Meaning
gynec/o	woman

Term	Term Analysis	Definition
gynecologist (**gye**-neh-**KOL**-oh-jist)	-logist = specialist	specialist in the study of diseases and treatment of the female genital tract

Root	Meaning
hyster/o (see also **metr/o** and **uter/o**)	uterus

Term	Term Analysis	Definition
hysterectomy (**hiss**-ter-**ECK**-toh-mee)	-ectomy = excision; removal	surgical removal of the uterus (Figure 18-6)

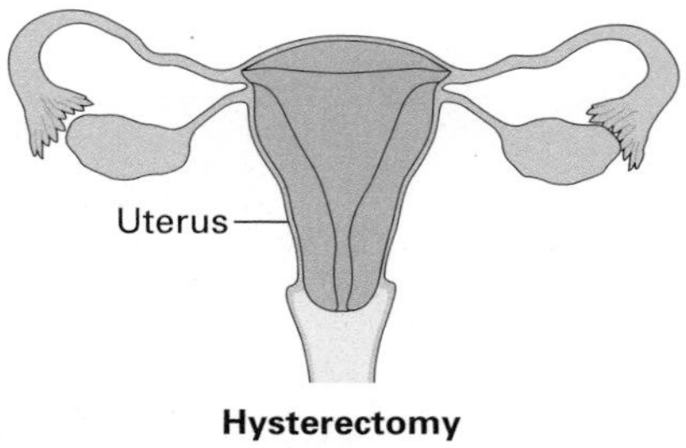

Uterus

Hysterectomy

FIGURE 18-6 Hysterectomy.

Root	Meaning
labi/o	lips

Term	Term Analysis	Definition
labial (**LAY**-bee-al)	-al = pertaining to	pertaining to the lips (of the vagina)

Root	Meaning
lact/o	milk

Term	Term Analysis	Definition
lactogenesis (**lack**-toh-**JEN**-ih-sis)	-genesis = production; formation	production and secretion of milk from the breast

Root	Meaning
ligati/o	binding; tying

Term	Term Analysis	Definition
tubal ligation (**TOO**-bal lye-**GAY**-shun)	-ion = process -al = pertaining to tub/o = tube; fallopian tube	female sterilization (Figure 18-7)

NOTE 1: This procedure involves blocking the fallopian tubes to prevent the sperm from meeting (fertilizing) the egg. If no fertilization occurs, the woman cannot become pregnant.

The tubes can be blocked by tying (ligating), cutting, burning, or a combination of these procedures.

NOTE 2: A tubal ligation does not involve removal of the uterus or any other organs. Menstruation continues.

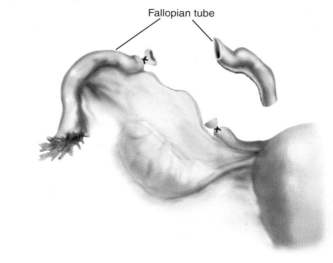

Fallopian tube

FIGURE 18-7 Tubal ligation.

Root	Meaning
mamm/o; mast/o	**breast**

Term	Term Analysis	Definition
mammary (**MAM**-ah-ree)	-ary = pertaining to	pertaining to the breast
mastopexy (**MAS**-toh-**peck**-see)	-pexy = surgical fixation	surgical fixation of the breast.
NOTE: Mastopexy is a type of plastic surgery performed on drooping breasts to improve their look and form.		

Root	Meaning
men/o	**menses; menstruation; month**

Term	Term Analysis	Definition
amenorrhea (ah-**men**-oh-**REE**-ah)	-rrhea = discharge; flow a- = no; not	no menstruation
dysmenorrhea (**dis**-men-oh-**REE**-ah)	-rrhea = discharge; flow dys- = painful; difficult; bad	painful menstruation
menorrhea (**men**-oh-**REE**-ah)	-rrhea = discharge; flow	normal menstruation
menorrhagia (**men**-oh-**RAY**-jee-ah)	-rrhagia = burst forth	excessive uterine bleeding during menstruation

Root	Meaning
metr/o	**uterus**

Term	Term Analysis	Definition
metrorrhagia (**meh**-troh-**RAY**-jee-ah)	-rrhagia = burst forth	uterine bleeding at times other than at the regular menstrual period

Root	Meaning
oophor/o (see also ovari/o)	ovary

Term	Term Analysis	Definition
oophororrhagia (oh-**of**-oh-**RAY**-jee-ah)	-rrhagia = burst forth	hemorrhaging from the ovary

Root	Meaning
ovari/o	ovary

Term	Term Analysis	Definition
ovarian cyst (oh-**VAR**-ree-an **SIST**)	-an = pertaining to cyst = closed sac or cavity	abnormal cystic growth on the ovary. A cyst is a closed sac or cavity containing fluid, semifluid, or solid material (see Figure 18-5)

Root	Meaning
perine/o	perineum (area between the vagina and the anus)

Term	Term Analysis	Definition
perineorrhaphy (**per**-ih-nee-**OR**-ah-fee)	-rrhaphy = suture	suturing of the perineum

NOTE: During delivery, the perineum may tear as the fetus exits the vaginal canal. A perineorrhaphy repairs the perineum.

Root	Meaning
salping/o (see also -salpinx)	fallopian tube; uterine tube

Term	Term Analysis	Definition
salpingo-oophorectomy sal-**ping**-goh-**oh**-of-oh-**RECK**-toh-mee)	-ectomy = excision; surgical removal oophor/o = ovary	excision of the fallopian tubes and ovaries

Root	Meaning
uter/o	uterus

Term	Term Analysis	Definition
intrauterine (in-trah-**YOO**-ter-in)	-ine = pertaining to intra- = within	within the uterus
uterine fibroids (**YOO**-ter-in **FYE**-broidz)	-ine = pertaining to fibroids = benign tumors	a benign muscle tumor of the uterus (see Figure 18-5); also known as fibroids, myomas, leiomyoma, or fibromyomas
uterovesical (**yoo**-ter-oh-**VES**-ih-kal)	-al = pertaining to vesic/o = bladder	pertaining to the uterus and bladder

Root	Meaning
vagin/o	vagina

Term	Term Analysis	Definition
vaginomycosis (**vaj**-ih-noh-mye-**KOH**-sis)	-osis = abnormal condition myc/o = fungus	fungal infection of the vagina

Root	Meaning
vulv/o	vulva; external genitalia; pudendum

Term	Term Analysis	Definition
vulvorectal (**vul**-voh-**RECK**-tal)	-al = pertaining to rect/o = rectum	pertaining to the vulva and rectum

Suffix	Meaning
-arche	beginning

Term	Term Analysis	Definition
menarche (men-**AR**-kee)	men/o = menses; menstruation; month	beginning of the regular menstrual cycle at approximately 13 years of age

Suffix	Meaning
-cele	**hernia** (protrusion of an organ from the structure that normally contains it)

Term	Term Analysis	Definition
cystocele (**SIS**-toh-seel)	cyst/o = bladder	hernia of the bladder that presses against the vaginal wall (Figure 18-8A, and 18B)

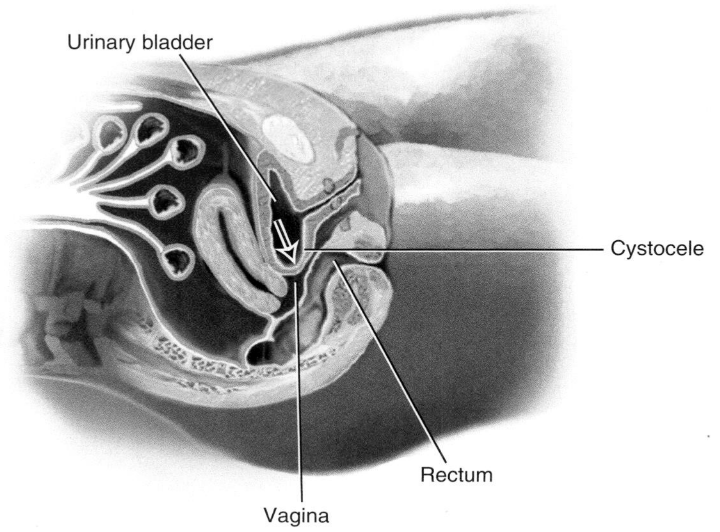

FIGURE 18-8 (A) Cystocele, lateral view.

(continued)

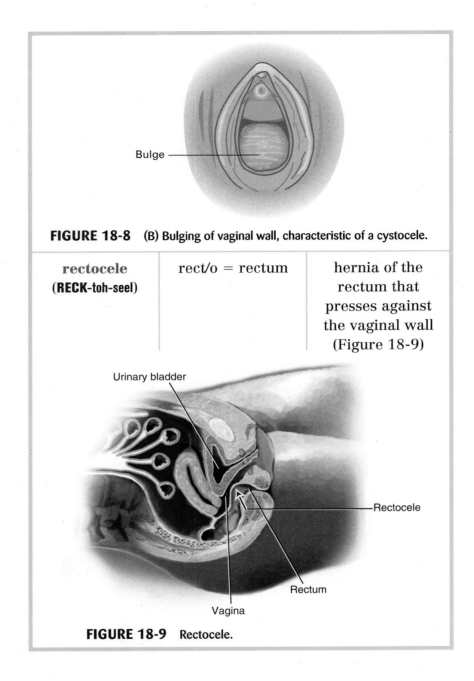

FIGURE 18-8 (B) Bulging of vaginal wall, characteristic of a cystocele.

rectocele (**RECK**-toh-seel)	rect/o = rectum	hernia of the rectum that presses against the vaginal wall (Figure 18-9)

FIGURE 18-9 Rectocele.

Suffix		Meaning
-salpinx		fallopian tube; uterine tube
Term	**Term Analysis**	**Definition**
hydrosalpinx (**high**-dro-**SAL**-pinks)	hydr/o = water	accumulation of a watery fluid in the fallopian tube

Prefix	Meaning
ante-	before

Term	Term Analysis	Definition
anteflexion (**an-tee-FLECK**-shun)	-ion = process flex/o = bending	bending forward of a part of an organ; normal position of the uterus as it bends forward over the bladder (Figure 18-10A)
anteversion (**an-tee-VER**-shun)	-ion = process versi/o = tilting; tipping	tilting forward of an organ or part of an organ; forward tilting of the uterus over the bladder (Figure 18-10B)

Prefix	Meaning
retro-	back; behind

Term	Term Analysis	Definition
retroflexion (**ret-roh-FLECK**-shun)	-ion = process flex/o = bending	bending back of a part of an organ; an abnormal position of the uterus as it bends backward toward the rectum (Figure 18-10C)
retroversion (**ret-roh-VER**-zhun)	-ion = process versi/o = tilting; tipping	tilting backward of an organ or part of an organ; an abnormal position of the uterus as it tilts backward toward the rectum (Figure 18-10D)

(continued)

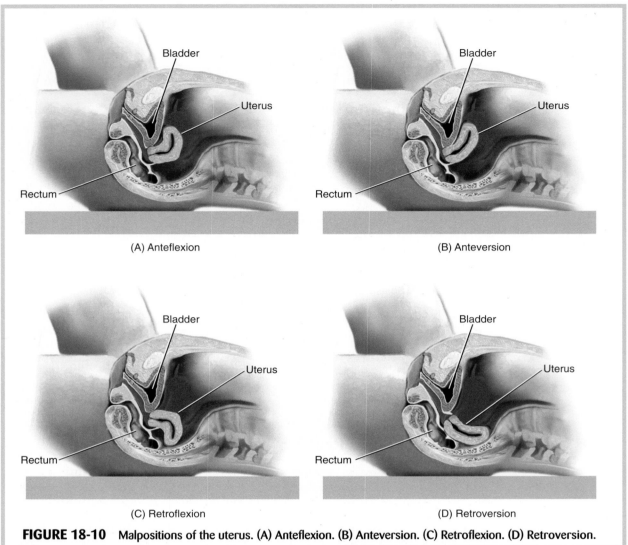

FIGURE 18-10 Malpositions of the uterus. (A) Anteflexion. (B) Anteversion. (C) Retroflexion. (D) Retroversion.

18.5 PATHOLOGY

Breast Cancer

Malignant tumor of the breast. If left untreated, the cancer can metastasize (**meh-TAS-tah-size**). This means that it spreads to the surrounding breast tissue and then to other parts of the body through the blood and lymph.

Endometriosis (**en-**doh-**mee-**tree-**OH-**sis**)

Endometrial tissue found at sites other than the uterus (refer to Figure 18-5). The ectopic (out of place) endometrial tissue finds its way into the pelvic cavity by moving out of the uterus and through the open fallopian tubes. Other abnormal sites where the endometrium can be found include the ovaries, tubes, and abdominal cavity.

Uterine (Endometrial) Cancer

Malignant tumor of the endometrium. Uterine cancer is the most common cancer of the reproductive organs.

Uterine Prolapse

Protrusion or displacement of the uterus through the vaginal canal. There are three stages (degrees) of prolapse depending on how far into the vaginal canal the uterus has fallen. These are illustrated in Figure 18-11.

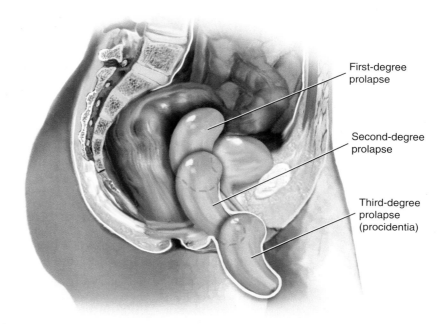

First-degree prolapse

Second-degree prolapse

Third-degree prolapse (procidentia)

FIGURE 18-11   Uterine prolapse. First degree: The cervix projects into the vaginal canal but does not project to the introitus (entrance to vagina). Second degree: The uterus projects further into the vaginal canal up to the introitus. Third degree: The uterus and cervix project through the introitus. This stage is also known as procidentia (**proh-sih-DEN**-shah)

Sexually Transmitted Diseases (STDs)

STDs include any disease that has been transmitted through any type of sexual activity, including vaginal, oral, and anal sex. AIDS is also an STD. Details about AIDS are in the chapter on the lymphatic and immune systems.

The most common types of STDs are chlamydia (**klah-MID**-ee-ah), genital herpes (Figure 18-12), genital warts (Figure 18-13), gonorrhea (**gon-oh-REE-ah**), and syphilis (**SIF-ih-lis**). In the early stages of these diseases, the patient is often asymptomatic (there are no symptoms). The patient may therefore spread the disease to other persons without knowing it. If left untreated, permanent damage to the reproductive organs may result.

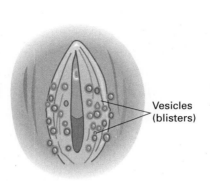

Vesicles (blisters)

Warts caused by human papillomavirus (HPV)

FIGURE 18-12 Genital herpes.

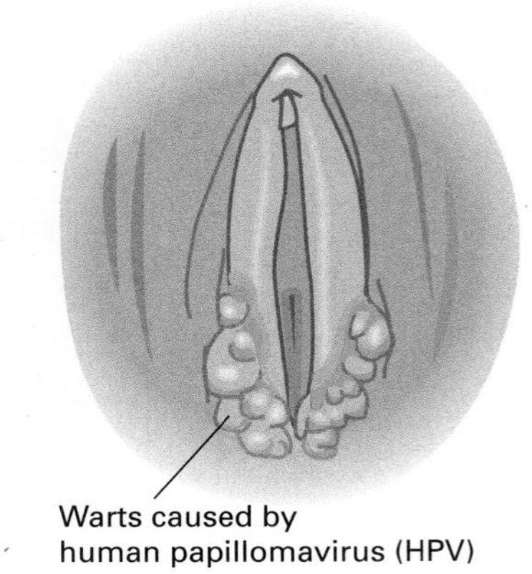

FIGURE 18-13 Genital warts.

18.6 REVIEW EXERCISES

Exercise 18-1 LOOK-ALIKE AND SOUND-ALIKE WORDS

Below is a list of look-alike and sound-alike words. Study the definitions of each set of words, then read the sentences carefully and circle the word in parentheses that correctly completes the meaning

menorrhagia	excessive uterine bleeding during menstruation
menorrhalgia	painful menstruation
metrorrhagia	uterine bleeding at times other than at the regular menstrual period
perineal	pertaining to the perineum
peritoneal	pertaining to the peritoneum
peroneal	pertaining to the fibula or outer side of the leg
parametrium	connective tissue located beside the uterus
perimetrium	outermost wall of the uterus

1. The patient was admitted with excessive menstrual bleeding. It was decided that a hysterectomy would be a permanent solution for her (**menorrhagia/metrorrhagia**).

2. Dysmenorrhea and (**menorrhagia/menorrhalgia/ metrorrhagia**) mean the same thing.

3. The third degree (**perineal/peritoneal/peroneal**) tear was a complication of delivery due to a very large fetal head.

4. The malignant cells have spread outside the uterine wall to the (**perimetrium/parametrium**).

Exercise 18-2 | MATCHING WORD PARTS WITH MEANING

Match the word part in Column A *with its meaning in* Column B.

Column A	Column B
_____ 1. ante-	A. vulva
_____ 2. episio-	B. uterus
_____ 3. colp/o	C. binding; tying
_____ 4. gynec/o	D. month
_____ 5. salping/o	E. ovary
_____ 6. ligati/o	F. breast
_____ 7. men/o	G. milk
_____ 8. -arche	H. bladder
_____ 9. metr/o	I. woman
_____ 10. oophor/o	J. vagina
_____ 11. -rrhaphy	K. before
_____ 12. lact/o	L. fallopian tube
_____ 13. mamm/o	M. tilting
_____ 14. cyst/o	N. suture
_____ 15. -versi/o	O. beginning

Exercise 18-3 | MATCHING—ANATOMY

Match the term in Column A *with its description in* Column B.

Column A	Column B
_____ 1. estrogen	A. discharge of endometrial tissue
_____ 2. ovum	B. neck of the uterus
_____ 3. fimbriae	C. inner lining of the uterus
_____ 4. cervix uteri	D. part of the external genitalia
_____ 5. endometrium	
_____ 6. rectouterine pouch	

(Exercise continues on page 396)

Column A	Column B
_____ 7. labia majora	E. hormone responsible for the growth of blood vessels in the endometrium
_____ 8. progesterone	
_____ 9. uterus	F. egg
_____ 10. menstruation	G. houses and protects the developing fetus
	H. cul-de-sac of Douglas
	I. hormone responsible for developing female secondary characteristics
	J. portion of the fallopian tube

Exercise 18-4 — MATCHING–PATHOLOGY

Match the following terms with its description that is written below. Not all terms are used.

metastasize _____

endometriosis _____

endometrial cancer _____

breast cancer _____

uterine prolapse _____

chlamydia _____

1. endometrial tissue found in the pelvic cavity

   _____

2. the spread of cancer from one organ to another

   _____

3. the most common cancer of the female reproductive system

   _____

4. displacement of the uterus through the vaginal canal

   _____

5. a sexually transmitted disease _____

| Exercise 18-5 | LABELING—FEMALE REPRODUCTIVE TRACT |

Write the name of each numbered structure on the corresponding line below the diagram (Figure 18-14). Use the body structures listed below.

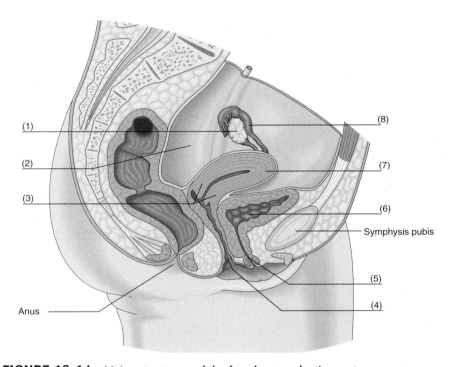

FIGURE 18-14   Major structures of the female reproductive system.

cervix
_____

fallopian tube
_____

ovary
_____

rectouterine pouch
_____

urethra
_____

urinary bladder
_____

uterus
_____

vagina
_____

1. _____

2. _____

3. _____

4. _____

5. _____

6. _____

7. _____

8. _____

Exercise 18-6 | DEFINITIONS—ANATOMY

Define the following terms:

1. estrogen _____

2. adnexa _____

3. myometrium _____

4. fertilization _____

5. lactiferous ducts _____

6. perimetrium _____

7. lactiferous sinus _____

8. ovulation _____

9. fetus _____

10. fundus of the uterus _____

Exercise 18-7 | PHYSIOLOGY

Write one function for each of the following.

1. ovaries _____

2. fimbriae _____

3. Bartholin's gland _____

4. mammary glands _____

5. estrogen _____

6. progesterone _____

7. fallopian tubes _____

8. uterus _____

9. vagina _____

| **Exercise 18-8** | **DEFINITIONS—LEARNING THE TERMS** |

Define the following terms.

1. cervical polyp _____

2. colporrhaphy _____

3. episiotomy _____

4. fibroadenoma _____

5. salpingo-oophorectomy _____

6. gynecologist _____

7. labial _____

8. lactogenesis _____

9. tubal ligation _____

10. mastopexy _____

11. menorrhea _____

12. menorrhagia _____

13. metrorrhagia _____

14. hysterectomy _____

15. vaginomycosis _____

16. cystocele _____

17. hydrosalpinx _____

18. anteflexion _____

19. retroversion _____

20. cervicitis _____

| Exercise 18-9 | **BUILDING MEDICAL WORDS** |

I. Use the combining form men/o to build medical words for the following definitions.

a. no menstruation _____

b. painful menstruation _____

c. normal menstruation _____

d. excessive uterine bleeding during menstruation

_____

II. Use the combining form metr/o to build medical words for the following definitions.

a. inner uterine wall _____

b. uterine bleeding at times other than regular menstrual periods _____

c. muscular uterine wall _____

d. outermost wall of the uterus _____

| Exercise 18-10 | **DEFINITIONS IN CONTEXT** |

Define the bolded terms in the spaces provided. Use your medical dictionary if necessary.

1. **Laparoscopic tubal ligation** was performed following delivery.

   a. laparoscopic tubal ligation _____

2. At laparoscopy, the **uterus** was small and normal in appearance. Both **fallopian tubes** were normal in appearance. The fallopian tubes were clamped and **ligated**.

   b. uterus _____

   c. fallopian tubes _____

   d. ligated _____

3. There was one area of **endometriosis** near the **fimbrial** aspect of the right fallopian tube.

   e. endometriosis _____

   f. fimbrial _____

4. On examination, the uterus was enlarged, and an ultrasound confirmed the presence of fibroids.

   g. ultrasound _____

   h. fibroids _____

Exercise 18-11 | SPELLING

Circle any words that are spelled incorrectly in the list below. Then correct the spelling in the space provided.

1. menstration _____

2. Bartolin's cyst _____

3. epiziorhaphy _____

4. dismenorrhea _____

5. pereniorrhaphy _____

6. rectroflection _____

7. endometriosis _____

8. sphylis _____

18.7 PRONUNCIATION AND SPELLING

1. Listen to each word on the audio CD.

2. Pronounce each word carefully.

3. Spell each word in the space provided.

Word	Pronunciation	Spelling
amenorrhea	ah-**men**-oh-**REE**-ah	
cervicitis	ser-vih-**SIGH**-tis	
chlamydia	klah-**MID**-ee-ah	
colporrhaphy	kohl-**POR**-ah-fee	
cystocele	**SIS**-toh-seel	
dysmenorrhea	dis-men-oh-**REE**-ah	

Word	Pronunciation	Spelling
endometriosis	en-doh-**mee**-tree-**OH**-sis	
endometrium	en-doh-**MEE**-tree-um	
episiorrhaphy	eh-**piz**-ee-**OR**-ah-fee	
estrogen	**ES**-troh-jen	
fallopian tubes	fal-**LOH**-pee-an **TOOBZ**	
fetus	**FEE**-tus	
genitalia	jen-ih-**TAIL**-yah	
gynecologist	**gye**-neh-**KOL**-oh-jist	
hysterectomy	hiss-ter-**ECK**-toh-mee	
menstruation	**men**-stroo-**AY**-shun	
myometrium	my-oh-**MEE**-tree-um	
oophorrhagia	oh-**of**-oh-**RAY**-jee-ah	
ovary	**OH**-vah-ree	
ovulation	**ahv**-yoo-**LAY**-shun	
perimetrium	per-ih-**MEE**-tree-um	
progesterone	pro-**JES**-ter-on	
retroflexion	ret-roh-**FLECK**-shun	
salpingo-oophorectomy	sal-**ping**-goh-**oh**-of-oh-**RECK**-toh-mee	
syphilis	**SIF**-ih-lis	
uterine fibroids	**YOO**-ter-in **FYE**-broidz	
uterovesical	**yoo**-ter-oh-**VES**-ih-kal	
uterus	**YOO**-ter-us	
vagina	vah-**JIGH**-nah	

CHAPTER 19

Endocrine System

LEARNING OBJECTIVES

After studying this chapter and completing the review exercises, you should be able to:

1. Define "endocrine glands" and "hormones."
2. Name the endocrine glands and their hormones.
3. Understand the function of these hormones in the body.
4. Pronounce, spell, define, and write the medical terms related to the endocrine system.
5. Describe common diseases related to the endocrine system.
6. Listen, read, and study so you can speak and write.

INTRODUCTION

The endocrine (**EN-doh-krin**) system consists of several glands. You can see them in Figure 19-1.

Glands are located in many areas of the body. They secrete powerful chemicals called hormones (**HOR-mohnz**) into the bloodstream. Hormones travel in the blood to various sites throughout the body. They regulate organ function and keep the body in a balanced, normal state no matter what is happening outside it. This balance is called homeostasis (**hoh-mee-oh-STAY-sis**). One example of homeostasis is the regulation of body temperature.

Hormones secreted by glands in the endocrine system maintain the body's normal temperature of about 98.6 degrees Fahrenheit (37 degrees Celsius) regardless of the outside temperature.

This chapter is organized under two major headings: peripheral endocrine glands and central endocrine glands. The peripheral endocrine glands are the thyroid (**THIGH**-royd), parathyroids (par-ah-**THIGH**-roydz), adrenals (ah-**DREE**-nalz), pineal (**PIN**-ee-al), and pancreas (**PAN**-kree-as). The first four have only one function: the

production of hormones. The pancreas not only produces hormones but also has important digestive functions. In this way, the pancreas is similar to other mixed-function organs, such as the kidneys, liver, ovaries, and testicles. The functions of these organs, except for the pancreas, have been taken up in their respective chapters.

There are only two central endocrine glands: the hypothalamus (high-poh-**THAL**-ah-mus) and the pituitary (pih-**TOO**-ih-tar-ee). They are both in the brain.

19.1 GLANDS OF THE ENDOCRINE SYSTEM

PRACTICE FOR LEARNING: GLANDS OF THE ENDOCRINE SYSTEM

Write the words below in the correct spaces on Figure 19-1. To help you, the number beside the word tells you where it goes on the figure. Be sure to pronounce each word as you write it. Repeat the pronunciation several times if you find the word hard to say.

1. pituitary gland (pih-**TOO**-ih-tar-ee)
2. hypothalamus (**high**-poh-**THAL**-ah-mus)
3. pineal gland (**PIN**-ee-al)
4. parathyroid gland (par-ah-**THIGH**-roid)
5. thymus gland (**THIGH**-mus)
6. ovaries (**OH**-vah-rees)
7. testicles (**TEST**-ick-els)
8. pancreas (**PAN**-kree-as)
9. adrenal glands (ah-**DREE**-nal)
10. thyroid gland (**THIGH**-royd)

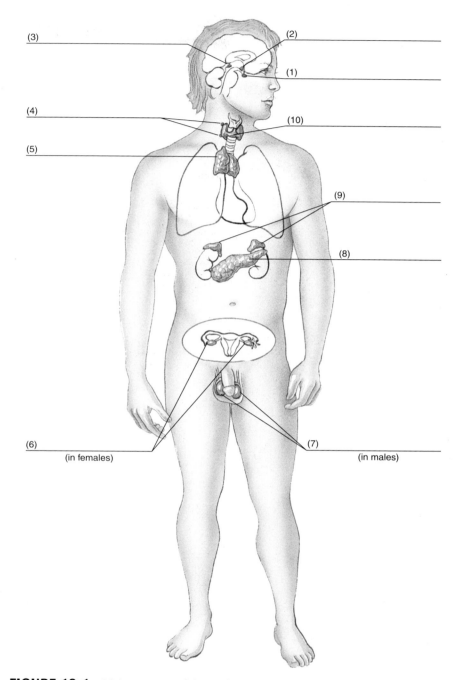

FIGURE 19-1 Major organs of the endocrine system.

19.2 PERIPHERAL ENDOCRINE GLANDS

Thyroid Gland

PRACTICE FOR LEARNING: THYROID GLAND

Write the words below in the correct spaces on Figure 19-2. To help you, the number beside the word tells you where it goes on the figure. Be sure to pronounce each word as you write it. Repeat the pronunciation several times if you find the word hard to say.

1. thyroid gland

2. right lobe

3. left lobe

4. isthmus (**ISS**-mus)

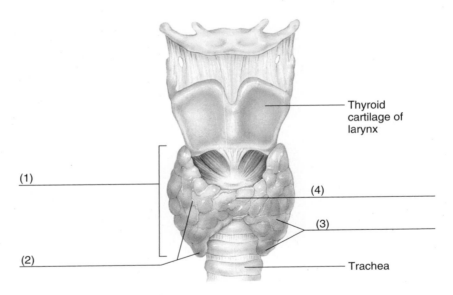

FIGURE 19-2   Thyroid gland.

Location and Structure

Figure 19-2 illustrates the thyroid gland. It is located in the neck below the larynx. It has right and left lobes connected by a structure called the isthmus.

Function

The thyroid secretes the hormones T₃ and T₄. T₃ is triiodothyronine (trigh-**eye**-oy-doh-**THIGH**-roh-nen). T₄ is thyroxine (thigh-**ROCK**-sin).

Thyroxine is also spelled thyroxin. These hormones regulate how much energy is used by the body's cells to perform their functions. This is called the metabolic rate. Iodine must be consumed in order for the thyroid to produce T_3 and T_4. A goiter (enlarged thyroid) will result if there is insufficient iodine in the diet.

Parathyroid Gland

PRACTICE FOR LEARNING: PARATHYROID GLAND

Write the words below in the correct spaces on Figure 19-3. To help you, the number beside the word tells you where it goes on the figure. Be sure to pronounce each word as you write it. Repeat the pronunciation several times if you find the word hard to say.

1. thyroid gland

2. parathyroid glands

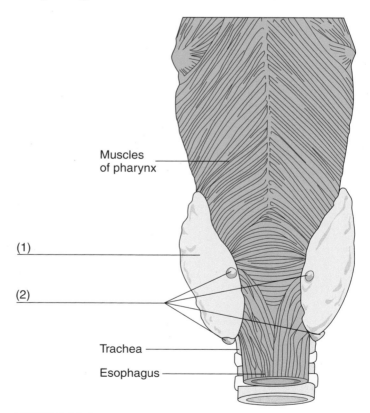

Muscles of pharynx

(1) _____

(2) _____

Trachea _____

Esophagus _____

FIGURE 19-3 Parathyroid glands.

IN BRIEF

Parathyroid gland secretes PTH

Location embedded in the thyroid gland

Function regulates calcium and phosphorus

Location and Structure

There are four parathyroid glands. As shown in Figure 19-3, there are two on each of the thyroid lobes. They are egg-shaped.

Function

These glands secrete **parathormone** (**par-ah-THOR-mohn**) (PTH).

PTH travels to the bone to help regulate calcium and phosphorus levels.

Adrenal Glands

PRACTICE FOR LEARNING: **ADRENAL GLANDS**

Write the words below in the correct spaces on Figure 19-4. To help you, the number beside the word tells you where it goes on the figure. Be sure to pronounce each word as you write it. Repeat the pronunciation several times if you find the word hard to say.

1. adrenal gland (**ad-DREE-nal**)

2. adrenal cortex (**KOR-tecks**)

3. adrenal medulla (**meh-DULL-ah**)

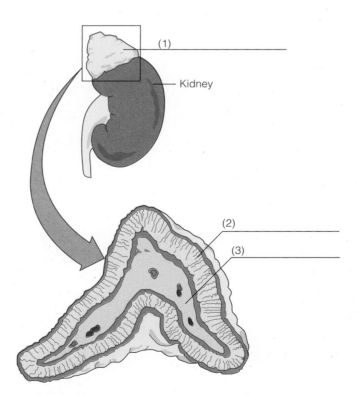

(1)

Kidney

(2)

(3)

FIGURE 19-4   Adrenal gland.

IN BRIEF

Adrenal medulla secretes adrenaline (epinephrine) and noradrenaline (norepinephrine)

Adrenal cortex secretes aldosterone, cortisol, and sex hormones

Location on top of the kidney

Function

aldosterone regulates sodium and potassium

cortisol regulates immune system

sex hormones regulates male and female secondary sexual characteristics

Location and Structure

The adrenal glands sit on top of the kidneys as shown in Figure 19-4. The outer and inner portions of each adrenal gland are actually separate glands. The outer portion is the adrenal cortex. The inner portion is the adrenal medulla. These glands are different in structure and function.

Function

The adrenal cortex secretes the following hormones: aldosterone (al-**DOS**-ter-ohn), cortisol (**KOR**-tih-sol), estrogen, and androgen (**AN**-droh-jen).

Aldosterone regulates sodium and potassium levels.

Cortisol (hydrocortisone) has several important functions. It regulates our immune system. It also plays a key role in how carbohydrates, fats, and proteins are used by the body.

Estrogens and androgens are the sex hormones. They are secreted in very small amounts to maintain secondary female and male characteristics such as hair growth and muscle bulk. These sex hormones are secreted in larger amounts by the ovaries and testicles.

The adrenal medulla produces adrenaline (ah-**DREN**-ah-len) (epinephrine) and noradrenaline (nor-ah-**DREN**-ah-len) (norepinephrine). These are called the "flight-or-fight" hormones. If a person is frightened enough to run away or angry enough to fight, these hormones prepare the body for the physical exertion needed during these times.

PRACTICE FOR LEARNING: THYROID, PARATHYROID, ADRENALS

Underline the correct word in each sentence.

1. Aldosterone is secreted by the (thyroid/parathyroid/adrenal) gland.

2. (T_4/Parathormone/Cortisol) regulates the metabolic rate.

3. (Aldosterone/Parathormone/Cortisol) regulates blood calcium.

4. (Aldosterone/Cortisol/Estrogen) regulates sodium and potassium levels.

5. (Epinephrine/Cortisol) prepares the body for fight-or-flight.

6. (Parathormone/Aldosterone/T₃) is secreted by the thyroid gland.

7. (Epinephrine/Estrogen/T₃) is secreted by the adrenal cortex.

8. The adrenal medulla secretes (aldosterone/sex hormones/norepinephrine/cortisol).

Answers: **1.** adrenal gland. **2.** T_4. **3.** parathormone. **4.** aldosterone. **5.** epinephrine. **6.** T_3. **7.** estrogen. **8.** norepinephrine.

Pineal Gland

Location and Structure

The pineal (**PIN-ee-al**) gland is shown in Figure 19-1. It looks like a pine cone and is located deep within the brain.

Function

The pineal gland secretes melatonin (**mel-ah-TOH-nin**). This hormone plays a role in telling us when it is time to go to sleep and when it is time to wake up. It is also connected to mood. It may be involved in determining when we commence puberty and in regulating the ovarian cycles.

Pancreas

Location and Structure

As described in the digestive system, the pancreas (**PAN-kree-as**) is a long, fish-shaped organ lying behind the stomach.

Function

The pancreas has both digestive and endocrine functions. The digestive function involves the secretion of substances to break down food.

The endocrine function involves cells in the pancreas called the islets of Langerhans (**LANG-er-hanz**). They produce and secrete the hormones insulin (**IN-suh-lin**) and glucagon (**GLOO-kah-gon**). Insulin and glucagon work together to regulate the amount of glucose (sugar) in the blood.

PRACTICE FOR LEARNING: PINEAL GLAND AND PANCREAS

1. Write the hormone secreted by the pineal gland.

_____

2. Write the hormones secreted by the pancreas.

_____

3. Name one function of the pineal gland.

_____

4. Name one function of the pancreatic hormones.

_____

> *Answers:* **1.** melatonin. **2.** insulin and glucagon. **3.** regulates sleeping and waking patterns; it is also connected to moods. **4.** regulates blood sugar levels.

19.3 CENTRAL ENDOCRINE GLANDS

Pituitary Gland

Location and Structure

The pituitary gland is about the size of a pea. It is located at the base of the brain. It hangs from the hypothalamus by a stalk called the **infundibulum (in-fun-DIB-yoo-lum)**. This is illustrated in Figure 19-5.

The pituitary gland has two lobes: anterior and posterior.

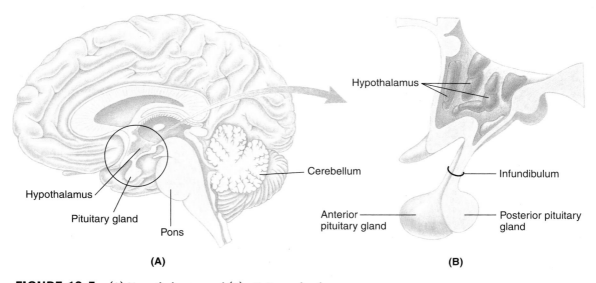

FIGURE 19-5 (A) Hypothalamus and (B) pituitary gland.

Function

The anterior lobe of the pituitary secretes several hormones. Many of these hormones stimulate other glands to secrete their own hormones. Because these hormones stimulate other glands, their names often end in the suffix **-tropic (TROP-ick)**, which means "to nourish" or "to stimulate." Following is a list of these hormones:

1. **Adrenocorticotropic** (ah-**dree**-noh-**kor**-tih-koh-**TROP**-ick) **hormone (ACTH)** stimulates the adrenal cortex.

2. **Somatotropic** (**soh**-mah-toh-**TROP**-ick) **hormone (STH)** or **growth hormone (GH)** stimulates growth in all body cells.

3. Thyroid-stimulating hormone (TSH) stimulates the thyroid gland.

4. **Gonadotropic** (**gon**-ah-doh-**TROP**-ick) hormones stimulate the gonads (ovaries and testicles). There are three gonadotropic hormones: **follicle-stimulating hormone (FSH), luteinizing** (**LOO**-tee-in-eye-zing) **hormone (LH)**, in the female, and interstitial cell-stimulating hormone (ICSH) in the male.

5. **Prolactin** (pro-**LACK**-tin) **(PRL)** stimulates breast development.

6. **Melanocyte-stimulating hormone (MSH)** stimulates the skin to produce melanocytes.

The **posterior lobe of the pituitary** is an extension of the hypothalamus. It stores and secretes two hormones produced by the hypothalamus:

1. **Antidiuretic** (an-tih-**dye**-yoo-**RET**-ick) **hormone (ADH)**. It prevents excessive loss of water.

2. **Oxytocin** (**ock**-see-**TOH**-sin). It stimulates uterine contractions during labor.

Hypothalamus

Location and Structure

The hypothalamus is illustrated in Figure 19-5. It works together with the pituitary gland. The hypothalamus is located deep in the central brain below the thalamus. It is made up of neurons. Some of the neurons in the hypothalamus secrete hormones and some do not. Thus, the hypothalamus is considered to be part of the endocrine system as well as the nervous system.

Function

The hypothalamus produces **neurohormones** (**NOO**-roh-**hor**-monz). They are called neurohormones because the hormones are produced by neurons. The hypothalamus produces the neurohormones oxytocin and the antidiuretic hormone (ADH). As well, the hypothalamus releases hormones that regulate the secretions of the pituitary gland.

PRACTICE FOR LEARNING: **HYPOTHALAMUS AND PITUITARY**

Underline the correct answer in each sentence.

1. The (hypothalamus/pituitary gland) produces oxytocin.

2. FSH and LH are (thyroid-stimulating hormones/adrenocorticotropic hormones/gonadotropic hormones).

3. The hormone responsible for milk production is (antidiuretic hormone/prolactin/oxytocin/gonadotropic hormone).

4. The adrenocorticotropic hormone is secreted by the (adrenal gland/posterior pituitary gland/anterior pituitary gland).

5. The thyroid-stimulating hormone is secreted by the (thyroid gland/anterior pituitary gland/posterior pituitary gland).

6. ADH is produced by the (hypothalamus/posterior pituitary gland/anterior pituitary gland) and stored in the (hypothalamus/posterior pituitary gland/anterior pituitary gland).

7. Gonadotropic hormones stimulate the (thyroid gland/adrenal cortex/ovaries/adrenal medulla).

Answers: **1.** hypothalamus. **2.** gonadotropic. **3.** prolactin. **4.** anterior pituitary gland. **5.** anterior pituitary gland. **6.** hypothalamus; posterior pituitary gland. **7.** ovaries.

19.4 ABBREVIATIONS OF MAJOR HORMONES

Hormones are commonly indicated by abbreviations. Table 19-1 lists the major hormones and their abbreviations.

TABLE 19-1   Abbreviations of Major Hormones

adrenocorticotropic hormone	ACTH
antidiuretic hormone	ADH
follicle-stimulating hormone	FSH
growth hormone	GH
interstitial cell-stimulating hormone	ICSH
luteinizing hormone	LH
parathormone	PTH
prolactin	PRL
somatotropic hormone	STH
thyroid-stimulating hormone	TSH
thyroxine	T_4
triiodothyronine	T_3

19.5 NEW ROOTS, SUFFIXES, AND PREFIX

Root	Meaning
calc/o	calcium
gonad/o	gonads (ovaries; testicles)
kal/o	potassium
natr/o	sodium
parathyroid/o	parathyroid
pituitar/o	pituitary

Suffix	Meaning
-dipsia	thirst
-genesis; -gen	production; producing
-ism	process; condition
-stasis	standing; stable

Prefix	Meaning
-eu	good

19.6 LEARNING THE TERMS

Following these steps will make it easier for you to learn medical terms:

1. Pronounce the term repeatedly until it is easy for you.

2. Write it down. Ensure the spelling is correct.

3. Also write the definition. If possible, relate the word to a word, thought, or picture that will help you remember it.

4. Analyze the term with the method taught in this text.

Root		Meaning	
acr/o		extremity; top	
Term	**Term Analysis**	**Definition**	
acromegaly (ack-roh-**MEG**-ah-lee)	-megaly = enlargement	enlargement of many skeletal structures, particularly the extremities.	

NOTE: Acromegaly is caused by increased secretions of growth hormone from the anterior pituitary gland.

Root		Meaning
andr/o		male
Term	**Term Analysis**	**Definition**
androgen (**AN**-droh-jen)	-gen = producing	substance producing male characteristics. An example is testosterone.

(continued)

Root	Meaning
crin/o	to secrete

Term	Term Analysis	Definition
endocrinologist (en-doh-krih-**NOL**-oh-jist)	-logist = specialist endo- = within	specialist in the study of the diagnosis and treatment of diseases of the endocrine glands and their hormonal secretions

Root	Meaning
estr/o	female

Term	Term Analysis	Definition
estrogen (**ESS**-troh-jen)	-gen = producing	female sex hormones

Root	Meaning
gluc/o; glyc/o	glucose; sugar

Term	Term Analysis	Definition
glucogenesis (**gloo**-koh-**JEN**-eh-sis)	-genesis = production	production of glucose
glycolysis (glye-**KOL**-ih-sis)	-lysis = breakdown; separation; destruction	breakdown of sugars

Root	Meaning
home/o	same

Term	Term Analysis	Definition
homeostasis (**hoh**-mee-oh-**STAY**-sis)	-stasis = standing; stable	a balanced, yet sometimes varied state.

NOTE: The function of the endocrine system is to regulate hormonal balance. It secretes more hormones when needed and fewer when there is an excess. In this way, a balance (homeostasis) is maintained.

Root	Meaning
thyr/o; thyroid/o	thyroid gland

Term	Term Analysis	Definition
euthyroid (**yoo**-**THIGH**-royd)	-oid = resembling eu- = good; normal	normal thyroid gland
hyperthyroidism (**high**-per-**THIGH**-royd-izm)	-ism = condition; process hyper- = excessive	condition characterized by excessive secretion of thyroid hormones

Suffix	Meaning
-tropic	stimulate

Term	Term Analysis	Definition
adrenocortico-tropic hormone (ah-**dree**-noh-**kor**-tih-koh-**TROP**-ick)	adren/o = adrenal gland cortic/o = cortex; outer layer	hormone secreted by the anterior pituitary that stimulates the adrenal cortex to secrete its own hormones

(continued)

gonadotropic hormones (**gon**-ah-doh-**TROP**-ick)	gonad/o = gonads; sex glands (ovaries and testicles)	hormones secreted by the anterior pituitary that stimulates the ovaries or testicles to secrete their own hormones
NOTE: Examples of gonadotropic hormones are LH, FSH, and ICSH.		

Prefix		Meaning
hyper-		increase; excessive
Term	**Term Analysis**	**Definition**
hypercalcemia (**high**-per-kal-**SEE**-mee-ah)	-emia = blood condition calc/o = calcium	excessive calcium in the blood
hyperkalemia (**high**-per-kah-**LEE**-mee-ah)	-emia = blood condition kal/o = potassium	excessive potassium in the blood
hyperglycemia (**high**-per-gligh-**SEE**-mee-ah)	-emia = blood condition glyc/o = sugar	excessive sugar in the blood

Prefix		Meaning
hypo-		decrease; deficient
Term	**Term Analysis**	**Definition**
hypopara-thyroidism (**high**-poh-**par**-ah-**THIGH**-roid-izm)	-ism = process; condition parathyroid/o = parathyroid	condition characterized by decreased secretions of the parathyroid hormone
hypopituitarism (**high**-poh-pih-**TOO**-ih-tar-izm)	-ism = process; condition pituitar/o = pituitary gland	condition characterized by decreased secretion of pituitary hormones

hyponatremia (**high**-poh-nah-**TREE**-mee-ah)	-emia = blood condition natr/o = sodium	decreased sodium in the blood

Prefix	Meaning
pan-	all

Term	Term Analysis	Definition
panhypopi-tuitarism (pan-**high**-poh-pih-**TOO**-ih-tar-izm)	-ism = condition; process hypo- = decrease; deficient pituitar/o = pituitary gland	a condition characterized by a deficiency of all pituitary hormones

Prefix	Meaning
poly-	many; much

Term	Term Analysis	Definition
polydipsia (**pol**-ee-**DIP**-see-ah)	-dipsia = thirst	excessive thirst
NOTE: Polydipsia is a symptom of diabetes mellitus.		
polyuria (**pol**-ee-**YOO**-ree-ah)	-uria = urination	excessive urination
NOTE: Polyuria is a symptom of diabetes mellitus.		

19.7 PATHOLOGY

Hypersecretion and Hyposecretion From the Endocrine Glands

Hypersecretion (excess secretion) and hyposecretion (inadequate secretion) may indicate pathology. Often, hypersecretion is caused by the growth of a tumor on the gland. Hyposecretion can indicate congenital absence of the gland, tumors large enough to take over the gland, and infections. As well, both hypersecretion and hyposecretion can be caused by autoimmune conditions (conditions in which the body turns against itself, thereby causing the disease).

Diabetes Mellitus (dye-ah-BEE-teez-MEL-ih-tus) DM

A disease in which the body is unable to use sugar to produce energy. One cause is insufficient insulin secreted from the pancreas. Another is the production of ineffective insulin. When either of these occurs, sugar is unable to move from the blood into body cells, where it is normally used to produce energy. The result is abnormally high levels of blood glucose. This is called hyperglycemia. It is a major symptom of diabetes.

When the body does not have enough glucose, it will break down fats and proteins for fuel. Over a long period of time, this results in the buildup of toxic wastes called ketones (**KEE**-tohnz). The condition is called ketoacidosis (**kee**-**toh**-**ass**-ih-**DOH**-sis). The excess sugars and ketones in the blood cause many diabetic complications such as blindness, heart attacks, and gangrene of the lower extremities.

There are two major types of diabetes.

Type 1 is an abrupt end to insulin production, often before the age of 25. The pancreatic cells do not produce enough insulin. This is thought to be due to an autoimmune reaction. The body's own antibodies destroy the pancreatic cells. Other causes may be environmental and viral.

Type 2 is a reduction in insulin production, often after the age of 40. Genetic factors and obesity play a role in the majority of the cases. Being overweight requires the pancreas to work harder to produce more insulin. Over time, the pancreatic cells secrete less insulin.

Graves' Disease

Graves' disease includes hyperthyroidism, goiter, and exophthalmia. Hyperthyroidism is excessive secretion of the thyroid hormones. It enlarges the thyroid gland (goiter) and has an affect on the tissues behind the eyeball, which pushes the eye outward (exophthalmia) (ex- = out; ophthalm/o = eye; -ia = condition).

Graves' disease is an autoimmune disorder. Antibodies that normally protect the body attack the thyroid gland. This causes increased secretion of the thyroid hormone.

19.8 REVIEW EXERCISES

| Exercise 19-1 | MATCHING WORD PARTS WITH MEANING |

Match the word part in Column A *with its meaning in* Column B.

Column A	Column B
_____ 1. home/o	A. male
_____ 2. estr/o	B. sugar
_____ 3. crin/o	C. female
_____ 4. natr/o	D. sodium
_____ 5. acr/o	E. thirst
_____ 6. -tropic	F. potassium
_____ 7. glyc/o	G. secrete
_____ 8. kal/o	H. same
_____ 9. andr/o	I. extremity
_____ 10. -dipsia	J. nourishment

| Exercise 19-2 | SHORT ANSWERS |

I. From the list below, select the endocrine gland that secretes the hormones that follow. The glands can be used more than once.

a. adrenal cortex
b. adrenal medulla
c. anterior pituitary
d. pancreas
e. posterior pituitary
f. thyroid

1. aldosterone _____

2. antidiuretic hormone _____

3. T_3 _____

4. cortisol _____

5. epinephrine _____

6. glucagon _____

7. follicle-stimulating hormone _____

(Exercise continues on page 422)

    8. insulin _____

    9. prolactin _____

    10. norepinephrine _____

II. *Match the hormone with its function (listed immediately below). One function can be used more than once.*

    a. plays a key role in the body's response to stress

    b. prevents excess loss of fluid

    c. regulates blood calcium and phosphorus

    d. regulates blood glucose levels

    e. regulates metabolic rate

    f. regulates sodium and potassium levels

    g. stimulates the adrenal cortex

    h. stimulates the development of the gonads

    i. stimulates uterine contractions

    1. adrenocorticotropic hormone

    _____

    2. oxytocin

    _____

    3. T_4

    _____

    4. parathormone

    _____

    5. aldosterone

    _____

    6. cortisol

    _____

    7. insulin

    _____

    8. glucagon

    _____

    9. antidiuretic hormone

    _____

    10. follicle-stimulating hormone

    _____

| **Exercise 19-3** | PATHOLOGY |

Answer the following questions on diabetes mellitus.

1. Write the major symptom of diabetes mellitus.

   _____

2. Why is glucose important to body cells?

   _____

3. Define "ketones."

   _____

4. What is the cause of diabetes mellitus?

   _____

5. Define type 1 diabetes.

   _____

   _____

6. Define type 2 diabetes.

   _____

   _____

| **Exercise 19-4** | DEFINITIONS |

Define the following:

1. **tropic hormones** _____

2. **neurohormones** _____

3. **homeostasis** _____

4. **acromegaly** _____

5. **glycolysis** _____

6. **euthyroid** _____

7. **polydipsia** _____

8. **glucogenesis** _____

9. **estrogen** _____

10. **hyperkalemia** _____

| Exercise 19-5 | BUILDING MEDICAL WORDS |

I. Using the suffix -emia, build the medical word meaning

   a. excessive calcium in the blood _____

   b. excessive blood sugar _____

   c. decreased sodium in the blood _____

   d. excessive potassium in the blood _____

II. Using the suffix -tropic, build the medical word meaning

   a. stimulating the adrenal cortex _____

   b. stimulating the gonads _____

| Exercise 19-6 | DEFINITIONS IN CONTEXT |

Define the bolded terms in context. Use your medical dictionary if necessary.

1. A 34-year-old was referred for **hyperthyroidism**. Patient was first found to be hyperthyroid one year ago. He has all the classic symptoms of **Graves' disease**, including **goiter, exophthalmia,** and weakness.

   a. hyperthyroidism _____

   b. Graves' disease _____

   c. goiter _____

   d. exophthalmia _____

2. Three days after admission, the diagnosis of **adrenal insufficiency** was confirmed. Apparently, **hypopituitarism** was ruled out.

   e. adrenal insufficiency _____

   f. hypopituitarism _____

3. This 64-year-old man was admitted because of a slowly growing mass in the right lobe of his **thyroid**. A **thyroid scan** showed regions of a nonfunctioning thyroid. Thyroid function was within normal limits. **Biopsy** of the thyroid confirmed a **benign adenoma**.

   g. thyroid _____

   h. thyroid scan _____

   i. biopsy _____

   j. benign adenoma _____

| **Exercise 19-7** | ## LABELING |

Write the name of each numbered structure on the corresponding line beside the diagram (Figure 19-6). Use the body structures listed on page 426.

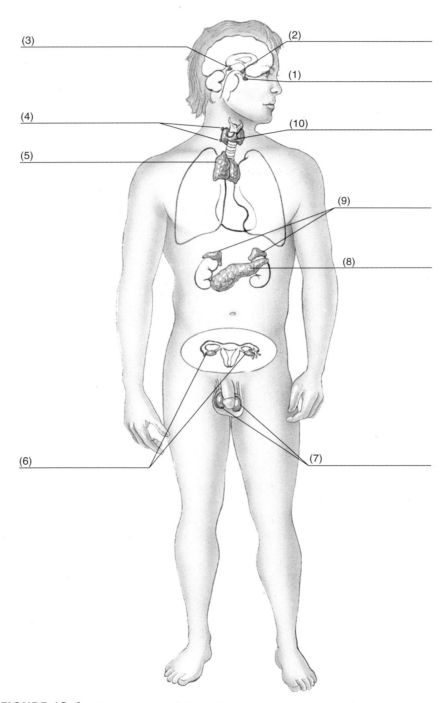

FIGURE 19-6 Major organs of the endocrine system.

adrenal glands _____

hypothalamus _____

ovaries _____

pancreas _____

parathyroid gland _____

pineal gland _____

pituitary gland _____

testicles _____

thymus gland _____

thyroid gland _____

1. _____

2. _____

3. _____

4. _____

5. _____

6. _____

7. _____

8. _____

9. _____

10. _____

Exercise 19-8 **SPELLING**

Circle any words that are spelled incorrectly in the list below.
Then correct the spelling in the space provided.

1. antidiretic _____

2. lutienizing _____

3. aldosterone _____

4. pancrease _____

5. diabetes _____

6. cortisal _____

7. hypopituitarism _____

8. homeostasis _____

9. hyperkalemia _____

10. polydipsia _____

19.9 PRONUNCIATION AND SPELLING

Listen, read, and study, so you can speak and write.

1. Listen to each word on the audio CD.

2. Pronounce each word carefully.

3. Spell each word in the space provided.

Word	Pronunciation	Spelling
acromegaly	**ack**-roh-**MEG**-ah-lee	
adrenocorticotropic hormone	ah-**dree**-noh-**kor**-tih-koh-**TROH**-pick	
aldosterone	al-**DOS**-ter-own	
androgen	**AN**-droh-jen	
antidiuretic	**an**-tih-**dye**-you-**RET**-ick	
cortisol	**KOR**-tih-sol	
endocrine	**EN**-doh-krin	
endocrinologist	en-doh-krih-**NOL**-oh-jist	
estrogen	**ESS**-troh-jen	
euthyroid	yoo-**THIGH**-royd	
glycolysis	glye-**KOL**-ih-sis	
homeostasis	**hoh**-mee-oh-**STAY**-sis	
hypercalcemia	**high**-per-kal-**SEE**-mee-ah	
hyperglycemia	**high**-per-glye-**SEE**-mee-ah	
hyperkalemia	**high**-per-kah-**LEE**-mee-ah	
hyperthyroidism	**high**-per-**THIGH**-royd-izm	
hyponatremia	**high**-poh-nah-**TREE**-mee-ah	

Word	Pronunciation	Spelling
hypopituitarism	**high**-poh-pih-**TOO**-ih-tar-izm	
isthmus	**ISS**-mus	
oxytocin	**ock**-see-**TOH**-sin	
pancreas	**PAN**-kree-as	
panhypopituitarism	pan-**high**-poh-pih-**TOO**-ih-tar-izm	
pineal	**PIN**-ee-al	
polydipsia	**pol**-ee-**DIP**-see-ah	
polyuria	**pol**-ee-**YOO**-ree-ah	
thyroxine	thigh-**ROCK**-sin	

Pronunciations

It is very important that you know how to pronounce the medical terms you learn. If you cannot pronounce a term, it will be difficult for you to remember how to spell it, and accurate spelling is very important. However, the proper pronunciation of a medical term is not always obvious. Therefore, all difficult terms in the first appearance are followed by a common pronunciation.

The system of pronunciation used is quite simple. Each term is re-spelled using combinations of letters that are commonly known to have a particular sound. For instance when *tion* appears in a word, the pronunciation will be written *shun*. The long "u" sound is made with *yoo*. So the word "cute" would be written as *kyoot*. Long "i," as in the word "hi," is usually written as *eye*. However, that is confusing in some words, and so sometimes the letters *ey* or *igh* are used instead. The goal is to provide an easy guide to pronunciation that fits the particular word. Further examples are listed in Table 1-1.

The syllables of the re-spelled term are separated by hyphens (-). The most strongly emphasized syllable is written bold type with capital letters (e.g., **BOLD**). Any syllable with secondary emphasis is written in bold but without capitals (e.g., **bold**). To help you put this all together, here are a few examples.

TABLE 1-1   Pronunciation of Medical Terms

a in *at* = **ah**
a in *rain* = **ay**
e in *pet* = **eh**
e in *meet* = **ee**
i in *skin* = **ih**
i in *pie* = **eye, ey,** or **igh**
o in *of* = **ah**
o in *boat* = **oh**
o in *boot* = **oo**
u in *under* = **uh**
u in *cute* = **yoo**
tion = **shun**

Plurals

Plurals are formed in various ways, depending on which letters are at the end of a term. To form the plural of singular terms ending in *is,* change the *i* to an *e,* as shown in the following examples:

Singular	Plural
diagnosis (dye-ag-**NOH**-sis)	diagnoses (dye-ag-**NOH**-seez)
pelvis (**PEL**-vis)	pelves (**PEL**-veez)
neurosis (noo-**ROH**-sis)	neuroses (noo-**ROH**-seez)

To form the plural of many singular words ending in *us,* change the *us* to an *i,* as shown in the following examples:

Singular	Plural
bronchus (**BRONG**-kus)	bronchi (**BRONG**-kye)
bacillus (bah-**SILL**-us)	bacilli (bah-**SILL**-eye)
calculus (**KAL**-kyoo-lus)	calculi (**KAL**-kyoo-lye)
embolus (**EM**-boh-lus)	emboli (**EM**-boh-lye)

There are a few exceptions. For example, the plural of *virus* (**VYE**-rus) is *viruses* (**VYE**-rus-ez), and the plural of *sinus* (**SIGH**-nus) is *sinuses* (**SIGH**-nus-ez).

The plural of singular words ending in *a* is formed by adding an *e* to the word, as shown in the following examples. Modifiers in Latin must agree with the noun. For example, the plural of *vena cava* is *venae cavae.*

Singular	Plural
sclera (**SKLEHR**-ah)	sclerae (**SKLEHR**-ee)
scapula (**SKAP**-yoo-lah)	scapulae (**SKAP**-yoo-lee)
vena cava (**VEE**-nah **CAV**-ah)	venae cavae (**VEE**-nee **CAV**-ee)

Singular terms ending in *um* are pluralized by changing the *um* to an *a,* as shown in the following examples:

Singular	Plural
acetabulum (**ass**-eh-**TAB**-yoo-lum)	acetabula (**ass**-eh-**TAB**-yoo-lah)
capitulum (kah-**PIT**-yoo-lum)	capitula (kah-**PIT**-yoo-lah)
septum (**SEP**-tum)	septa (**SEP**-tah)
diverticulum (**dye**-ver-**TICK**-yoo-lum)	diverticula (**dye**-ver-**TICK**-yoo-lah)

To form the plural of singular words ending in *ix* or *ex,* change the ending to *ices,* as shown in the following examples:

Singular	Plural
calix (**KAY**-licks)	calices (**KAY**-lih-seez)
cervix (**SER**-vicks)	cervices (**SER**-vih-seez)
index (**IN**-decks)	indices (**IN**-dih-seez)
varix (**VAR**-icks)	varices (**VAR**-ih-seez)

Singular words ending in *oma* are made plural by the addition of a *ta* or *s,* as shown in the following examples:

Singular	Plural
adenoma (**ad**-eh-**NOH**-mah)	adenomata or adenomas (**ad**-eh-no-**MAT**-ah) (**ad**-eh-**NOH**-mahz)
carcinoma (**kar**-sih-**NOH**-mah)	carcinomata or carcinomas (**kar**-sin-oh-**MAT**-ah) (**kar**-sin-**OH**-mahz)
fibroma (figh-**BROH**-mah)	fibromata or fibromas (figh-broh-**MAT**-ah) (figh-**BROH**-mahz)

To form the plural of singular words ending in *nx,* change the *x* to *g* and add *es,* as shown in the following examples:

Singular	Plural
larynx (**LAR**-inks)	larynges (**LAR**-in-jeez)
phalanx (**FAH**-lanks)	phalanges (fah-**LAN**-jeez)

To form the plural of singular words ending in *on,* change the *on* to an *a* or simply add an *s,* as shown in the following example:

Singular	Plural
ganglion (**GANG**-glee-on)	ganglia or ganglions (**GANG**-glee-ah) (**GANG**-glee-onz)

To form the plural of singular words ending in *ax,* change the *ax* to *aces,* as shown in the following example:

Singular	Plural
thorax (**THOH**-racks)	thoraces (**THOH**-rah-sees)

Word Part to Definition

Word Part — Definition

A

Word Part	Definition
a(n)-	inadequate; no; not; lack of
ab-	away from
abdomin/o	abdomen
-ac	pertaining to
acetabul/o	acetabulum; hip socket
acr/o	extremity; top
acromi/o	acromion
ad-	toward
aden/o	gland
adenoid/o	adenoids
adip/o	fat
adren/o	adrenal gland
adrenal/o	adrenal gland
-al	pertaining to
albin/o	white
albumin/o	albumin (a blood protein)
-algia	pain
alveol/o	air sacs; alveolus
ambly/o	dull; dim
amni/o	amnion; sac in which the fetus lies in the uterus
an/o	anus
ana-	apart; up
andr/o	male; man
angi/o	vessel
anis/o	unequal size
ankyl/o	fusion of parts; bent; crooked
ante-	before
anter/o	front
anti-	against
aort/o	aorta
append/o	appendix

Word Part	Definition
aque/o	water
-ar	pertaining to
-arche	beginning
arteri/o	artery
arthr/o	joint
articul/o	joint
-ary	pertaining to
-assay	analysis of a mixture to identify its contents
-asthenia	no strength
atel/o	imperfect
ather/o	fatty debris; fatty plaque
atri/o	atrium (upper chambers of the heart)
audi/o	hearing
audit/o	hearing
aur/o	ear
auto-	self
axill/o	armpit

B

Word Part	Definition
bacteri/o	bacteria
balan/o	glans penis
bi/o	life
bil/i	bile
bilirubin/o	bilirubin (a bile pigment)
-blast	immature, growing thing
blephar/o	eyelid
brachi/o	arm
brady-	slow
bronch/o	bronchus
bronchi/o	bronchus
bronchiol/o	bronchioles; small bronchi

Word Part	Definition
bucc/o	cheek
burs/o	bursa (sac filled with synovial fluid located around joints)

Word Part	Definition
calc/o	calcium
calcane/o	heel
calic/o; calyc/o	calix/calyx
-capnia	carbon dioxide
capsul/o	capsule
carcin/o	cancer; cancerous
cardi/o	heart
carp/o	wrist
cartilagin/o	cartilage
catheter/o	something inserted
caud/o	tail
cec/o	cecum
-cele	hernia (protrusion of an organ from the structure that normally contains it)
cellul/o	cell
-centesis	surgical puncture to remove fluid
cephal/o	head
cerebell/o	cerebellum
cerebr/o	brain
cervic/o	cervix; neck; neck of uterus; cervix uteri
-chalasia	relaxation
cheil/o	lips
chol/e	bile; gall
cholangi/o	bile ducts
cholecyst/o	gallbladder
choledoch/o	common bile duct
cholesterol/o	cholesterol
chondr/o	cartilage
chori/o	choroid
chrom/o	color
-cidal	to kill
cili/o	hair
-clasis	surgical fracture or refracture
-clast	breakdown
clavicul/o	clavicle; collarbone
-clonus	turmoil
-clysis	washing; irrigation
coagulati/o	to condense; to clot
coccyg/o	coccyx; tailbone
cochle/o	cochlea

Word Part	Definition
col/o	colon; large intestine
colon/o	colon
colp/o	vagina
coni/o	dust
conjunctiv/o	conjunctiva
constrict/o	to draw together
-continence	to stop
-conus	cone-shaped
core/o	pupil
corne/o	cornea
coron/o	crown
corpor/o	body
cortic/o	cortex; outer covering; outer layer
cost/o	ribs
crani/o	skull
crin/o	to secrete
-crine	to secrete
-crit	separate
cry/o	cold
crypt/o	hidden
culd/o	cul-de-sac
-cusis	hearing
cutane/o	skin
cycl/o	ciliary body
-cyesis	pregnancy
cyst/o	bladder; sac
cyt/o	cell
-cyte	cell
-cytosis	increase in the number of cells

Word Part	Definition
dacry/o	tears; lacrimal duct
de-	lack of; removal
dent/o	tooth
derm/o	skin
-derma	skin
dermat/o	skin
-dermis	skin
-desis	surgical binding; surgical fusion
di-	two
dia-	complete; through
diaphor/e	profuse sweating
dilat/o	dilation; dilatation; to expand; widen
dipl/o	double

Word Part	Definition
-dipsia	thirst
don/o	donates
dors/o	back
dorsi-	back
duct/o	to draw
duoden/o	duodenum (proximal portion of small intestine)
dur/o	dura mater (outermost membrane surrounding the brain)
-dynia	pain
dys-	bad; difficult; painful; poor

E

Word Part	Definition
e-	out; outside; outward; without
-eal	pertaining to
-ear	pertaining to
ec-	out
ech/o	sound
-ectasis	dilation; dilatation; stretching
-ectomy	excision; surgical removal
-edema	accumulation of fluid
electr/o	electric
-emesis	vomit; vomiting
-emia	blood condition
emmetr/o	in proper measure
en-	inward
encephal/o	brain
endo-	with; within
enter/o	small intestine
epi-	above; on; upon
epididym/o	epididymis
episi/o	vulva; external genitalia; pudendum
epitheli/o	covering
-er	specialist; one who specializes; specialist in the study of
erythemat/o	red
erythr/o	red
eso-	inward
esophag/o	esophagus
-esthesia	sensation
estr/o	female
ethm/o	ethmoid bone; sieve
eu-	normal; good
ex-	out; outside; outward

Word Part	Definition
exo-	out; outside; outward
extra-	out; outside; outward

F

Word Part	Definition
faci/o	face
fasci/o	fascia
femor/o	femur; thigh bone
fibr/o	fibers; fibrous tissue
fibul/o	fibula
flex/o	bending
-flux	flow
front/o	frontal bone

G

Word Part	Definition
galact/o	milk
gastr/o	stomach
-gen	producing
-genesis	development; production
-genic	producing; produced by
gingiv/o	gums
glen/o	socket; pit; glenoid cavity
gli/o	glue
glomerul/o	glomerulus
gloss/o	tongue
gluc/o	sugar
glycogen/o	glycogen (storage form of sugar)
gonad/o	gonads; sex glands
goni/o	angle (especially of the anterior chamber)
-grade	to step; to go
-gram	record; writing
granul/o	granules
-graph	instrument used to record
-graphy	process of recording; producing images
-gravida	pregnancy
gynec/o	female; woman

H

Word Part	Definition
hem/o	blood
hemat/o	blood
hemi-	half

Word Part / Definition

Word Part	Definition
hepat/o	liver
herni/o	hernia
hiat/o	hiatus, opening
hidr/o	sweat
hist/o	tissue
histi/o	tissue
home/o	same
humer/o	humerus; upper arm
hydr/o	water
hyper-	abnormal increase; above; above normal; excessive
hypo-	abnormal decrease; below; below normal; under
hyster/o	uterus

I

Word Part	Definition
-ia	condition; state of
-iasis	abnormal condition; process
-ic	pertaining to
-ician	specialist; one who specializes; expert
ile/o	ileum (distal portion of the small intestine)
ili/o	hip
immun/o	immunity; safe
in-	no; not
-ine	pertaining to
infer/o	below; downward
infra-	within
inguin/o	groin
insulin/o	insulin
inter-	between
intestin/o	intestine
intra-	within
-ion	process
-ior	pertaining to
ir/o	iris
irid/o	iris
is/o	equal
isch/o	hold back
ischi/o	ischium (posterior portion of the hip bone)
-ism	condition; process; state of
-ist	specialist; one who specializes; specialist in the study of

Word Part	Definition
-itis	inflammation (the redness, swelling, heat, and pain that occur when the body protects itself from injury)
-ium	structure

J

Word Part	Definition
jejun/o	jejunum (medial portion of small intestine)

K

Word Part	Definition
kal/o	potassium
kerat/o	cornea; hard; hornlike
keratin/o	hard; hornlike
kinesi/o	movement
-kinesia	movement; motion
-kinesis	movement; motion
kyph/o	humpback

L

Word Part	Definition
labi/o	lip
labyrinth/o	inner ear; labyrinth
lacrim/o	lacrimal apparatus; tears
lact/o	milk
lapar/o	abdominal wall; abdomen
laryng/o	larynx; voice box
lei/o	smooth
leuk/o	white
ligati/o	binding; tying
lingu/o	tongue
lip/o	fat
lipid/o	fat
-lith	calculus; stone
lith/o	stone
lob/o	lobe
-logist	specialist; one who specializes; specialist in the study of
-logy	study of; process of study
lord/o	swayback
lumb/o	lower back; loins

Word Part	Definition
lymph/o	lymph (clear, watery fluid)
lymphaden/o	lymph glands; lymph nodes
lymphangi/o	lymph vessels
-lysis	breakdown; destruction; separate; separation
-lytic	pertaining to destruction, separation, or breakdown

M

Word Part	Definition
magnet/o	magnet
-malacia	softening
malleol/o	malleolus (bony projection on the distal aspects of the tibia and fibula)
mamm/o	breast
mandibul/o	mandible; lower jaw
mast/o	breast
maxill/o	maxilla; upper jaw
meat/o	meatus
medi/o	middle
medull/o	marrow; medulla; inner portion of an organ
-megaly	enlargement
melan/o	black
men/o	menses; menstruation; month
mening/o	membrane; meninges
metacarp/o	metacarpals (bones of the hand)
metatars/o	metatarsals (bones of the foot)
-meter	instrument used to measure;
metr/o	uterus
-metrist	specialist in the measurement of
-metry	process of measuring; to measure; measurement
mi/o	contraction; less
mono-	one
muc/o	mucus (a bodily secretion, of the mucous membrane, sometimes sticky and frequently thick)
multi-	multiple
muscul/o	muscle
my/o	muscle

Word Part	Definition
myc/o	fungus
mydri/o	dilation (dilatation); wide
-myein	to shut
myel/o	bone marrow; spinal cord
myelin/o	myelin sheath
myos/o	muscle
myring/o	tympanic membrane; eardrum

N

Word Part	Definition
nas/o	nose
nat/i	birth
natr/o	sodium
necr/o	death
neo-	new
nephr/o	kidney
neur/o	nerve
noct/o	night
norm/o	normal
nulli-	none

O

Word Part	Definition
o/o	egg
occipit/o	occiput (back part of the head)
ocul/o	eye
odont/o	teeth; tooth
-oid	resembling
-ole	small
olecran/o	elbow; olecranon
oligo-	deficient; few; scanty
-oma	mass; tumor
onych/o	nail
oophor/o	ovary
ophthalm/o	eye
-opia	visual condition; vision
-opsia	visual condition; vision
-opsy	to view
-opt/o	vision; sight
-or	one who; person or thing that does something
or/o	mouth
orchi/o	testicle; testis
orchid/o	testicle; testis
orex/i	appetite

Word Part | Definition

Word Part	Definition
ortho-	straight
-ory	pertaining to
-ose	pertaining to
-osis	abnormal condition
oste/o	bone
ot/o	ear
-ous	pertaining to
ov/o	egg
ovari/o	ovary
ox/o	oxygen
oxy-	quick; sharp

P

Word Part	Definition
palpebr/o	eyelid
pan-	all
pancreat/o	pancreas
papill/o	nipple-like; optic disc
para-	abnormal; beside; near
-para	give birth; near; part with child; to part with
parathyroid/o	parathyroid gland
pariet/o	parietal bone; wall
-partum	labor; delivery; childbirth
patell/a	patella; kneecap
patell/o	patella; kneecap
path/o	disease
-pathy	disease
-pause	stoppage; cessation
pector/o	chest
ped/o	child
pelv/i	pelvis
pelv/o	pelvis
-penia	decrease; deficiency
-pepsia	digestion
peri-	around
perine/o	perineum
peritone/o	peritoneum
-pexy	surgical fixation
phac/o	lens
-phagia	swallow; to eat
phalang/o	phalanx (one of three bones making up each finger or toe)
phall/o	penis
pharmac/o	drug
pharyng/o	pharynx; throat
-phasia	speech
phleb/o	vein
-phobia	fear; irrational fear

Word Part	Definition
-phonia	voice
-phoresis	transmission; carry
phot/o	light
phren/o	diaphragm
physi/o	nature
-physis	to grow
pil/o	hair
pine/o	pineal gland
pituitar/o	pituitary gland
-plakia	patches
-plasia	development; formation
-plasm	development; formation
-plasty	surgical repair or reconstruction
-plegia	paralysis (loss or impairment of motor function)
pleur/a	pleura; pleural cavity
pleur/o	pleura; pleural cavity
-pnea	breathing
pneum/o	air; respiration; lungs
pneumat/o	air; respiration; lungs
pneumon/o	lungs
-poiesis	production; manufacture; formation
-poietin	a hormone that stimulates the production of blood cells
poikil/o	variation; irregular
poli/o	gray matter
poly-	many
-porosis	porous
post-	after
poster/o	back
practition/o	practice
-prandial	meal
presby-	old age
primi-	first
proct/o	rectum
pronati/o	pronation
prostat/o	prostate; prostate gland
proxim/o	near; close
pseudo-	false
-ptosis	downward displacement; drooping; falling; prolapse; sagging
-ptysis	spitting
pub/o	pubis (portion of the hip bone)
pulmon/o	lungs
pupill/o	pupil
py/o	pus

Word Part	Definition
pyel/o	renal pelvis (upper dilated portion of the ureter)
pylor/o	pylorus (distal portion of the stomach); pyloric sphincter

Word Part	Definition
quadri-	four

Word Part	Definition
radi/o	radius (one of the bones of the lower arm)
radicul/o	nerve roots
re-	back
rect/o	rectum
ren/o	kidney
reticul/o	network
retin/o	retina
retro-	backward; back; behind
rhabd/o	rod-shaped; striped; striated
rhin/o	nose
rhythm/o	rhythm
-rrhage	bursting forth
-rrhagia	bursting forth
-rrhaphy	suture; sew
-rrhea	flow; discharge
-rrhexis	rupture

Word Part	Definition
sacr/o	sacrum
salping/o	eustachian tube; fallopian tubes; uterine tubes
-salpinx	fallopian tube; uterine tube
-sarcoma	malignant tumor of connective tissue
scapul/o	scapula
-schisis	cleft; splitting
-sclerosis	hardening
scoli/o	curved
-scope	instrument used to visually examine (a body cavity or organ)
-scopy	process of visually examining (a body cavity or organ)
seb/o	sebum

Word Part	Definition
sect/o	to cut
secundi-	second
sial/o	saliva
sialaden/o	salivary glands
sigmoid/o	sigmoid colon
sinus/o	sinuses
-sis	state of; condition
skelet/o	skeleton
somat/o	body
son/o	sound
-spadias	opening; split
-spasm	sudden, involuntary contraction
sperm/o	spermatozoa; sperm
spermat/o	spermatozoa; sperm
sphen/o	sphenoid bone; wedge
spin/o	spine; spinal column; backbone
splen/o	spleen
spondyl/o	vertebra
staped/o	stapes
-stasis	standing; stable; stoppage; stopping; controlling
steat/o	fat
-stenosis	narrowing; stricture
stern/o	sternum; breastbone
steth/o	chest
stomat/o	mouth
-stomy	new opening
sub-	tongue; under
super/o	above; toward the head
supinati/o	supination
supra-	above; beyond; excessive
sym-	together; with
synovi/o	synovium; synovial membrane

Word Part	Definition
tachy-	fast
-taxia	order
tempor/o	temporal bone
ten/o	tendon
tend/o	tendon
tendin/o	tendon
tenosynovi/o	tendon sheath (covering of a tendon)
tens/o	stretch
tensi/o	tension
test/o	testicle; testis

Word Part	Definition
testicul/o	testicle; testis
tetra-	four
thalam/o	thalamus
thel/o	nipple
-therapy	treatment
-thermy	heat
thorac/o	chest; thorax
-thorax	chest
thromb/o	clot
thym/o	thymus; thymus gland
thyr/o	thyroid gland; shield
thyroid/o	thyroid gland; shield
tibi/o	tibia; shin
-tic	pertaining to
-tocia	labor
-tocin	labor
tom/o	to cut
-tome	instrument used to cut
-tomy	to cut; incise; process of cutting; incision
ton/o	tension
tonsill/o	tonsils
top/o	place
trabecul/o	trabecula (strands of connective tissue)
trache/o	trachea; windpipe
trans-	across
trigon/o	trigone
-tripsy	crushing
-trophic	pertaining to development, growth, or nourishment
-trophy	development; growth; nourishment
-tropia	turning
-tropic	stimulating
-tropion	turning
tub/o	fallopian tube
tympan/o	tympanic membrane; eardrum

U

Word Part	Definition
-ule	small
uln/o	ulnar (one of the bones of the lower arm)
ultra-	excess; beyond
-um	structure
ungu/o	nail
ur/o	urinary tract; urine; urination

Word Part	Definition
ure/o	urea (end product of protein breakdown and is found in urine)
ureter/o	ureters
urethr/o	urethra
-uria	urine; urination
urin/o	urine
-us	condition; thing
uter/o	uterus
uve/o	uvea (includes the choroid, ciliary body, and iris)

V

Word Part	Definition
vagin/o	vagina
valvul/o	valve
varic/o	varicose vein; dilated, twisted vein
vas/o	vas deferens; vessel
vascul/o	vessel
ven/o	vein
ventr/o	front
ventricul/o	ventricle (lower chambers of the heart)
versi/o	turning; tilting; tipping
vertebr/o	vertebra
vesic/o	bladder
viscer/o	internal organs
vitre/o	glasslike; gel-like
vulv/o	vulva; external genitalia; pudendum

X

Word Part	Definition
xer/o	dry
xiph/o	sword

Y

Word Part	Definition
-y	process

Z

Word Part	Definition
zygomat/o	cheekbone

Definition to Word Part

Definition	Word Part
A	
abdomen	abdomin/o; lapar/o
abdominal wall	lapar/o
abnormal	para-
abnormal condition	-iasis; -osis
abnormal increase	hyper-
above	epi-; hyper-; super/o; supra-
accumulation of a fluid	-edema
acetabulum	acetabul/o
acromion	acromi/o
across	trans-
adenoids	adenoid/o
adrenal gland	adren/o; adrenal/o
after	post-
against	anti-
air	pneum/o; pneumat/o
air sacs	alveol/o
albumin (a blood protein)	albumin/o
all	pan-
alveolus	alveol/o
amnion	amni/o
analysis of a mixture to identify its contents	-assay
angle (especially of the anterior chamber)	goni/o
anus	an/o
aorta	aort/o
apart	ana-
appendix	append/o
appetite	orex/i
arm	brachi/o

Definition	Word Part
armpit	axill/o
around	circum-; peri-
artery	arteri/o
aspiration	-centesis
atrium	atri/o
away from	ab-
B	
back	dorsi-; dors/o; poster/o; re-; retro-
back part of the head (occiput)	occipit/o
backbone	spin/o
backward	retro-
bacteria	bacteri/o
bad	dys-
bear (to)	-para
before	ante-
beginning	-arche
behind	retro-
below	hypo-; infer/o; sub-
below normal	hypo-
bending	flex/o
bent	ankyl/o
beside	para-
between	inter-
beyond	supra-; ultra-
bile	bil/i; chol/e
bile vessel	cholangi/o
bilirubin (a bile pigment)	bilirubin/o
binding	ligati/o
birth	nat/o
black	melan/o
bladder	cyst/o; vesic/o
blood	hem/o; hemat/o
blood condition	-emia

Definition	Word Part	Definition	Word Part
body	corpor/o; somat/o	close	proxim/o
bone	osse/o; oste/o	clot	thromb/o
bone marrow	myel/o	clot (to)	coagulati/o
bony projection on the distal aspects of the tibia and fibula	malleol/o	coccyx	coccyg/o
		cochlea	cochle/o
		cold	cry/o
		collarbone	clavicul/o
brain	cerebr/o; encephal/o	colon	col/o; colon/o
breakdown	-clast; -lysis	color	chrom/o
breast	mamm/o; mast/o	common bile duct	choledoch/o
breastbone	stern/o	complete	dia-
breathing	-pnea	condense (to)	coagulati/o
bronchioles	bronchiol/o	condition	-ia; -ism; -sis
bronchus	bronchi/o; bronch/o	cone-shaped	-conus
bursa	burs/o	contraction	mi/o
bursting forth	-rrhage; -rrhagia	controlling	-stasis
		cornea	corne/o; kerat/o
		cortex	cortic/o
		covering	epitheli/o
		covering of a tendon	tenosynovi/o
		crooked	ankyl/o

C

Definition	Word Part	Definition	Word Part
calcium	calci/o; calc/o	crown	coron/o
calculus	-lith	crushing	-tripsy
calix	calic/o; calyc/o	cul-de-sac	culd/o
calyx	calic/o; calyc/o	curved	scoli/o
cancer	carcin/o	cut (to)	cis/o; sect/o; tom/o; -tomy
cancerous	carcin/o		
capsule	capsul/o		
carbon dioxide	-capnia		
carry	-phoresis		
cartilage	cartilagin/o; chondr/o		

D

Definition	Word Part
cecum	cec/o
cell	cellul/o; cyt/o; -cyte
cerebellum	cerebell/o
cervix	cervic/o
cervix uteri	cervic/o
cessation	-pause
cheek	bucc/o
cheekbone	zygomat/o
chest	pector/o; steth/o; thorac/o; -thorax
child	ped/o
childbirth	-partum
cholesterol	cholesterol/o
choroid	chori/o
ciliary body	cycl/o
clavicle	clavicul/o
clear, watery fluid	lymph/o
cleft	-schisis

Definition	Word Part
death	necr/o
decrease	hypo-; -penia
deficiency	-penia
deficient	oligo-
delivery	-partum
destruction	-lysis
development	-plasia; -plasm -trophy; -genesis
diaphragm	phren/o
difficult	dys-
digestion	-pepsia
dilated, twisted vein	varic/o
dilation (dilatation)	dilat/o; -ectasis; mydri/o
dim	ambly/o
discharge	-rrhea
disease	path/o; -pathy
donates	don/o

Definition	Word Part	Definition	Word Part
double	dipl/o	fallopian tube	salping/o; -salpinx; tub/o
downward	infer/o		
downward displacement	-ptosis	false	pseudo-
		fascia (band of tissue surrounding a muscle)	fasci/o
draw (to)	duct/o		
draw together (to)	constrict/o		
drooping	-ptosis	fast	tachy-
drug	pharmac/o	fat	adip/o; lip/o; lipid/o; steat/o
dry	xer/o		
dull	ambly/o	fatty debris	ather/o
duodenum (proximal portion of small intestine)	duoden/o	fatty plaque	ather/o
		fear	-phobia
		female	estr/o; gynec/o
		femur	femor/o
dura mater (outermost membrane surrounding the brain)	dur/o	few	oligo-
		fibers	fibr/o
		fibrous tissue	fibr/o
		fibula	fibul/o
		first	primi-
		flow	-flux; -rrhea
		formation	-plasia; -plasm -poiesis

E

ear	aur/o; ot/o	formed in	-genic
eardrum	myring/o; tympan/o	four	quadri-; tetra-
eat (to)	-phagia	front	anter/o; ventr/o
egg	o/o; ov/o	frontal bone	front/o
elbow	olecran/o	fungus	myc/o
electric	electr/o	fusion of parts	ankyl/o
enlargement	-megaly		
epididymis	epididym/o		
equal	is/o		
esophagus	esophag/o		
ethmoid bone	ethm/o		

G

eustachian tube	salping/o	gall	chol/e
excess	ultra-	gallbladder	cholecyst/o
excessive	hyper-; supra-	gel-like	vitre/o
excision	-ectomy	give birth	-para
expand (to)	dilat/o	gland	aden/o
expert	-ician	glans penis (tip of penis)	balan/o
external genitalia	episi/o; vulv/o		
extremity	acr/o	glasslike	vitre/o
eye	ocul/o; ophthalm/o	glenoid cavity	glen/o
eyelid	blephar/o; palpebr/o	glomerulus	glomerul/o
		glycogen (storage form of sugar)	glycogen/o

face	faci/o	go (to)	-grade
falling	-ptosis	gonads	gonad/o
		good	eu-
		granules	granul/o
		gray matter	poli/o
		groin	inguin/o

Definition	Word Part	Definition	Word Part
grow (to)	-physis	incise	-tomy
growing thing	-blast	incision	-tomy
growth	-trophy	increase in the number of cells	-cytosis
gums	gingiv/o		
		inflammation (redness, swelling, heat, and pain that occur when the body protects itself from injury)	-itis

H

Definition	Word Part
hair	cili/o; pil/o
half	hemi-
hard	kerat/o; keratin/o
hardening	-sclerosis; scler/o
head	cephal/o
hearing	audi/o; -cusis
heart	cardi/o
heat	-thermy
heel	calcane/o
hernia (protrusion of an organ from the structure that normally contains it)	-cele; herni/o
hiatus	hiat/o
hidden	crypt/o
hip	ili/o
hip socket	acetabul/o
hold back	isch/o
hormone that stimulates the production of blood cells	-poietin
hornlike	kerat/o; keratin/o
humerus	humer/o
humpback	kyph/o

Definition	Word Part
inner ear	labyrinth/o
instrument used to cut	-tome
instrument used to measure	-meter
instrument used to record	-graph
instrument used to visually examine (a body cavity or organ)	-scope
insulin	insulin/o
internal organ	viscer/o
intestine	ile/o; intestin/o
inward	en-; eso-
iris	irid/o; ir/o
irrational fear	-phobia
irregular	poikil/o
irrigation	-clysis
ischium	ischi/o

I

Definition	Word Part
ileum (distal portion of the small intestine)	ile/o
immature	-blast
immunity	immun/o
imperfect	atel/o
in proper measure	emmetr/o
inadequate	a(n)-

J

Definition	Word Part
jejunum (medial portion of small intestine)	jejun/o
joint	arthr/o; articul/o

K

Definition	Word Part
kidney	nephr/o; ren/o
kill (to)	-cidal
kneecap	patell/a; patell/o

Definition	Word Part	Definition	Word Part
		manufacture	-poiesis
		many	poly-
	L	marrow	medull/o
		mass	-oma
labor	-partum; -tocia; -tocin	maxilla	maxill/o
		meal	-prandial
labyrinth	labyrinth/o	measure (to)	-metry
lack of	de-	meatus	meat/o
lacrimal apparatus	lacrim/o	medulla	medull/o
lacrimal duct	dacry/o	membrane	chori/o; mening/o
large intestine	col/o	meninges	mening/o
larynx	laryng/o	menses	men/o
lens	phac/o; phak/o	menstruation	men/o
less	mi/o	metacarpals (bones of the hand)	metacarp/o
life	bi/o		
light	phot/o	metatarsals (bones of the foot)	metatars/o
lips	cheil/o; labi/o		
little bronchi	bronchiol/o	middle	medi/o
liver	hepat/o	milk	galact/o; lact/o
lobe	lob/o	month	men/o
loins	lumb/o	motion	-kinesia; -kinesis
loss or impairment of motor function	-plegia	mouth	or/o; stomat/o
		movement	-kinesia; -kinesis
lower back	lumb/o	mucus (a bodily secretion, of the mucous membrane, sometimes sticky and frequently thick)	muc/o
lower jaw	mandibul/o		
lungs	pneum/o; pneumat/o; pneumon/o; pulmon/o		
		multiple	multi-
lymph (clear, watery fluid)	lymph/o	muscle	muscul/o; myos/o
		myelin sheath	myelin/o
lymph gland	lymphaden/o		
lymph node	lymphaden/o		**N**
lymph vessel	lymphangi/o		
		nail	onych/o; ungu/o
	M	narrowing	-stenosis
		nature	physi/o
magnet	magnet/o	near	proxim/o; para-
male	andr/o	neck	cervic/o
malignant tumor of connective tissue	-sarcoma	neck of uterus	cervic/o
		nerve	neur/o
		nerve roots	radicul/o
malleolus	malleol/o	network	reticul/o
man	andr/o	new opening	-stomy
mandible	mandibul/o	night	noct/o

Definition	Word Part	Definition	Word Part
nipple	thel/o	pelvis	pelv/i; pelv/o
nipple-like	papill/o	penis	phall/o
no	a(n)-; in-	perineum	perine/o
no strength	-asthenia	peritoneum	peritone/o
none	nulli-	person or thing that does something	-or
normal	eu-; norm/o	pertaining to	-ac; -al; -ar; -ary; -eal; -ear; -ic; ine; -ior; -or; -ory; -ose; -ous; -tic
nose	nas/o; rhin/o		
not	a(n)-; in-		
nourishment	-trophy		
nutrition	-trophy	pertaining to destruction, separation, or breakdown	-lytic

O

Definition	Word Part	Definition	Word Part
occiput (back part of the head)	occipit/o	pertaining to nourishment; development or growth	-trophic
old age	presby-		
olecranon	olecran/o		
on	epi-	phalanges (one of three bones making up each finger or toe)	phalang/o
one	mono-		
one who	-or		
one who specializes; specialist	-er; -or; -ician; -ist; -logist	pharynx	pharyng/o
opening	-spadias; hiat/o	pineal gland	pine/o
optic disc	papill/o	pit	glen/o
order	-taxia	pituitary gland	pituitar/o
out	e-; ec-; ex-; exo-; extra-	place	top/o
		pleura	pleur/a; pleur/o
outer layer	cortic/o	pleural cavity	pleur/a; pleur/o
outside	e-; ec-; ex-; exo-; extra-	poor	dys-
		porous	-porosis
outward	e-; ec-; ex-; exo-; extra-	posterior portion of the hip bone	ischi/o
		potassium	kal/o
ovary	oophor/o; ovari/o	practice	practition/o
oxygen	ox/o	pregnancy	-cyesis; -gravida
		process	-iasis; -ion; -ism; -y
		process of cutting	-tomy

P

Definition	Word Part	Definition	Word Part
		process of measuring	-metry
pain	-algia; -dynia	process of producing images	-graphy
painful	dys-		
pancreas	pancreat/o	process of recording	-graphy
paralysis	-plegia	process of study	-logy
parathyroid gland	parathyroid/o	process of visually examining (a body cavity or organ)	-scopy
parietal bone	pariet/o		
part with child	-para		
patches	-plakia	produced by	-genic
patella	patell/a; patell/o	producing	-gen; -genic

Definition	Word Part	Definition	Word Part
production	genesis; -poiesis	sac in which the fetus lies in the uterus	amni/o
profuse sweating	diaphor/e		
prolapse	-ptosis		
pronation	pronati/o	sagging	-ptosis
prostate	prostat/o	saliva	sial/o
protrusion	-cele	salivary gland	sialaden/o
pubis (a portion of the hip bone)	pub/o	same	home/o
		scanty	oligo-
pudendum	episi/o; vulv/o	scapula	scapul/o
pupil	core/o; pupill/o	sebum	seb/o
pus	py/o	second	secundi-
pyloric sphincter	pylor/o	secrete (to)	crin/o; -crine
pylorus	pylor/o	self	auto-
		sensation	-esthesia
		separate	-crit; -lysis
		sew	-rrhaphy

Q

Definition	Word Part
quick	oxy-

... continued ...

		sex glands	gonad/o
		sharp	oxy-
		shield	thyr/o; thyroid/o
		shin	tibi/o
		shut (to)	-myein
		sieve	ethm/o
		sight	opt/o
		sigmoid colon	sigmoid/o
		sinuses	sinus/o
		skeleton	skelet/o

R

Definition	Word Part
radius (bone of lower arm)	radi/o
reconstruction	-plasty
record	-gram
rectum	proct/o; rect/o
red	erythemat/o; erythr/o
relaxation	-chalasis
removal	de-
renal pelvis	pyel/o
resembling	-oid
respiration	pneumat/o; pneum/o
retina	retin/o
rhythm	rhythm/o
ribs	cost/o
rod-shaped	rhabd/o
rupture	-rrhexis

skin	cutane/o; derm/o; -derma; dermat/o; -dermis
skull	crani/o
small	-ole; -ule
small bronchial tubes	bronchiol/o
small intestine	enter/o
smooth	lei/o
socket	glen/o
sodium	natr/o
softening	-malacia
something inserted	catheter/o
sound	ech/o; son/o
specialist	-ician; -logist
specialist in the measurement of	-metrist
specialist in the study of; one who specializes; specialist	-er; -or; -ician; -ist; -logist
speech	-phasia
spermatozoa (sperm)	sperm/o; spermat/o

S

Definition	Word Part
sac	cyst/o
sac filled with synovial fluid located around joints	burs/o

Definition	Word Part		Definition	Word Part
sphenoid bone	sphen/o			
spinal column	spin/o			
spinal cord	myel/o			
spine	spin/o		**T**	
spitting	-ptysis			
spleen	splen/o		tail	caud/o
split	-spadias		tailbone	coccyg/o
splitting	-schisis		tears	dacry/o; lacrim/o
stable	-stasis		teeth	odont/o
standing	-stasis		temporal bone	tempor/o
stapes	staped/o		tendon	tend/o; tendin/o
state of	-ia; -ism; -sis		tendon sheath	tenosynovi/o
step (to)	-grade		tension	tensi/o; ton/o
sternum	stern/o		testicle	orchi/o; orchid/o;
stimulating	-tropic			test/o; testicul/o
stomach	gastr/o		testis	orchi/o; orchid/o;
stone	-lith; lith/o			test/o; testicul/o
stop (to)	-continence		thalamus	thalam/o
stoppage	-pause; -stasis		thigh bone	femor/o
straight	ortho-		thing	-us
stretching	-ectasis		thirst	-dipsia
striated	rhabd/o		thorax	thorac/o
stricture	-stenosis		throat	pharyng/o
striped	rhabd/o		thymus gland	thym/o
structure	-ium; -um		thyroid gland	thyr/o; thyroid/o
study of	-logy		tibia	tibi/o
sudden, involuntary	-spasm		tilting	versi/o
contraction			tip of penis	balan/o
sugar	gluc/o		tipping	versi/o
supination	supinati/o		tissue	hist/o; histi/o
surgical binding	-desis		together	sym-
surgical fixation	-pexy		tone	ton/o
surgical fracture	-clasis		tongue	gloss/o; lingu/o
surgical fusion	-desis		tonsils	tonsill/o
surgical puncture to	centesis		tooth	dent/o; odont/o
remove fluid			top	acr/o
surgical reconstruction	-plasty		toward	ad-
surgical refracture	-clasis		toward the head	super/o
surgical removal	-ectomy		trabecula (strands of	trabecul/o
surgical repair	-plasty		connective tissue)	
suture (to sew)	-rrhaphy		trachea	trache/o
swallow	-phagia		transmission	-phoresis
swayback	lord/o		treatment	-therapy
sweat	hidr/o		trigone	trigon/o
sword	xiph/o		tube	tub/o
synovial membrane	synovi/o		tumor	-oma
synovium	synovi/o		turmoil	-clonus

Definition	Word Part	Definition	Word Part
turning	-tropia; -tropion; versi/o	varicose vein	varic/o
two	di-	vas deferens	vas/o
tying	ligati/o	vein	phleb/o; ven/o
tympanic membrane	tympan/o; myring/o	ventricle (lower chambers of the heart)	ventricul/o
		vertebra	vertebr/o; spondyl/o

Definition	Word Part
ulna (bone of lower arm)	uln/o
umbilicus	umbilic/o
under	hypo-; sub-
unequal size	anis/o
up	ana-
upon	epi-
upper arm	humer/o
upper dilated portion of the ureter	pyel/o
upper jaw	maxill/o
urea (end product of protein breakdown and is found in urine)	ure/o
ureter	ureter/o
urethra	urethr/o
urinary tract	ur/o
urination	ur/o; -uria
urine	ur/o; -uria; urin/o
uterine tube	salping/o; -salpinx
uterus	uter/o; hyster/o; metr/o
uvea	uve/o

Definition	Word Part
vessel	angi/o; vas/o; vascul/o
view (to)	-opsy
vision	-opia; -opsia; opt/o
visual condition	-opia; -opsia
voice	-phonia
voice box	laryng/o
vomit	-emesis
vulva	episi/o; vulv/o

Definition	Word Part
wall	pariet/o
washing	-clysis
water	aque/o; hydr/o
wedge	sphen/o
white	albin/o; leuk/o
wide	mydri/o
widen	dilat/o
windpipe	trache/o
with	endo; sym-
within	endo-; infra-; intra-
without	e-
woman	gynec/o
wrist	carp/o
writing	-gram

Definition	Word Part
vagina	colp/o; vagin/o
valve	valvul/o
variation	poikil/o

Abbreviations, Acronyms, and Symbols

A

^{99m}Tc	technetium 99m
AAT	alpha$_1$ antitrypsin
Ab	antibody
ABG	arterial blood gases
ABR	auditory brainstem response
ACh	acetylcholine
ACL	anterior cruciate ligament
ACTH	adrenocorticotropic hormone
AD	right ear
AED	automatic external defibrillator
AF	atrial fibrillation
AFB	acid-fast bacillus
AF; A-fib	atrial fibrillation
Ag	antigen
ALP	alkaline phosphatase
ALS	amyotrophic lateral sclerosis
ALT	alanine transaminase
AM; a.m.	morning
AMD	age-related macular degeneration
ANA	antinuclear antibody
AP	anteroposterior
aPTT	activated partial thromboplastin time
ARF	acute renal failure
AS	left ear
AST	aspartate transaminase
ATP	adenosine triphosphate
AV	atrioventricular

B

BBB	blood-brain barrier
BM	bowel movement
BPH	benign prostatic hypertrophy
BSE	breast self-examination
BSO	bilateral salpingo-oophorectomy
BUN	blood urea nitrogen

C

C	cervical
C&S	culture and sensitivity
Ca	calcium
CABG	coronary artery bypass graft
CAD	coronary artery disease
CAPD	continual ambulatory peritoneal dialysis
CBC	complete blood count
CD	Crohn's disease
CF	cystic fibrosis
CHD	coronary heart disease
CHF	congestive heart failure
mCi	millicurie
μCi	microcurie
CK	creatine kinase
CNS	central nervous system
CO_2	carbon dioxide
CPAP	continuous positive airway pressure
CPK	creatine phosphokinase
CPR	cardiopulmonary resuscitation
CRF	chronic renal failure
CS	cesarean section
CSF	cerebrospinal fluid
CT	computed tomography
CTS	carpal tunnel syndrome
CVA	cerebrovascular accident
CVS	cardiovascular system; chorionic villus sampling
CXR	chest x-ray

D

D	dorsal
D&C	dilation and curettage
dB	decibels
DCIS	ductal carcinoma in situ
dL	deciliter
DRE	digital rectal exam
Dx	diagnosis

E

EBV	Epstein-Barr virus
ECCE	extracapsular cataract extraction
ECG; EKG	electrocardiogram
EDB	estimated date of birth
EECP	enhanced external counterpulsation
EEG	electroencephalography
EENT	eyes, ears, nose, and throat
ELISA	enzyme-linked immunosorbent assay
EMG	electromyography
endo	endoscopy
ENT	ears, nose, and throat
EOM	extraocular muscles
ER	emergency room
ERCP	endoscopic retrograde cholangiopancreatography
ERS	endoscopic retrograde sphincterotomy
ESL	extracorporeal shockwave lithotripsy
ESR	erythrocyte sedimentation rate
ESRD	end-stage renal disease
EUA	examination under anesthesia
EXU	excretory urogram

F

FB	foreign body
FBS	fasting blood glucose
FEV_1	forced expiratory volume
FSH	follicle-stimulating hormone
FVC	forced vital capacity

G

g	gram
μg	microgram
G	gravida
GB	gallbladder
GGT	gamma-glutamyl transpeptidase
GH	growth hormone
GI	gastrointestinal
GIT	gastrointestinal tract
GTT	glucose tolerance test
GU	genitourinary

H

HAV	hepatitis A virus
HBV	hepatitis B virus
HCT	hematocrit
HCV	hepatitis C virus
HD	hemodialysis; Hodgkin's disease
HDL	high density lipoprotein
HDN	hemolytic disease of the newborn
HEENT	head, eyes, ears, nose, and throat
HF	heart failure
Hgb, Hb	hemoglobin
HGH	human growth hormone
H_pSA	*Helicobacter pylori* stool antigen
HSV	herpes simplex virus
Hz	Hertz

I

IBS	irritable bowel syndrome
ICD	implantable cardioverter-defibrillator
I&D	incision and drainage
ICSH	interstitial cell-stimulating hormone
ICU	intensive care unit
IM	intramuscular
IOL	intraocular lens
IOP	intraocular pressure
IP	interphalangeal
IPD	intermittent peritoneal dialysis
IPPA	inspection, palpation, percussion, and auscultation
IPPB	intermittent positive pressure breathing
IUD	intrauterine device
IV	intravenous
IVP	intravenous pyelogram
IVU	intravenous urography

K

KKUB	kidney, kidney, ureter, bladder
KUB	kidney, ureter, bladder

L

L	lumbar; liter
LAP	leucine aminopeptidase

LAVH	laparoscopic assisted vaginal hysterectomy
lb	pound
LCIS	lobular carcinoma in situ
LDH	lactic dehydrogenase
LDL	low density lipoprotein
LEEP	loop electrocautery excision procedure
LFT	liver function tests
LH	luteinizing hormone
LLQ	left lower quadrant
LNMP	last normal menstrual period
LOC	level of consciousness
LP	lumbar puncture
LRT	lower respiratory tract
LUQ	left upper quadrant
LUTS	lower urinary tract symptoms

M

m	meter; milli
MA	mental age
MBJ	muscles, bones, and joints
mcg	microgram
mcL	microliter
MCP	metacarpophalangeal
MD	muscular dystrophy
mEq	milliequivalent
mg	milligram (1/1000 gram)
mg%	milligram percent
mg/dL	milligrams per deciliter
mL	milliliter
mm	millimeter (1/1000 meter)
mμ	millimicron (1/1000 micron)
mmol	millimole
MRI	magnetic resonance imaging
MS	multiple sclerosis
MSH	melanocyte stimulating hormone
MSS	musculoskeletal system
MUGA	multiple-gated acquisition scan (of heart)

N

NAD	no appreciable disease
NB	newborn
ng	nanogram
NG	nasogastric
NHL	non-Hodgkin's lymphoma
NOS	not otherwise specified

NS	nervous system
NSAID	nonsteroidal anti-inflammatory drugs
NTP	normal temperature and pulse
NYD	not yet diagnosed

O

O_2	oxygen
OA	osteoarthritis
OD	overdose; right eye
ORIF	open reduction and internal fixation
OS	left eye
os	opening bone
OSS	organs of special sense
oz	ounce

P

P	para; pulse; phosphorus
PA	posteroanterior
PaCO$_2$	partial pressure of carbon dioxide
PaO$_2$	partial pressure of oxygen
PCL	posterior cruciate ligament
PCP	*Pneumocystis carinii*
PD	Parkinson's disease; peritoneal dialysis
PEEP	positive end-expiratory pressure
PERRLA	pupils equal, round, react to light and accommodation
PET	positron-emission tomography
PFT	pulmonary function test
pH	a measure of the alkalinity or acidity of a substance
physio	physiotherapy
PID	pelvic inflammatory disease
PIP	proximal interphalangeal (joint)
PM; p.m.	afternoon
PMI	point of maximum impulse; point of maximum intensity
PMN	polymorphonuclear
PNS	peripheral nervous system
PPD	purified protein derivative
PT	prothrombin time
PTA	prior to admission
PTC	percutaneous transhepatic cholangiography
PTH	parathormone
PYO	pyrexia of unknown origin

R

R	respiration
RA	rheumatoid arthritis
RBC	red blood cell
RDS	respiratory distress syndrome
RF	rheumatoid factors
Rh	Rhesus
RIA	radioimmunoassay
RICE	rest, ice, compression, elevation
RLQ	right lower quadrant
ROM	range of motion
RP	retrograde pyelogram
RS	respiratory system
RUQ	right upper quadrant

S

S	sacral
s	second
SAP	serum alkaline phosphatase
SIADH	syndrome of inappropriate antidiuretic hormone
SLR	straight leg raising
SOB	shortness of breath
sp gr	specific gravity
stat	immediately

T

T	thoracic; temperature
T_3	triiodothyronine
T_4	thyroxine; thyroxin
TAH	total abdominal hysterectomy
TFT	thyroid function test
TLC	tender loving care
TM	tympanic membrane
TMJ	temporomandibular joint
TPR	temperature, pulse, and respiration
TRUS	transrectal ultrasound
TSH	thyroid-stimulating hormone
TUR	transurethral resection
TURP	transurethral resection of prostate
Tx	treatment

U

UA	urinalysis
URT	upper respiratory tract
US	ultrasound
UTI	urinary tract infection

V

VD	vomiting and diarrhea; venereal disease
V/Q scan	ventilation/perfusion scan (Q stands for quotient)
VF; V-fib	ventricular fibrillation

W

WBC	white blood cell
wt	weight

Symbols

=	equal
≠	unequal
+	plus; positive
−	minus; negative
↑	above; increase
↓	below; decrease
♂	male
♀	female
>	is greater than
<	is less than
%	percent
:	ratio
′	foot
″	inches
$\bar{c}$	with
$\bar{s}$	without
#	pound

Glossary of Diagnostic Tests

A

abdominal x-ray: x-ray of the kidneys, ureters, and bladder (KUB) without the use of contrast medium. Also known as **flat plate of abdomen.**

Achilles jerk; ankle jerk: a test in which a tap on the Achilles tendon causes plantar flexion of the foot.

allergy testing: skin tests that show the body's response to foreign substances (antigens).

anteroposterior (AP) view: x-rays enter the body from the front to the back.

antiglobulin test (Coombs' test) (KOOMZ): laboratory test used to detect abnormal antibodies on the surface of red blood cells.

antinuclear antibody (ANA): a blood test used to detect unusual antibodies called antinuclear antibodies, which cause tissue damage and are an indicator of autoimmune disease.

arterial blood gases (ABG): a laboratory test that measures the amount of oxygen and carbon dioxide in the blood.

arthroscopy: a surgical method of looking into a joint without making a large incision. A small incision is made near the joint and an arthroscope is inserted. The arthroscope has a video camera attached, which allows the surgeon to view the entire joint cavity. Surgery is performed by inserting surgical instruments into additional small incisions. Recovery time is minimal and hospital stay is reduced.

aspiration biopsy: tissue is removed without a surgical incision. A needle is placed into tissue such as bone marrow, and the material is aspirated (withdrawn) into the needle. The tissue is then examined.

audiometry: a test that measures hearing ability.

auditory brainstem response (ABR): a test that helps determine the cause of hearing loss by measuring nervous impulses to the brainstem after the cochlea is stimulated by sound.

B

Babinski's reflex: dorsiflexion (backward flexion) of the toes when the sole of the foot is stimulated. This is a normal response in newborns and infants but it indicates nerve dysfunction in others.

barium enema: barium is placed into the rectum as a contrast medium followed by x-rays of the large bowel.

barium studies: an x-ray procedure used to diagnose digestive-tract problems. Barium sulfate is used as a contrast medium. As barium settles in the organs, it will appear white on the x-ray film.

barium swallow: barium is taken by mouth, followed by x-rays of the pharynx and esophagus.

biopsy: removal of a piece of tissue for examination under a microscope.

bleeding time: a test used to measure the time it takes for bleeding to stop following a small puncture wound to the skin.

blood glucose levels: a test used to determine the amount of glucose (sugar) in the blood. It is also known as serum glucose level. The amount of glucose in the blood is expressed as milligrams per deciliter (mg/dL). Normal blood glucose level is 70 to 100 mg/dL.

blood urea nitrogen (BUN): a test that measures the amount of urea in the blood. Urea is a waste product that is carried in the blood to the kidney, where it is filtered by the nephrons and excreted in urine.

bone scan: a picture of the bone is produced using a special camera after the patient has been injected with radioactive phosphate. The radioactive phosphate is picked up by the diseased bone and shows up as dark areas called "hot spots" on the scan.

breath test: a procedure used to diagnose ulcers caused by the bacteria *Helicobacter pylori.*

cardiac count: a catheter is inserted into a vein in the arm or femur and pushed upward into the heart. An x-ray of the blood vessels of the heart (angiocardiography) is performed at the same time as the catheterization so that the placement of the catheter can be monitored. Diagnostic information such as levels of oxygen and carbon dioxide, or indicators of coronary artery disease and disorders of the heart valves, is obtained.

cardiac enzymes: a test for myocardial infarction by measuring cardiac enzymes such as creatine phosphokinase (CPK) and lactate dehydrogenase (LDH). During a myocardial infarction, the damaged cells release CPK and LDH into the bloodstream. High levels of these enzymes in the blood are a good indicator of myocardial infarction.

Cardiolite scan: this test uses a radiopharmaceutical, known as a tracer, to produce images of the heart muscle. An exercise test is used with it to diagnose coronary heart disease. While the patient is exercising on a treadmill, the tracer is injected into a vein in the arm. The tracer travels through the blood, to the coronary arteries, and is picked up by the heart muscle. Healthy areas of the heart that have sufficient blood supply pick up the tracer immediately and appear as "hot spots" on the scan. Areas that do not have sufficient

blood supply pick up the tracer slowly and appear as "cold spots" on the scan.

catheter: a tube-shaped, flexible, surgical instrument that can be inserted into a body cavity for the withdrawal or introduction of fluid.

catheterization: the process of passing a catheter into a body cavity.

chest x-ray: an image is taken of the internal structures of the chest. The pictures can be taken in different body positions.

cholangiography: x-ray of the bile ducts following injection of a contrast medium.

coagulation time: measurement of the time it takes blood to clot in a test tube. Also known as clotting time.

cold spot: a term used to describe areas on a scan where there is low uptake into the tissues of a radioactive substance that has been injected into the body.

colposcopy (kol-POS-koh-pee): process of visually examining the vagina and cervix using a special magnifying device called a colposcope.

complete blood count (CBC): a general screening test during routine physical examinations. Several tests are done on a sample of blood including hematocrit, hemoglobin, white blood cell count, and platelet count.

computed tomography (kom-PYOO-ted toh-MOG-rah-fee): a procedure utilizing an x-ray beam passing through a body part. The beam visually cuts the part into many slices at various depths. This information is computer analyzed and a series of pictures is assembled into one image of the part. CT scans allow for clearer visualization than conventional x-ray. Common body parts studied in this fashion include the brain, abdomen, kidneys, and chest. Abbrev. **CT scan.**

contrast medium: a dye that is placed into the patient's body to improve the visibility of an x-ray.

count: any test that involves the calculation of the total number of something in a sample.

creatine kinase (CK); creatine phosphokinase (CPK): a laboratory test to evaluate the levels of CPK in the blood. CPK is an enzyme found in cardiac and skeletal muscle tissue. When muscle is damaged, the cells release CPK. CPK spills into the blood, elevating normal blood levels.

creatinine clearance: a test of blood and urine to assess kidney function. It measures the kidney's ability to clear creatinine from the blood. Creatinine is a waste product produced by the breakdown of creatine (a protein found in muscle). Creatinine is excreted in the urine.

culture: a method of identifying bacteria. Microorganisms or living tissue cells are placed in an environment that stimulates growth. As the microorganism multiples, it can be easily identified.

culture and sensitivity (C&S): a test to measure a microorganism's sensitivity to antibiotics. The microorganism is cultured and exposed to various antibiotics. The antibiotic that is most effective in killing the microorganism is the one used to treat the patient.

culture specimen: a sample of microorganisms or living tissue cells taken from an area of the body for laboratory examination. Culture specimens can be taken from sputum (mucus and other material brought up through the respiratory tract), blood, urine, throat, cervix uteri, and stool.

cystoscopy: visual examination of the bladder using a cystoscope. The cystoscope is placed through the urethra and into the bladder with or without anesthetic. A tiny camera inside the cystoscope shows the inside of the organs on a television monitor. Other instruments can be used with the cystoscope to perform biopsies, remove calculi, or burn (cauterize) abnormal tissue.

D

differential; white blood cell differential: a count of each different type of white blood cell (eosinophils, basophils, neutrophils, lymphocytes, and monocytes).

digital rectal exam (DRE): palpation (feeling) of the prostate and other structures by placing a gloved finger through the anal canal and into the rectum.

dilation and curettage (dye-LAY-shun and kyoo-reh-TAZH): a surgical procedure used to determine the cause of uterine bleeding or other conditions. The cervical opening is widened with an instrument called a dilator. This is followed by the insertion of a second instrument called a **curet (kyoo-RET)**, which has jagged edges on one side. The curet is used to scrape the endometrial lining from the uterine wall so that it may be examined. Abbrev. **D&C,**

Doppler ultrasound: the use of ultrasound to measure the speed and direction of blood flow through a blood vessel.

drawer test: a test to determine the stability of the anterior and posterior cruciate ligaments that support and stabilize the knee joint.

E

echocardiography: a procedure that produces an image of the heart using ultrasound waves.

electrocardiography (ECG; EKG): a measurement of the electrical activity of the heart. The record produced is called an electrocardiogram. It is a "snapshot" of how well the conduction system is working.

electrocochleography (ee-leck-troh-kock-lee-OG-rah-fee): a process for recording the electrical activity of the cochlea.

electroencephalography (ee-leck-troh-en-sef-ah-LOG-rah-fee): a procedure used to record the electrical impulses of the brain. Abbre. **EEG.**

electrolytes: substances capable of producing an electrical charge. They are found in blood, body tissues, and urine. They are important in muscle and nerve function. Examples include calcium, sodium, potassium, chloride, and magnesium.

electromyography (ee-leck-troh-my-OG-rah-fee): a procedure used to record the electrical impulses produced by a muscle when it is at rest and when it is moving. This is done by inserting tiny needle electrodes into the muscle. Abbrev. **EMG**.

electrophoresis: a test on blood or urine that utilizes an electrical current to separate proteins in a mixture. This allows different protein components and quantities to be determined.

ELISA (enzyme-linked immunosorbent assay): blood test to screen patients for antibodies to HIV.

endoscope: any instrument utilizing a narrow flexible tube with a tiny video camera attached to view inside body organs and cavities. Endoscopes are named using the root of the organ or cavity being viewed. Examples include *gastroscope*, instrument used to view the inside of the stomach; *bronchoscope*, instrument used to view the inside of the bronchus; *laparoscope*, instrument used to view the inside of the abdominal cavity; and *cystoscope*, instrument used to view the bladder.

endoscopic retrograde cholangiopancreatography (ERCP): the bile ducts and pancreas are studied using an endoscope. The endoscope is inserted through the mouth, into the stomach, and into the duodenum. A contrast medium is introduced through the endoscope. It flows backward (retrograde) and highlights the biliary ducts and pancreas. X-rays are taken.

endoscopy: the process of visually examining a body cavity or organ using an instrument called an endoscope. Biopsies and tissue repair can also be done by inserting cutting devices through the endoscope. Endoscopies are named using the root of the organ or cavity being viewed.

enzymes: proteins within cells that act as a catalyst in chemical reactions.

erythrocyte count: see red blood cell count.

erythrocyte sedimentation rate (ESR): a test that measures the time it takes for red blood cells to settle out of plasma to the bottom of a test tube.

excretory urography (EXU): examination of the kidneys, ureters, and bladder following injection of a contrast medium into a vein.

Also known as **intravenous urography (IVU)** or **intravenous pyelography (IVP)**.

exercise stress test: an electrocardiogram obtained while the patient is exercising.

exophthalmometry: the process of measuring the forward protrusion of the eyeball as seen in exophthalmia.

fasting blood sugar (FBS): laboratory test that measures blood glucose levels after the patient has fasted for at least eight hours.

fluoroscopy (floo-ROSS-kah-pee): an x-ray of moving structures, such as the movement of substances through the digestive tract. The image is produced on a fluorescent screen rather than on a single x-ray film. This procedure has the advantage of allowing observation of structures as they move. Fluoroscopy is used with barium studies to observe how well barium flows through the gastrointestinal tract.

frozen section: during surgery, a piece of tissue is removed and quickly frozen for microscopic examination. Frozen sections are done when a quick diagnosis is needed to eliminate the need for two operations, one for diagnosis and one for treatment.

funduscopy (fun-DOS-ka-pee); ophthalmoscopy: the process of visually examining the back of the eye.

gastric analysis: contents of the stomach are analyzed for acid levels, appearance, and volume.

glucose tolerance test (GTT) : a test that monitors the body's ability to utilize glucose after a measured amount of a sweet drink has been taken by the patient. The blood sugar is measured before and after the drink. Blood sugar should return to normal after three hours.

glycated hemoglobin test: a test that measures the amount of glucose attached to hemoglobin. The more glucose attached to hemoglobin, the higher the blood glucose level.

Heaf test: see tuberculin skin test

hematocrit (HCT): a laboratory test to determine the percentage of erythrocytes per volume of blood.

hemoccult (hee-moh-KULT) test: an examination of stool for blood. It is called a hemoccult (hem/o = blood; occult = hidden) because the blood is difficult to see. A small amount of stool is placed on a special hemoccult card. Guaiac (GWEE-ack), a special substance, is then added to the stool to reveal any hidden blood.

hemoglobin (Hgb, Hb): a test to determine the total amount of hemoglobin in a sample of blood.

HIDA scan: a procedure used to produce an image of the liver, gallbladder, and biliary ducts following injection of radiopharmaceutical into a vein. The radiopharmaceutical travels to the liver, and is excreted by the biliary ducts. It is traced by a special scanner that takes the images.

Holter monitor: an electrocardiogram taken while the patient is going about a typical daily routine.

hot spot: a term used to identify areas on a scan where there is high uptake into the tissue of the radiopharmaceutical that has been injected into the body.

immunoelectrophoresis (ih-myoo-noh-ee-leck-troh-for-EE-sis): a procedure utilizing an electric current to identify and measure immunoglobulins in a sample of blood. Immunoglobulins are proteins that function as antibodies. Under normal conditions, they are present in the blood in predictable amounts. They are classified into IgG, IgA, IgM, IgD, and IgE.

jerk: a sudden, involuntary response to a stimulus; a sudden reflex.

knee jerk: see reflex, patellar

lateral decubitus view: an x-ray position; x-rays enter the body from the side while the patient is lying down.

lateral view: an x-ray position; x-rays enter the body from either the right or left side of the chest.

leukocyte count: see white blood cell count.

lipid tests: a measurement of the amount of lipids (fats) in a sample of blood. Types of lipids are cholesterol, triglycerides, phospholipids, high-density lipoprotein, and low-density lipoproteins.

liver function tests (LFTs): a group of blood tests measuring the level of liver enzymes in the blood. These enzymes are normally in hepatic cells, but are released when the liver is diseased or damaged. ALT, AST, ALP, and LDH are some of the more common enzymes. The enzymes are known by their abbreviations. Look at the Abbreviation Glossary for the meanings of these abbreviations.

lumbar puncture (LP); spinal tap: an examination of the cerebrospinal fluid for microorganisms or blood. A needle is inserted into the subarachnoid space below the third lumbar vertebra. Cerebrospinal fluid is withdrawn and analyzed.

lung perfusion and ventilation scan: a type of nuclear medicine test that produces an image of blood and air flow to the lungs. A radiopharmaceutical is injected into a vein and eventually settles in the arterioles of the lungs. A special camera is used to detect the radiopharmaceutical, and a series of pictures are made of the thorax. These pictures are seen on a special screen called an oscilloscope. A normal scan will show even distribution of the radiopharmaceutical throughout the lungs. An abnormal scan will show no radiopharmaceutical, which suggests decreased blood flow to that part of the lung.

lymphangiography: an x-ray of the lymphatic system following injection of a contrast medium into the feet. A fluoroscope (a type of x-ray that displays movement onto a television monitor) is used. The flow of the contrast medium is followed as it travels from the feet upward toward the abdomen. Once the dye has been completely injected, x-rays are taken of the lymphatic system.

magnetic resonance imaging (MRI): a picture of a body structure produced by the use of electromagnetic energy rather than conventional x-ray, ultrasound, or radioactive substances. No contrast medium is used. MRIs provide clear pictures of soft-tissue abnormalities such as edema and tumors.

mammography: process of taking x-rays of the breast.

Mantoux test: see tuberculin skin test

MUGA scan (multiple-gated acquisition scan): an image is produced of the heart muscle following injection of technetium 99m (^{99m}Tc), a radioactive substance. It can provide information on blood flow through the heart and how well the ventricles pump blood out of the heart.

myelogram: x-ray of the spinal cord following injection of a contrast media into the subarachnoid space.

oblique view: an x-ray position; x-rays enter the body on a slant in order to visualize behind structures.

otoscopy (oh-**TOSS**-kah-pee): the process of viewing the middle and inner ear using an otoscope. Video otoscopy is a recent

advancement providing color images of the ear that can be copied and enlarged.

Pap smear: a laboratory test that allows examination of cells from the cervix uteri for disease, especially cancerous cells.

patch test: a test in which a small amount of a substance called an **allergen** (**AL**-er-jen) is placed on the skin and covered with a patch. If the patient is sensitive to the allergen, there will be an allergic reaction. The patient will develop a raised, itchy bump called a **wheal** (**WEEL**). A wheal looks like a mosquito bite. It may be redder or paler than the surrounding skin.

patellar reflex: extension of the lower leg when the area below the patella (kneecap) is tapped; also called knee jerk.

pelvic ultrasound: the use of ultrasound to obtain an image of the abdomen and pelvis. This procedure is used during pregnancy to assess fetal size and development as well as placental location. As well, ovarian tumors and other pelvic masses can be detected using ultrasound.

percutaneous transhepatic cholangiography (PTC): the bile ducts undergo an x-ray exam following injection of a contrast medium through the skin and into the liver.

PET scan; positron emission tomography (**POZ**-ee-tron ee-**MISH**-un toh-**MOG**-rah-fee) (**PET** scan): a procedure in which a picture is taken of internal body structures to study how cells function in certain body areas. A radioactive substance is injected into a vein and traced as it travels through the body. PET scans are helpful in diagnosing and treating such diseases as cancer, Alzheimer's, schizophrenia, and stroke.

plantar reflex: toes curl under when the sole of the foot (plantar aspect) is stroked.

platelet count: a test that measures the number of platelets in a sample of blood. The normal value is 150,000 to 400,000 per microliter of blood.

posteroanterior (PA) view: x-rays enter the body from back to front.

prostate-specific antigen (PSA): a test to determine the level of PSA in the blood. PSA is a protein produced by the prostate gland. PSA is removed from the body in semen, although a small amount enters the bloodstream and can be measured. An elevated PSA level may indicate prostatic cancer, benign prostatic hypertrophy, or prostatitis.

prothrombin time (PT): a laboratory test that measures the time it takes for a clot to form.

pulmonary arteriography: a procedure in which images of the pulmonary blood vessels are taken following injection of a contrast medium into the vascular system.

pulmonary function test (PFT): a series of tests on lung performance using a spirometer, an instrument to record breathing ability. It measures total lung capacity (TLC), which is the total volume of air the lungs can hold. Some of the test measurements are obtained by normal, quiet breathing, and other tests require forced inhalation or exhalation.

pulse oximetry (PULSS-ock-SIM-eh-tree): a procedure used to measure the percentage of hemoglobin saturated with oxygen. An instrument called an oximeter (ock-SIM-eh-ter) is used. It has a probe that attaches to the patient's fingertip. The probe is linked to a computerized unit. The probe emits a light that is absorbed by hemoglobin in various degrees, depending upon the amount of oxygen present. The computerized unit can then calculate the percentage of hemoglobin that is oxygenated.

punch biopsy: a circular piece of tissue is removed with a sharp instrument.

R

radioactive iodine uptake: a test used to assess thyroid function. Radioactive iodine is taken orally. Eventually, it is taken up by the thyroid. A high uptake of radioactive iodine indicates too much thyroxine is being produced.

radioimmunoassay (RIA): a test used to identify antibodies the immune system has formed in response to the presence of antigens.

radiopharmaceutical: a radioactive substance combined with a chemical that is easily absorbed by the target organ.

range of motion (ROM): an assessment of the degree to which a joint can be moved in any direction, including adduction, abduction, flexion, extension, dorsiflexion, and plantar flexion. Range is measured in degrees. Limited joint movement may be 55 degrees, or full-range movement, 360 degrees.

red blood cell count (RBC): a test that measures the number of red blood cells in a sample of blood. The normal value is 4.7 to 6.1 million cells per microliter for men and 4.2 to 5.4 million cells per microliter for women.

red blood cell morphology: a study of red blood cells to determine abnormalities of size, shape, color, and structure.

reflex: a sudden, involuntary response to a stimulus.

refraction test: a common test used to study the bending of light rays as they pass through the eye, in order to clearly identify errors of refraction. The unit of measurement of the refractive power of the lens is diopter (dye-OP-ter).

retrograde urography: an x-ray of the urinary structures following injection of a contrast medium into the bladder through the urethra. The contrast medium flows backward (retrograde) highlighting urinary structures.

rheumatoid factors (RF): proteins present in the blood of patients with rheumatoid arthritis.

Romberg's (ROM-bergz) sign: swaying or loss of balance when the patient is asked to stand erect with the feet together and the eyes closed. Indicates nerve dysfunction.

S

scan (nuclear medicine): an image of a body organ is taken after a radiopharmaceutical has been introduced into the body. The radiopharmaceutical is known as a tracer.

The tracer travels through the bloodstream to the body organ being studied. An area where there is high uptake of the radiopharmaceutical is known as a "hot spot." An area where there is little or no uptake of the radiopharmaceutical is called a "cold spot." The tracer gives off small amounts of radiation that is detected using a special camera (gamma camera). Images of the radioactivity are produced. The image is called a scan. Scans are commonly taken on bone, brain, liver, lung, thyroid, and heart.

scratch test: test to identify substances a person is allergic to. Potential allergens are applied to scratches made on the skin surface. If there is an allergic reaction, the patient will develop a raised, red area on the skin.

scrotal transillumination: a bright light is held behind the scrotum. A scrotum filled with watery fluid will shine red because the light will pass through it. More solid abnormalities such as testicular tumors are seen as dark shadows because the light will not pass through.

semen analysis: a laboratory test to evaluate infertility. Semen is collected in a specimen container and analyzed microscopically. The sperm in the semen is counted and examined for size, shape, and mobility. Semen is examined for pH (balance of acids and bases), thickness, appearance, and volume.

serum alkaline phosphatase (SAP): a blood test used to measure the levels of alkaline phosphatase, which is important in the building of new bone.

serum calcium (Ca) and serum phosphorus (P): measurement of calcium or phosphorus in the blood (serum).

shave biopsy: tissue that extends above the level of its surroundings is removed with a scalpel (**SKAL-pel**), a sharp knife.

skeletal x-ray: x-ray of the bone without the use of a contrast medium. The bone shows up clearly as a white object against a black background.

small bowel series: barium is taken by mouth, followed by x-rays of the small bowel (duodenum, jejunum, and ileum).

smear: a laboratory test used to identify microorganisms. The specimen is placed on a slide and stained using the **Gram stain** method. The Gram stain will highlight the microorganism so that it is visible and can be identified.

spirometry (speye-ROM-eh-tree): the process of measuring breathing ability using a spirometer.

stool analysis: an examination of stool (feces) to identify fats, microorganisms, occult (hidden) blood, and other abnormal substances.

thallium scan: an image of the heart and its blood vessels is obtained following injection of a radioactive substance that includes thallium-201. Normal myocardial tissue absorbs the radioactive substance while diseased tissue does not.

thrombocyte count: see platelet count.

thyroid function test (TFT): this laboratory test measures thyroxine, triiodothyronine, and thyroid-stimulating hormone in the blood.

tine test: see tuberculin skin test.

transillumination (tranz-ih-loo-mih-NAY-shun): passing light through body tissues for the purpose of examining the part.

transrectal ultrasound (TRUS): the use of ultrasound to produce an image of the prostate. The well-lubricated transducer (instrument that emits the sound waves) is inserted into the rectum. An image is produced as the transducer is moved along the prostate.

transvaginal ultrasound: a procedure in which the transducer (instrument that emits the sound waves) is placed inside the vagina. The echogram is clearer and the details are sharper.

tuberculin skin test: tuberculin such as *PPD* (purified protein derivative of *mycobacterium tuberculosis*) is injected intradermally. This is called the *Mantoux test*. Another method is to apply the tuberculin to the skin. This is done by making many punctures in the skin. These are called the *Heaf* and *tine tests*. An inflammatory reaction will occur if the patient is sensitive to the tuberculin. This causes the localized area of skin to become red and swollen. This positive reaction means the persons has prior or present contact with *Mycobacterium tuberculosis*.

tuning fork test: a vibrating tuning fork is placed against the bones of the skull sending vibrations that can be heard if there is no hearing loss. Types include Weber and Rinne (**RIN-ay**).

tympanometry (**tym-pah-NOM-eh-tree**): measures how well sound can pass through the eardrum to the middle ear.

ultrasound/ultrasonography (US): an image is produced using high frequency sound waves rather than x-rays, magnetic fields, or radioisotopes. An instrument called a transducer passes sound waves through the organ. These waves are reflected back from the organ and recorded on an oscilloscope (special screen). Because tissues of different density will be reflected at different rates, an image is formed. No contrast medium is placed into the body. The record of the ultrasound is called an echogram or sonogram.

upper gastrointestinal series: barium is taken by mouth, followed by x-rays of the upper digestive tract, from the pharynx to the ileum.

uric acid: a measurement of uric acid in the urine. Uric acid is a waste product of protein breakdown that is removed from the body in the urine. High amounts of uric acid in the urine can cause kidney stones.

urinalysis (**yoo-rih-NAL-ih-sis**) **(UA):** laboratory urinalysis of urine. It is one of the most common tests performed to evaluate the general health of a person. This test includes macroscopic (seen with the naked eye) observations of the urine and microscopic (seen with the help of a microscope) observations. The urine is

analyzed for the presence of such elements as albumin (a protein), bacteria, bilirubin, blood, ketones, glucose, pus, white blood cells, and casts (clumps of cellular matter that have formed as if in a mold). The color, pH (balance between acids and bases), and specific gravity (the amount of wastes, minerals, and other substances) are also noted in urine.

urinary catheterization: insertion of a catheter into the urethra for the removal of urine.

visual acuity (**ah-KYOO-eh-tee**): a noninvasive method of judging how good the patient's eyesight is. A **Snellen** (**SNEL-en**) chart is used. This chart contains different letters of different sizes. The patient stands 20 feet from the chart, covers one eye, and reads each letter. How well the patient sees the letters is an indication of visual acuity. It is measured as a fraction; 20/20 vision is normal.

visual fields: a noninvasive test used to examine the patient's peripheral vision.

voiding cystography (**sis-TOG-raf-fee**): a procedure in which x-rays of the bladder and urethra are taken while the patient is voiding. A contrast medium is placed directly into the urinary structures.

Western Block: a blood test to screen patients for antibodies to HIV.

white blood cell count (WBC): a test used to measure the number of white blood cells in a sample of blood. The normal value is 5000 to 10,000 cells per microliter of blood.

x-ray: an image taken of internal structures using x-rays.

A

F

T

U

V

AUDIO CDs TO ACCOMPANY
ILLUSTRATED GUIDE TO MEDICAL TERMINOLOGY
Juanita J. Davies

DUPLICATION POLICY